# Evidence-Based Diagnosis

*Evidence-Based Diagnosis* is a textbook about diagnostic, screening, and prognostic tests in clinical medicine. The authors' approach is based on many years of experience teaching physicians in a clinical research training program. Although requiring only a minimum of mathematics knowledge, the quantitative discussions in this book are deeper and more rigorous than those in most introductory texts. The book includes numerous worked examples and 60 problems (with answers) based on real clinical situations and journal articles. The book will be helpful and accessible to anyone looking to select, develop, or market medical tests. Topics covered include:

- The diagnostic process
- Test reliability and accuracy
- Likelihood ratios
- ROC curves
- Testing and treatment thresholds
- Critical appraisal of studies of diagnostic, screening, and prognostic tests
- Test independence and methods of combining tests
- Quantifying treatment benefits using randomized trials and observational studies
- Bayesian interpretation of P-values and confidence intervals
- Challenges for evidence-based diagnosis

**Thomas B. Newman** is Chief of the Division of Clinical Epidemiology and Professor of Epidemiology and Biostatistics and Pediatrics at the University of California, San Francisco. He previously served as Associate Director of the UCSF/Stanford Robert Wood Johnson Clinical Scholars Program and Associate Professor in the Department of Laboratory Medicine at UCSF. He is a co-author of *Designing Clinical Research* and a practicing pediatrician.

**Michael A. Kohn** is Associate Clinical Professor of Epidemiology and Biostatistics at the University of California, San Francisco, where he teaches clinical epidemiology and evidence-based medicine. He is also an emergency physician with more than 20 years of clinical experience, currently practicing at Mills–Peninsula Medical Center in Burlingame, California.

# Evidence-Based Diagnosis

Thomas B. Newman
University of California, San Francisco

Michael A. Kohn
University of California, San Francisco

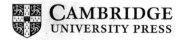
CAMBRIDGE
UNIVERSITY PRESS

CAMBRIDGE UNIVERSITY PRESS

Cambridge, New York, Melbourne, Madrid, Cape Town, Singapore, São Paulo, Delhi

Cambridge University Press
32 Avenue of the Americas, New York, NY 10013-2473, USA

www.cambridge.org
Information on this title: www.cambridge.org/9780521714020

First published 2009

Printed in the United States of America

*A catalog record for this publication is available from the British Library*

*Library of Congress Cataloging in Publication data*

Newman, Thomas B.
Evidence-based diagnosis / Thomas B. Newman, Michael A. Kohn.
    p.   ;   cm.
Includes bibliographical references and index.
ISBN 978-0-521-88652-9 (hardback) – ISBN 978-0-521-71402-0 (pbk.)
1. Diagnosis.   2. Evidence-based medicine.   3. Function tests (Medicine) – Evaluation.
4. Diagnosis – Research.   I. Kohn, Michael A.   II. Title.
[DNLM: 1. Diagnostic Techniques and Procedures – Problems and Exercises.   2. Clinical Medicine –
methods – Problems and Exercises.   3. Evidence-Based Medicine – Problems and Exercises.
WB 18.2 N555e 2009]
RC71.3.N49   2009
616.07′5–dc22        2008044178

ISBN    978-0-521-88652-9 hardback
ISBN    978-0-521-71402-0 paperback

# Contents

# Preface

This is a book about diagnostic testing. It is aimed primarily at clinicians, particularly those who are academically minded, but it should be helpful and accessible to anyone involved with selection, development, or marketing of diagnostic, screening, or prognostic tests. Although we admit to a love of mathematics, we have restrained ourselves and kept the math to a minimum – a little simple algebra and only three Greek letters, $\kappa$ (kappa), $\alpha$ (alpha), and $\beta$ (beta). Nonetheless, quantitative discussions in this book go deeper and are more rigorous than those typically found in introductory clinical epidemiology or evidence-based medicine texts.

Our perspective is that of skeptical consumers of tests. We want to make proper diagnoses and not miss treatable diseases. Yet, we are aware that vast resources are spent on tests that too frequently provide wrong answers or right answers of little value, and that new tests are being developed, marketed, and sold all the time, sometimes with little or no demonstrable or projected benefit to patients. This book is intended to provide readers with the tools they need to evaluate these tests, to decide if and when they are worth doing, and to interpret the results.

The pedagogical approach comes from years of teaching this material to physicians, mostly Fellows and junior faculty in a clinical research training program. We have found that many doctors, including the two of us, can be impatient when it comes to classroom learning. We like to be shown that the material is important and that it will help us take better care of our patients, understand the literature, and improve our research. For this reason, in this book we emphasize real-life examples. When we care for patients and read journal articles, we frequently identify issues that the material we teach can help people understand. We have decided what material to include in this book largely by creating homework problems from patients and articles we have encountered, and then making sure that we covered in the text the material needed to solve them. This explains the disproportionate number of pediatric and emergency medicine examples, and the relatively large portion of the book devoted to problems and answers – the parts we had the most fun writing.

Although this is primarily a book about diagnosis, two of the twelve chapters are about evaluating treatments – both using randomized trials (Chapter 9) and observational studies (Chapter 10). The reason is that evidence-based diagnosis requires not only being able to evaluate tests and the information they provide, but also the *value* of that information – how it will affect treatment decisions, and how those decisions will affect patients' health. For this reason, the chapters about treatments emphasize quantifying risks and benefits. Other reasons for including the material about treatments, which also apply to the material about P-values and confidence intervals in Chapter 11, are that we love to teach it, have lots of good examples, and are able to focus on material neglected (or even wrong) in other books.

After much deliberation, we decided to include in this text answers to all of the problems. However, we strongly encourage readers to think about and even write out the answers to the problems before looking at the answers at the back of the book. The disadvantage of including all of the answers is that instructors wishing to use this book for a course will have to create new problems for any take-home or open-book examinations. Because that includes us, we will continue to write new problems, and will be happy to share them with others who are teaching courses based on this book. We will post the additional problems on the book's Web site: http://www. epibiostat.ucsf.edu/ebd. Several of the problems in this book are adapted from problems our students created in our annual final examination problem-writing contest. Similarly, we encourage readers to create problems and share them with us. With your permission, we will adapt them for the second edition!

# Acknowledgments & Dedication

This book started out as the syllabus for a course TBN first taught to Robert Wood Johnson Clinical Scholars and UCSF Laboratory Medicine Residents beginning in 1991, based on the now-classic textbook *Clinical Epidemiology: A Basic Science for Clinical Medicine* by Sackett, Haynes, Guyatt, and Tugwell (Sackett et al. 1991). Although over the years our selection of and approach to the material has diverged from theirs, we enthusiastically acknowledge their pioneering work in this area.

We thank our colleagues in the Department of Epidemiology and Biostatistics, particularly Steve Hulley for his mentoring and steadfast support. We are particularly indebted to Dr. Andrea Marmor, a stellar clinician, teacher, and colleague at UCSF, and Lauren Cowles, our editor at Cambridge University Press, both of whom made numerous helpful suggestions on every single chapter. We also thank our students, who have helped us develop ways of teaching this material that work best, and who have enthusiastically provided examples from their own clinical areas that illustrate the material we teach.

TBN: I would like to thank my wife, Johannah, and children, David and Rosie, for their support on the long road that led to the publication of this book. I dedicate this book to my parents, Ed and Carol Newman, in whose honor I will donate my share of the royalties to Physicians for Social Responsibility, in support of its efforts to rid the world of nuclear weapons.

MAK: I thank my wife, Caroline, and children, Emily, Jake, and Kenneth, and dedicate this book to my parents, Martin and Jean Kohn.

Sackett, D. L., R. B. Haynes, et al. (1991). *Clinical epidemiology: a basic science for clinical medicine*. Boston, MA, Little Brown.

# Abbreviations/Acronyms

| | |
|---|---|
| AAA | abdominal aortic aneurysm |
| ACI | acute cardiac ischemia |
| ALT | alanine transaminase |
| ANOVA | analysis of variance |
| ARR | absolute risk reduction |
| AST | aspartate transaminase |
| AUROC | area under the ROC curve |
| B | net benefit of treating a patient with the disease |
| BMD | bone mineral density |
| BNP | B-type natriuretic peptide |
| C | net cost of treating a patient without the disease |
| CACS | Coronary Artery Calcium Score |
| CCB | calcium channel blocker |
| CDC | Centers for Disease Control |
| CHD | congenital heart disease |
| CHF | congestive heart failure |
| CI | confidence interval |
| CK | creatine kinase |
| CK-MB | creatine kinase–MB fraction |
| CMV | cytomegalovirus |
| CP | chest pain |
| CSF | cerebrospinal fluid |
| CT | computed tomography |
| CV | coefficient of variation |
| D− | disease negative |
| D+ | disease positive |
| DFA | direct fluorescent antibody |
| dL | deciliter |
| DRE | digital rectal examination |

| | |
|---|---|
| DS | Down syndrome |
| DXA | dual-energy x-ray absorptiometry |
| EBM | evidence-based medicine |
| ECG | electrocardiogram |
| ESR | erythrocyte sedimentation rate |
| FRS | Framingham Risk Score |
| GCS | Glasgow Coma Scale |
| GP | general practitioner |
| $H_0$ | null hypothesis |
| $H_A$ | alternative hypothesis |
| HAART | highly active antiretroviral therapy |
| HBsAg | hepatitis B surface antigen |
| HCG | human chorionic gonadotropin |
| HEDIS | Health Plan Employer Data and Information Set |
| HHS | Health and Human Services |
| HPF | high power field |
| ICD-9 | International Classification of Diseases, 9th revision |
| IU | international unit(s) |
| IV | intravenous |
| IVIG | intravenous immune globulin |
| LD | lactate dehydrogenase |
| ln | natural logarithm |
| LR | likelihood ratio |
| mg | milligram(s) |
| MI | myocardial infarction |
| mm | millimeter(s) |
| MS | multiple sclerosis |
| NBA | nasal bone absent |
| NEXUS | National Emergency X-Radiology Utilization Study |
| NIH | National Institutes of Health |
| NNH | number needed to harm |
| NNT | number needed to treat |
| NPV | negative predictive value |
| NS | not significant |
| NSAID | non-steroidal anti-inflammatory drug |
| NT | nuchal translucency |
| OIA | optical immunoassay |
| OM | otitis media |
| OME | otitis media with effusion |
| OR | odds ratio |
| $pCO2$ | partial pressure of carbon dioxide |
| PCR | polymerase chain reaction |
| PE | pulmonary embolism |
| PPV | positive predictive value |

| PSA | prostate-specific antigen |
|---|---|
| $P_{TT}$ | treatment threshold probability |
| PVC | premature ventricular contraction |
| qCT | quantitative computed tomography |
| ROC | receiver operating characteristic |
| RR | relative risk |
| RRR | relative risk reduction |
| SK | streptokinase |
| SROC | summary receiver operating characteristic |
| T | total cost of testing |
| tPA | tissue plasminogen activator |
| TSA | Transportation Safety Administration |
| UA | urinalysis |
| US | ultrasound |
| UTI | urinary tract infection |
| V/Q | ventilation/perfusion |
| VCUG | voiding cystourethrogram |
| WBC | white blood cell |
| WHO | World Health Organization |

## Greek letters

| $\alpha$ | alpha |
|---|---|
| $\beta$ | beta |
| $\kappa$ | kappa |

# Introduction: understanding diagnosis and diagnostic testing

## Two areas of evidence-based medicine: diagnosis and treatment

The term "evidence-based medicine" (EBM) was coined by Gordon Guyatt and colleagues of McMaster University around 1992 (Evidence-Based Medicine Working Group 1992). Oversimplifying greatly, EBM is about using the best available evidence to help in two related areas:

- Diagnosis: How to evaluate a test and then use it to estimate the probability that a patient has a given disease.
- Treatment: How to determine whether a treatment is beneficial in patients with a given disease, and if so, whether the benefits outweigh the costs and risks.

The two areas of evidence-based diagnosis and treatment are closely related. Although a diagnosis can be useful for prognosis, epidemiologic tracking, and scientific study, it may not be worth the costs and risks of testing to diagnose a disease that has no effective treatment. Even if an effective treatment exists, there are probabilities of disease so low that it is not worth testing for the disease. These probabilities depend not only on the cost and accuracy of the test, but also on the effectiveness of the treatment. As suggested by the title, this book focuses more intensively on the diagnosis area of EBM.

## The purpose of diagnosis

When we think about diagnosis, most of us think about a sick person going to the health care provider with a collection of signs and symptoms of illness. The provider, perhaps with the help of some tests, identifies the cause of the patient's illness, then tells the patient the name of the disease and what to do to treat it. Making the diagnosis can help the patient by explaining what is happening, predicting the prognosis, and determining treatments. In addition, it can benefit others by establishing the level of infectiousness to prevent the spread of disease, tracking the burden of disease and the success of disease control efforts, discovering etiologies to prevent future cases, and advancing medical science.

Assigning each illness a diagnosis is one way that we attempt to impose order on the chaotic world of signs and symptoms, grouping them into categories that share various characteristics, including etiology, clinical picture, prognosis, mechanism of transmission, and response to treatment. The trouble is that homogeneity with respect to one of these characteristics does not imply homogeneity with respect to the others. So if we are trying to decide how to diagnose a disease, we need to know why we want to make the diagnosis, because different purposes of diagnosis can lead to different disease classification schemes.

For example, entities with different etiologies or different pathologies may have the same treatment. If the goal is to make decisions about treatment, the etiology or pathology may be irrelevant. Consider a child who presents with puffy eyes, excess fluid in the ankles, and a large amount of protein in the urine – a classic presentation of the nephrotic syndrome. When the authors were in medical school, we dutifully learned how to classify nephrotic syndrome in children by the appearance of the kidney biopsy. There were minimal change disease, focal segmental glomerulosclerosis, membranoproliferative glomerulonephritis, and so on. "Nephrotic syndrome" was not considered a *diagnosis*; a kidney biopsy to determine the type of nephrotic syndrome was felt to be necessary.

However, minimal change disease and focal segmental glomerulosclerosis make up the overwhelming majority of nephrotic syndrome cases in children, and both are treated with corticosteroids. So, although a kidney biopsy would provide prognostic information, current recommendations suggest skipping the biopsy initially, starting steroids, and then doing the biopsy later only if the symptoms do not respond or there are frequent relapses. Thus, if the purpose of making the diagnosis is to guide treatment, the pathologic classification that we learned in medical school is usually irrelevant. Instead, nephrotic syndrome is classified as "steroid responsive or non-responsive" and "relapsing or non-relapsing." If, as is usually the case, it is "steroid-responsive and non-relapsing," we will never know whether it was minimal change disease or focal segmental glomerulosclerosis, because it is not worth doing a kidney biopsy to find out.

There are many similar examples where, at least at some point in an illness, an exact diagnosis is not necessary to guide treatment. We have sometimes been amused by the number of different Latin names there are for certain similar skin conditions, all of which are treated with topical steroids, which makes distinguishing between them rarely necessary from a treatment standpoint. And, although it is sometimes interesting for an emergency physician to determine which knee ligament is torn, "acute ligamentous knee injury" is a perfectly adequate emergency department diagnosis, because the treatment is immobilization, ice, analgesia, and orthopedic follow-up, regardless of the specific ligament injured.

Disease classification systems sometimes have to expand as treatment improves. Before the days of chemotherapy, a pale child with a large number of blasts (very immature white blood cells) on the peripheral blood smear could be diagnosed simply with leukemia. That was enough to determine the treatment (supportive) and the prognosis (grim) without any additional tests. Now, there are many different types of leukemia based, in part, on cell surface markers, each with a specific prognosis and treatment schedule. The classification based on cell surface markers has no *inherent* value; it is valuable only because careful studies have shown that these markers predict prognosis and response to treatment.

If one's purpose is to keep track of disease burden rather than to guide treatment, different classification systems may be appropriate. Diseases with a single cause (e.g., the diseases caused by premature birth) may have multiple different treatments. A classification system that keeps such diseases separate is important to clinicians, who will, for example, treat necrotizing enterocolitis very differently from hyaline membrane disease. On the other hand, epidemiologists and health services researchers looking at neonatal morbidity and mortality may find it most advantageous to group these diseases with the same cause together, because if we can successfully prevent prematurity, then the burden from all of these diseases should decline. Similarly, an epidemiologist in a country with poor sanitation might only want to group together diarrheal diseases by mode of transmission, rather than keep separate statistics on each of the responsible organisms, in order to track success of sanitation efforts. Meanwhile, a clinician practicing in the same area might only need to sort out whether a case of diarrhea needs antibiotics, an antiparasitic drug, or just rehydration.

In this text, when we are discussing how to quantify the information and usefulness of diagnostic tests, it will be helpful to clarify why a diagnostic test is being considered – what decisions is it supposed to help us with?

## Definition of "disease"

In the next several chapters, we will be discussing tests to diagnose "disease." What do we mean by that term? We use the term "disease" for *a health condition that is either already causing illness or is likely to cause illness relatively quickly in the absence of treatment*. If the disease is not currently causing illness, it is presymptomatic. For most of this book, we will assume that the reason for diagnosis is to make treatment decisions, and that diagnosing disease is important for treatment decisions because there are treatments that are beneficial in those who have a disease and not beneficial in those who do not.

For example, acute coronary ischemia is an important cause of chest pain in patients presenting to the emergency department. Its short-term mortality is 25% among patients discharged from the emergency department and only 12.5% among patients who are hospitalized (presumably for monitoring, anticoagulation, and possibly thrombolysis or angioplasty) (Lee and Goldman 2000). Patients presenting to the emergency department with nonischemic chest pain do not have high short-term mortality and do not benefit from hospitalization. Therefore, a primary purpose of diagnosing acute coronary ischemia is to help with the treatment decision about whom to hospitalize.

The distinction between a disease and a risk factor depends on what we mean by "likely to cause illness relatively quickly." Congenital hypothyroidism, if untreated, will lead to severe retardation, even though this effect is not immediate. This is clearly a disease, but because it is not already causing illness, it is considered presymptomatic. On the other hand, mild hypertension is asymptomatic and is important mainly as a risk factor for heart disease and stroke, which are diseases. At some point, however, hypertension can become severe enough that it is likely to cause illness relatively quickly (e.g., a blood pressure of 280/140) and is a disease. Similarly, diseases like hepatitis C, ductal carcinoma in situ of the breast, and prostate cancer illustrate that there is a continuum between risk factors, presymptomatic diseases, and diseases that depends on the likelihood and timing of subsequent illness. For the first five chapters of this book we will be focusing on "prevalent" disease – that is, diseases that patients either do or do not have at the time we test them. In Chapter 6 on screening, we will distinguish between screening for unrecognized symptomatic disease[1], presymptomatic disease, and risk factors. In Chapter 7 on prognostic testing, we will also consider incident diseases and outcomes of illness – that is, diseases and other outcomes (like death) that are not yet present at the time of the test, but have some probability of happening later, that may be predicted by the results of a test for risk factors or prognosis.

Relative to patients without the disease, patients with the disease have a high risk of bad outcomes and will benefit from treatment. We still need to quantify that benefit so we can compare it with the risks and costs of treatment. Because we often cannot be certain that the patient has the disease, there may be some threshold probability of disease at which the projected benefits of treatment will outweigh the risks and costs. In Chapters 3 through 8, we will sometimes assume that such a treatment threshold probability exists. In Chapter 9, when we discuss quantifying the benefits (and harms) of treatments, we will show how they determine the treatment threshold probability of disease.

## Dichotomous disease state (D+/D−): a convenient oversimplification

Most discussions of diagnostic testing, including this one, simplify the problem of diagnosis by assuming a dichotomy between those with a particular disease and those without the disease. The patients with disease, that is, with a positive diagnosis, are denoted "D+," and the patients without the disease are denoted "D−." This is an oversimplification for two reasons. First, there is usually a spectrum of disease. Some patients we label D+ have mild or early disease, and other patients have severe or advanced disease; so instead of D+, we should have D+, D++, and D+++. Second, there is usually a spectrum of those who do not have the disease (D−) that includes other diseases as well as varying states of health. Thus for symptomatic patients, instead of D+ and D−, we should have D1, D2, and D3, each potentially at varying levels of severity, and for asymptomatic patients we will have D− as well.

---

[1] It is possible for patients with a disease (e.g., depression, deafness, anemia) to have symptoms that they do not recognize.

For example, a patient with prostate cancer might have early, localized cancer or widely metastatic cancer. A test for prostate cancer, the prostate-specific antigen, is much more likely to be positive in the case of metastatic cancer. Or consider the patient with acute headache due to subarachnoid hemorrhage. The hemorrhage may be extensive and easily identified by computed tomography scanning, or it might be a small sentinel bleed, unlikely to be identified by computed tomography and identifiable only by lumbar puncture.

Even in patients who do not have the disease in question, a multiplicity of potential diagnoses of interest may exist. Consider a young woman with lower abdominal pain and a positive urine pregnancy test. The primary concern is ectopic pregnancy, but women without ectopic pregnancies may have either normal or abnormal intrauterine pregnancies. One test commonly used in these patients, the $\beta$-HCG, is unlikely to be normal in patients with abnormal intrauterine pregnancies, even though they do not have ectopic pregnancies (Kohn et al. 2003). For patients presenting to the emergency department with chest pain, acute coronary ischemia is not the only serious diagnosis to consider; aortic dissection and pulmonary embolism are among the other serious causes of chest pain, and these have very different treatments from acute coronary ischemia.

Thus, dichotomizing disease states can get us into trouble because the composition of the D+ group (which includes patients with differing severity of disease) as well as the D− group (which includes patients with differing distributions of other diseases) can vary from one study and one clinical situation to another. This, of course, will affect results of measurements that we make on these groups (like the distribution of prostate-specific antigen results in men with prostate cancer or of $\beta$-HCG results in women who do not have ectopic pregnancies). So, although we will generally assume that we are testing for the presence or absence of a single disease and can therefore use the D+/D− shorthand, we will occasionally point out the limitations of this assumption.

## Generic decision problem: examples

We will start out by considering an oversimplified, generic medical decision problem in which the patient either has the disease (D+) or doesn't have the disease (D−). If he has the disease, there is a quantifiable benefit to treatment. If he doesn't have the disease, there is an equally quantifiable cost associated with treating unnecessarily. A single test is under consideration. The test, although not perfect, provides information on whether the patient is D+ or D−. The test has two or more possible results with different probabilities in D+ individuals than in D− individuals. The test itself has an associated cost. The choice is to treat without the test, do the test and determine treatment based on the result, or forego treatment without testing.

Here are several examples of the sorts of clinical scenarios that material covered in this book will help you understand better. In each scenario, the decision to be made includes whether to treat without testing, to do the test and treat based on testing results, or to do nothing (neither test nor treat). We will refer to these scenarios throughout the book.

---

**Clinical scenario: febrile infant**

A 5-month-old boy has a fever of 39.7°C with no obvious source. You are concerned about a bacterial infection in the blood (bacteremia), which could be treated with an injection of an antibiotic. You have decided that other tests, such as a lumbar puncture or chest x-ray, are not indicated, but you are considering drawing blood to use his white blood cell count to help you decide whether or not to treat.

*Disease in question*: Bacteremia.
*Test being considered*: White blood cell count.
*Treatment decision*: Whether to administer an antibiotic injection.

**Clinical scenario: screening mammography**

A 45-year-old economics professor from a local university wants to know whether she should get screening mammography. She has not detected any lumps on breast self-examination. A positive screening mammogram would be followed by further testing, possibly including biopsy of the breast.

*Disease in question*: Breast cancer.
*Test being considered*: Mammogram.
*Treatment decision*: Whether to pursue further evaluation for breast cancer.

**Clinical scenario: flu prophylaxis**

It is the flu season, and your patient is a 14-year-old girl who has had fever, muscle aches, cough, and a sore throat for two days. Her mother has seen a commercial for Tamiflu® (oseltamivir) and asks you about prescribing it for the whole family so they don't catch the flu. You are considering testing the patient with a rapid bedside test for influenza A and B.

*Disease in question*: Influenza.
*Test being considered*: Bedside influenza test for 14-year-old patient.
*Treatment decision*: Whether to prescribe prophylaxis for others in the household. (You assume that prophylaxis is of little use if your 14-year-old patient does not have the flu but rather some other viral illness.)

**Clinical scenario: sonographic screening for fetal chromosomal abnormalities**

In late first-trimester pregnancies, fetal chromosomal abnormalities can be identified definitively using chorionic villus sampling, but this is an invasive procedure that entails some risk of accidentally terminating the pregnancy. Chromosomally abnormal fetuses tend to have larger nuchal translucencies (a measurement of fluid at the back of the fetal neck) and absence of the nasal bone on 13-week ultrasound, which is a noninvasive test. A government perinatal screening program faces the question of who should receive the screening ultrasound examination and what combination of nuchal translucency and nasal bone examination results should prompt chorionic villus sampling.

*Disease in question*: Fetal chromosomal abnormalities.
*Test being considered*: Prenatal ultrasound.
*Treatment decision*: Whether to do the definitive diagnostic test, chorionic villus sampling.

## Preview of coming attractions: criteria for evaluating diagnostic tests

In the next several chapters, we will consider four increasingly stringent criteria for evaluating diagnostic tests:

1. *Reliability.* The results of a test should not vary based on who does the test or where it is done. This consistency must be maintained whether the test is repeated by the same observer or by different observers and in the same location or different locations. To address this question for tests with continuous results, we need to know about things like the within-subject standard deviation, within-subject coefficient of variation, correlation coefficients (i.e., why they can be misleading), and Bland–Altman plots. For tests with categorical results (e.g., normal/abnormal), we should understand kappa and its alternatives. These measures of reliability are discussed in Chapter 2. If you find that repetitions of the test do not agree any better than would be expected by chance alone, you might as well stop: the test cannot be informative or useful. But simply performing better than would be expected by chance, although necessary, is not sufficient to establish that the test is worth doing.

2. *Accuracy.* The test must be able to distinguish between those with disease and those without disease. We will measure this ability using sensitivity and specificity, test-result distributions in D+ and D− individuals, Receiver Operating Characteristic curves, and likelihood ratios. These are covered in Chapters 3 and 4. Again, if a test is not accurate, you can stop; it cannot be useful. It is also important to be able to tell how much new information a test gives. For this we will need to address the concept of "test independence" (Chapter 8).

3. *Usefulness.* In general, this means that the test result should have a reasonable probability of changing decisions (which we have assumed will, on average, benefit the patient).[2] To determine this, we need to know how to combine our test results with other information to estimate the probability of disease, and at what probability of disease different treatments are indicated (Chapters 3, 4, 7, and 8).

   The best proof of a test's usefulness is a randomized trial showing that clinical outcomes are better in those who receive the test than in those who do not. Such trials are mainly practical to evaluate certain screening tests, which we will discuss in Chapter 6. If a test improves outcomes in a randomized trial, we can infer that it meets the three preceding criteria (reliability, accuracy, and usefulness). Similarly, if it clearly does not meet these criteria, there is no point in doing a randomized trial. More often, tests provide some information and their usefulness will vary depending on specific characteristics of the patient that determine the prior probability of disease.

---

[2] This discussion simplifies the situation by focusing on value provided by affecting management decisions. In fact, there may be some value to providing information even if it does not lead to changes in management (as demonstrated by peoples' willingness to pay for testing). Just attaching a name to the cause of someone's suffering can have a therapeutic effect. However, giving tests credit for these effects, like giving drugs credit for the placebo effect, is problematic.

4. *Value.* Even if a test is potentially useful, it may not be worth doing if it is too expensive, painful, or difficult to do. Although we will not formally cover cost-effectiveness analysis or cost-benefit analysis in this text, we will informally show (in Chapters 3 and 9) how the cost of a test can be weighed against possible benefits from better treatment decisions.

## Summary of key points

1. There is no single best way to classify people into those with different diagnoses; the optimal classification scheme depends on the purpose for making the diagnosis.
2. We will initially approach evaluation of diagnostic testing by assuming that the patient either does or does not have a particular disease, and that the purpose of diagnosing the disease is to decide whether or not to treat. We must recognize, in doing this, that dichotomization of disease states may inaccurately represent the spectrum of both disease and nondisease, and that diagnosis of disease may have purposes other than treatment.
3. Increasingly stringent criteria for evaluating tests include reliability, accuracy, usefulness, and value.

## References

Evidence-Based Medicine Working Group (1992). "Evidence-based medicine. A new approach to teaching the practice of medicine." *JAMA* **268**(17): 2420–5.

Kohn, M. A., K. Kerr, et al. (2003). "Beta-human chorionic gonadotropin levels and the likelihood of ectopic pregnancy in emergency department patients with abdominal pain or vaginal bleeding." *Acad Emerg Med* **10**(2): 119–26.

Lee, T. H., and L. Goldman (2000). "Evaluation of the patient with acute chest pain." *N Engl J Med* **342**(16): 1187–95.

## Chapter 1 Problems: understanding diagnosis

1. In children with apparent viral gastroenteritis (vomiting and diarrhea), a test for rotavirus is often done. No specific antiviral therapy for rotavirus is available, but rotavirus is the most common cause of hospital-acquired diarrhea in children and is an important cause of acute gastroenteritis in children attending child care. A rotavirus vaccine is recommended by the CDC's Advisory Committee on Immunization Practices. Why would we want to know if a child's gastroenteritis is caused by rotavirus?
2. Randomized trials (Campbell 1989; Forsyth 1989; Lucassen et al. 2000) suggest that about half of formula-fed infants with colic respond to a change from cow's milk formula to formula in which the protein has been hydrolyzed. Colic in these studies (and in textbooks) is generally defined as crying at least 3 hours per day at least three times a week in an otherwise well infant. You are seeing a distressed mother of a formula-fed 5-week-old who cries inconsolably for about 1 to 2 hours

daily. Your physical examination is normal. Does this child have colic? Would you recommend a trial of hydrolyzed-protein formula?

3. An 86-year-old man presents with weight loss for 2 months and worsening shortness of breath for 2 weeks. An x-ray shows a left pleural effusion; thoracocentesis shows undifferentiated carcinoma. History, physical examination, and routine laboratory tests do not disclose the primary cancer. Could "metastatic undifferentiated carcinoma" be a sufficient diagnosis, or are additional studies needed? Does your answer change if he is demented?

4. Your patient, an otherwise healthy 20-month-old girl, was diagnosed with a urinary tract infection at an urgent care clinic where she presented with fever last week. At this writing, the American Academy of Pediatrics recommends a voiding cystourethrogram (VCUG, an x-ray preceded by putting a catheter through the urethra into the bladder to instill contrast) to evaluate the possibility that she has vesicoureteral reflux (reflux of urine from the bladder up the ureters to the kidneys) (AAP 1999). A diagnosis of vesicoureteral reflux typically leads to two alterations in management: 1) prophylactic antibiotics and 2) additional VCUGs. However, there is no evidence that prophylactic antibiotics are effective at decreasing infections or scarring in this setting (Hodson et al. 2007), and they may even be harmful (Garin et al. 2006, Newman 2006). How does this information affect the decision to do a VCUG in order to diagnose reflux?

## References for problem set

AAP (1999). "Practice parameter: the diagnosis, treatment, and evaluation of the initial urinary tract infection in febrile infants and young children. American Academy of Pediatrics. Committee on Quality Improvement. Subcommittee on Urinary Tract Infection." *Pediatrics* **103**(4 Pt 1): 843–52.

Campbell, J. P. (1989). "Dietary treatment of infant colic: a double-blind study." *J R Coll Gen Pract* **39**(318): 11–4.

Forsyth, B. W. (1989). "Colic and the effect of changing formulas: a double-blind, multiple-crossover study." *J Pediatr* **115**(4): 521–6.

Garin, E. H., F. Olavarria, et al. (2006). "Clinical significance of primary vesicoureteral reflux and urinary antibiotic prophylaxis after acute pyelonephritis: a multicenter, randomized, controlled study." *Pediatrics* **117**(3): 626–32.

Hodson, E. M., D. M. Wheeler, et al. (2007). "Interventions for primary vesicoureteric reflux." *Cochrane Database Syst Rev 3*: CD001532.

Lucassen, P. L., W. J. Assendelft, et al. (2000). "Infantile colic: crying time reduction with a whey hydrolysate: a double-blind, randomized, placebo-controlled trial." *Pediatrics* **106**(6): 1349–54.

Newman, T. B. (2006). "Much pain, little gain from voiding cystourethrograms after urinary tract infection." *Pediatrics* **118**(5): 2251.

# Reliability and measurement error

## Introduction

A test cannot be useful unless it gives the same or similar results when administered repeatedly to the same individual within a time period too short for real biological changes to take place. Consistency must be maintained whether the test is repeated by the same measurer or by different measurers. This desirable characteristic of a test is generally called "reliability," although some authors prefer "reproducibility." In this chapter, we will look at several different ways to quantify reliability of a test. Measures of reliability depend on whether the test is being administered repeatedly by the same observer, or by different people or different methods, as well as what type of variable is being measured. Intra-rater reliability compares results when the test is administered repeatedly by the same observer, and inter-rater reliability compares the results when measurements are made by different observers. Standard deviation and coefficient of variation are used to determine reliability between multiple measurements of a continuous variable in the same individual. These differences can be random or systematic. We usually assume that differences between repeated measurements by the same observer and method are purely random, whereas differences between measurements by different observers or by different methods can be both random and systematic. The term "bias" refers to systematic differences, distinguishing them from "random error." The Bland–Altman plot describes reliability in method comparison, in which one measurement method (often established, but invasive, harmful, or expensive) is compared with another method (often newer, easier, or cheaper).

As we discuss these measures of reliability, we are generally comparing measurements with each other, not with the "truth" as determined by a reference "gold standard." Comparing a test result with a gold standard assesses its accuracy or validity, something we will cover in Chapters 3 and 4. However, sometimes one of the continuous measurements being compared in a Bland–Altman plot is considered the gold standard. In this case, the method comparison is called "calibration."

## Types of variables

How we assess intra- or inter-rater reliability of a measurement depends on whether the scale of measurement is categorical, ordinal, or continuous. Categorical variables can take on a limited number of separate values. Categorical variables with only two possible values, for example, present/absent or alive/dead, are dichotomous. Categorical variables with more than two possible values are nominal or ordinal. Nominal variables, for example, blood type, race, or cardiac rhythm, have no inherent order. Ordinal variables have an inherent order, such as pain that is rated "none," "mild," "moderate," or "severe." Many scores or scales used in medicine, such as the Glasgow Coma Score, are ordinal variables.

Continuous variables, such as weight, serum glucose, or peak expiratory flow, can take on an infinite number of possible values. In contrast, discrete variables, like parity, the number of previous hospitalizations, or the number of sexual partners, can take on only a finite number of values. If discrete variables take on many possible values, they behave like continuous variables. Either continuous variables or discrete variables that take on many values can be grouped into categories to create ordinal variables.

In this chapter, we will learn about the kappa statistic for measuring intra- and inter-rater reliability of a nominal measurement and about the weighted kappa statistic for ordinal measurements. Assessment of intra-rater or intra-method reliability of a continuous test requires measurement of either the within-subjects standard deviation or the within-subjects coefficient of variation (depending on whether the random error is proportional to the level of the measurement). A Bland–Altman plot can help estimate both systematic bias and random error. While correlation coefficients are often used to assess intra- and inter-rater reliability of a continuous measurement, we will see that they are inappropriate for assessing random error and useless for assessing systematic bias.

## Measuring inter-observer agreement for categorical variables

### Agreement

When there are two observers or when the same observer repeats a measurement on two occasions, the agreement can be summarized in a "k by k" table, where k is the number of categories that the measurement can have. The simplest measure of inter-observer agreement is the concordance or observed agreement rate, that is, the proportion of observations on which the two observers agree. This can be obtained by summing the numbers along the diagonal of the "k by k" table from the upper left to the lower right and dividing by the total number of observations.

We start by looking at some simple 2 × 2 ("yes or no") examples. Later in the chapter, we will look at examples with more categories.

**Example 2.1** Suppose you wish to measure inter-radiologist agreement at classifying 100 x-rays as either "normal" or "abnormal." Because there are two possible values, you can put the results in a 2 × 2 table.

**Classification of 100 X-rays by 2 Radiologists**

| | | Radiologist #2 | | |
| --- | --- | --- | --- | --- |
| | | Abnormal | Normal | Total |
| Radiologist #1 | Abnormal | 20 | 15 | 35 |
| | Normal | 10 | 55 | 65 |
| | Total | 30 | 70 | 100 |

In this example, out of 100 x-rays, there were 20 that both radiologists classified as abnormal (upper left) and 55 that both radiologists classified as normal (lower right), for an observed agreement rate of $(20 + 55)/100 = 75\%$.

When the observations are not evenly distributed among the categories (e.g., when the proportion "abnormal" on a dichotomous test is substantially different from 50%), the observed agreement rate can be misleading.

**Example 2.2** If two radiologists each rate only five of 100 x-rays as abnormal, but do not agree on which ones are abnormal, their observed agreement will still be $(0 + 90)/100 = 90\%$.

**Prevalence of "Abnormal" Only 5%**

| | | Radiologist #2 | | |
| --- | --- | --- | --- | --- |
| | | Abnormal | Normal | Total |
| Radiologist #1 | Abnormal | 0 | 5 | 5 |
| | Normal | 5 | 90 | 95 |
| | Total | 5 | 95 | 100 |

In fact, if two observers both know an abnormality is uncommon, they can have nearly perfect agreement just by never or rarely saying that it is present.

**Kappa for dichotomous variables**

To address this problem, another measure of inter-observer agreement, called kappa (the Greek letter $\kappa$), is sometimes used. Kappa measures the extent of agreement inside a table, such as the ones in Examples 2.1 and 2.2, beyond what would be expected from the observers' overall estimates of the frequency of the different categories. The observers' estimated frequency of observations in each category is found from the totals for each row and column on the outside of the table. These outside totals are called the "marginals" in the table. Kappa measures agreement beyond what would be expected from the marginals. Kappa ranges from $-1$ (perfect disagreement) to 1 (perfect agreement). A kappa of 0 indicates that the amount of agreement was exactly that expected from the marginals. Kappa is calculated as:

$$\text{Kappa} = \frac{\text{Observed \% agreement} - \text{Expected \% agreement}}{100\% - \text{Expected \% agreement}} \qquad \text{(Eq. 2.1)}$$

Observed % agreement is the same as the concordance rate.

**Table 2.1.** Formula for kappa

|          |     | Rater #2 | | |
|----------|-----|-----|-----|--------|
|          |     | $+$ | $-$ | Total  |
| Rater #1 | $+$ | a   | b   | $R_1$  |
|          | $-$ | c   | d   | $R_2$  |
| Total    |     | $C_1$ | $C_2$ | N  |

| | |
|---|---|
| Observed % Agreement (sum along diagonal and divide by N): | $(a+d)/N$ |
| Expected number for $+/+$ cell: | $R_1/N \times C_1$ |
| Expected number for $-/-$ cell: | $R_2/N \times C_2$ |
| Expected % Agreement (sum expected numbers along diagonal and divide by N) : | $(R_1/N \times C_1 + R_2/N \times C_2)/N$ |

$$\text{Kappa} = \frac{\text{Observed \% agreement} - \text{Expected \% agreement}}{100\% - \text{Expected \% agreement}}$$

## Calculating expected agreement

We obtain expected agreement by adding the expected agreement in each cell along the diagonal. For each cell, the number of agreements expected from the marginals is the proportion of total observations found in that cell's row (the row total divided by the sample size) times the number of observations found in that cell's column (the column total). We will illustrate why this is so later.

In Example 2.1, the expected number in the "Abnormal/Abnormal" cell is $30/100 \times 35 = 0.3 \times 35 = 10.5$. The expected number in the "Normal/Normal" cell is $70/100 \times 65 = 0.7 \times 65 = 45.5$. So the total expected number of agreements is $10.5 + 45.5 = 56$, and the expected % agreement is $56/100 = 56\%$. In contrast, in Example 2.2, in which both observers agree that abnormality was uncommon, the expected % agreement is much higher: $[(5/100 \times 5) + (95/100 \times 95)]/100 = [0.25 + 90.25]/100 = 90.5\%$.

## Understanding expected agreement

The expected agreement used in calculating kappa is sometimes referred to as the agreement expected by chance alone. We prefer to call it agreement expected from the marginals, because it is the agreement expected by chance only under the assumption that the marginals are fixed and known to the observers, which is generally not the case.

To understand where the expected agreement comes from, consider the following experiment. After the initial reading that resulted in Table 2.1, suppose our 2 radiologists are each given back their stack of 100 films with a jellybean jar containing numbers of red and green jelly beans corresponding to their initial readings. For example, since Radiologist #1 rated 35 of the films abnormal and 65 normal, he would get a jar with exactly 35 red and 65 green jellybeans. His instruction is then to close his eyes and draw out a jellybean for each x-ray in the stack. If the jellybean is red, he calls the film abnormal. If the jellybean is green, he calls the film normal. After he has "read" the film, he eats the jellybean. (This is known in statistical terms as sampling without replacement.) When he is finished, he takes the stack of 100 films to Radiologist #2. She is given the same instructions; only her bottle has the numbers of colored jellybeans in proportion to her initial reading, that is, 30 red jellybeans and 70 green ones. The average agreement between the 2 radiologists over many repetitions of the jellybean method is the expected agreement, given their marginals.

If both of them have mostly green or mostly red jellybeans, their expected agreement will be more than 50%. In fact, in the extreme example, where both observers call all of the films normal or abnormal, they will be given all green or all red jellybeans, and their "expected" agreement will be 100%. Kappa addresses the question: How well did the observers do compared with how well they would have done if they had jars of colored jelly beans in proportion to their totals (marginals), and they had used the jellybean color to read the film?

Now, why does multiplying the proportion in each cell's row by the number in that cell's column give you the expected number in that cell? Because if Radiologist #1 thinks 35% of the films are abnormal, and agrees with Radiologist #2 no more than at a level expected from that, then he should think 35% of the films rated by Radiologist #2 are abnormal, regardless of how they are rated by Radiologist #2.[1]

"Wait a minute!" we hear you cry, "In real life studies, the marginals are seldom fixed." In general, no one tells the participants what proportion of the subjects are normal. You might think that, if they manage to agree on the fact that most are normal, they should get some credit. This is, in fact, what can be counter-intuitive about kappa. But that's how kappa is defined, so if you want to give credit for agreement on the marginals, you will need to use another statistic.

### Understanding the kappa formula

Before we calculate some values of kappa, let us make sure you understand Equation 2.1. The numerator is how much better agreement was than what would be expected from the marginals. The denominator is how much better it could have been, if it were perfect. So kappa can be understood as how far from the expected agreement to perfect agreement the observed agreement was.

**Example 2.3** Fill in the blanks: If expected agreement is 60% and observed agreement is 90%, then kappa would be___because 90% is __% of the way from 60% to 100% (see Figure 2.1).
    *Answers: 0.75, 75.*

**Example 2.4** Fill in the blanks: If expected agreement is 70% and observed agreement is 80%, then kappa would be ___ because 80% is __% of the way from 70% to 100%.
    *Answers: 0.33, 33*

Returning to Example 2.1, because the observed agreement is 75% and expected agreement 56%, kappa is $(75\% - 56\%)/(100\% - 56\%) = 0.43$. That is, the agreement beyond expected, $75\% - 56\% = 19\%$, is 43% of the maximum

---

[1] In probability terms, if the two observers are *independent* (that is, not looking at the films, just guessing using jellybeans), the probability that a film will receive a particular rating by Radiologist # 1 and another particular rating by radiologist #2 is just the product of the probabilities.

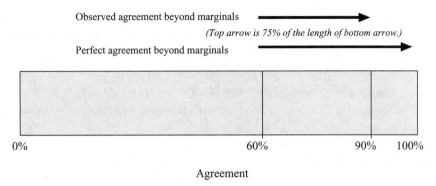

Figure 2.1  Visualizing kappa as the proportion of the way from expected to perfect agreement the observed agreement was for Example 2.3.

agreement beyond expected, 100% − 56% = 44%. This is respectable, if somewhat less impressive than 75% agreement. Similarly, in Example 2.2, kappa is (90% − 90.5%)/(100% − 90.5%) = −0.5%/9.5% = −0.05, indicating that the degree of agreement was a tiny bit worse than what would be expected based on the marginals.

### Impact of the marginals and balanced versus unbalanced disagreement

If the percent agreement stays roughly the same, kappa will decrease as the proportion of positive ratings becomes more extreme (farther from 50%). This is because, as the expected agreement increases, the room for agreement beyond expected is reduced. Although this has been called a paradox (Feinstein and Cicchetti 1990), it only feels that way because of our ambivalence about whether two observers should get credit for recognizing how rare or common a finding is.

**Example 2.5** Yen et al. (2005) compared abdominal exam findings suggestive of appendicitis, such as tenderness to palpation and absence of bowel sounds, between pediatric emergency physicians and pediatric surgical residents. Abdominal tenderness was present in roughly 60% of the patients, and bowel sounds were absent in only about 6% of patients. The physicians agreed on the presence or absence of tenderness only 65% of the time, and the kappa was 0.34. In contrast, they agreed on the presence or absence of bowel sounds an impressive 89% of the time, but because absence of bowel sounds was rare, kappa was essentially zero (−0.04). They got no credit for agreeing that absence of bowel sounds was a rare finding.

Similarly, if observers disagree markedly on the prevalence of a finding, kappa will tend to be higher than if they agree on the prevalence, even though the observed agreement stays the same. When observers disagree on the prevalence of a finding, it suggests that they may have different thresholds for saying that it is present – for example, one needs be more certain than the other. This sort of systematic, unbalanced disagreement is best assessed, not by looking at the marginals (where it is diluted by agreement), but by looking for asymmetry across the diagonal. If there are a lot more or fewer observations above the diagonal than below, it suggests this sort of systematic disagreement. Kappa is not particularly useful in assessing systematic disagreement.

One final point: We generally assume that systematic differences in ratings occur only in studies of inter-rater reliability (comparing two different observers), not intra-rater reliability (comparing the same observer at different time points). However, imagine a radiologist re-reviewing the same set of x-rays before and after having been sued for missing an abnormality. We might expect the readings to differ systematically, with unbalanced disagreements favoring abnormality on the second reading that were normal on the first reading.

## Kappa for three or more categories

### Unweighted

So far, our examples for calculating kappa have been dichotomous ratings, like abnormal versus normal radiographs or presence or absence of right lower quadrant tenderness on abdominal exam. The calculation of expected agreement works the same with three or more categories.

**Example 2.6** Suppose two pediatricians independently evaluate 100 eardrums, and classify each as Normal, Otitis Media with Effusion (OME), or Acute Otitis Media (Acute OM).

**Classification by 2 Pediatricians of 100 Eardrums into 1 of 3 Categories**

|  |  | Normal | OME | Acute OM | Total |
|---|---|---|---|---|---|
|  |  | **Pediatrician #2** | | | |
| Pediatrician #1 | Normal | 38 | 7 | 5 | **50** |
|  | OME | 8 | 11 | 11 | **30** |
|  | Acute OM | 14 | 2 | 4 | **20** |
|  | **Total** | **60** | **20** | **20** | **100** |

In this case, the observed number of agreements is:

$38 + 11 + 4 = 53.$

And the observed % agreement is:

$53/100 = 53\%.$

The expected numbers along the diagonal are:

$(50/100)(60) + (30/100)(20) + (20/100)(20) = 30 + 6 + 4 = 40.$

So, the expected % agreement is:

$40/100 = 40\%.$

And kappa is:

$(53\% - 40\%)/(100\% - 40\%) = 0.22.$

This is not particularly impressive agreement. However, the pediatricians agreed better in differentiating between normal and abnormal eardrums, as can be seen by collapsing the two otitis categories to make a 2 × 2 table:

### Collapsing Two Categories, OME and Acute OM, into One, Abnormal

|  |  | Pediatrician #2 | | |
|---|---|---|---|---|
|  |  | Normal | Abnormal | Total |
| Pediatrician #1 | Normal | 38 | 12 | 50 |
|  | Abnormal | 22 | 28 | 50 |
|  | Total | 60 | 40 | 100 |

Kappa for this table is 0.32 (check this for yourself[2]). So the pediatricians agreed slightly better when differentiating between normal and abnormal eardrums. Collapsing similar categories together often improves kappa.

## Linear weights

When there are more than two categories, it is important to distinguish between ordinal variables and nominal variables. For ordinal variables, kappa fails to capture all the information in the data, because it does not give partial credit for ratings that are similar, but not exactly the same. Weighted kappa allows for such partial credit. The formula for weighted kappa is the same as that for regular kappa, except that observed and expected agreement are calculated by summing cells, not just along the diagonal, but for the whole table, with each cell first multiplied by a weight for that cell.

The weights for partial agreement can be anything you want, as long as they are used to calculate both the observed and expected levels of agreement. The most straightforward way to do the weights (and the default for most statistical packages) is to assign a weight of 0 when the two raters are maximally far apart (i.e., the upper right and lower left corners of the k × k table), a weight of 1 when there is exact agreement, and weights proportionally spaced in between for intermediate levels of agreement. Because a plot of these weights against the number of categories between the ratings of the two observers yields a straight line, these are sometimes called "linear weights." We will give you the formula below, but it is easier to just look at some examples and see what we mean.

In Example 2.6, there are three categories. Complete disagreement is two categories apart, partial agreement is one category apart, and complete agreement is zero categories apart. So with linear weights, these get weighted 0, 1/2, and 1, respectively.

Similar logic holds for larger numbers of categories. As shown in Table 2.3, if there are four categories, the weights would be 0, 1/3, 2/3, and 1.

Now for the formula: If there are k ordered categories, then take the number of categories between the two raters, divide by k − 1 (the farthest they could be apart) and subtract from 1. That is,

$$\text{Linear Weight for the Cell in "Row i, Column j"} = 1 - \frac{|i - j|}{k - 1} \qquad \text{(Eq. 2.2)}$$

Along the diagonal, $i = j$ and the weight is 1, for perfect agreement. At the upper right and lower left corners, $|i - j| = (k - 1)$, and the weights are 0.

---

[2] Observed % agreement = $(38 + 28)/100 = 66\%$.
 Expected % agreement = $(30 + 20)/100 = 50\%$.
 Kappa = $(66\% - 50\%)/(100\% - 50\%) = 0.32$.

**Table 2.2.** Linear weights for three categories

|  |  | Rater #2 | | |
|---|---|---|---|---|
|  |  | Category 1 | Category 2 | Category 3 |
|  | Category 1 | 1 | 1/2 | 0 |
| Rater #1 | Category 2 | 1/2 | 1 | 1/2 |
|  | Category 3 | 0 | 1/2 | 1 |

**Example 2.7** Gill et al. (2004) examined the reliability of the individual components of the Glasgow Coma Scale score, including the eye opening component. They compared the eye opening score of two emergency physicians independently assessing the same patient. They do not provide the raw data, but the results were something like this:

**Eye-Opening Scores of 2 Emergency Physicians on 116 Patients**

|  |  | Emergency Physician #2 | | | | |
|---|---|---|---|---|---|---|
|  |  | None | To Pain | To Command | Spontaneous | Total |
|  | **None** | 11 | 2 | 0 | 4 | 17 |
| **Emergency** | **To Pain** | 4 | 1 | 2 | 0 | 7 |
| **Physician #1** | **To Command** | 0 | 3 | 8 | 3 | 14 |
|  | **Spontaneous** | 2 | 1 | 7 | 68 | 78 |
|  | **Total** | 17 | 7 | 17 | 75 | 116 |

We will calculate unweighted kappa, weighted kappa using linear weights, and weighted kappa using the custom weights that the authors used. Because we will be calculating weighted kappa, we will need the expected numbers for each cell in the $4 \times 4$ table, not just for the diagonal cells that indicate complete agreement. As an example, consider the highlighted cell in the third column of the fourth row of the table. Looking at the row total, we see that Emergency Physician #1 thought that 78 out of the 116 patients had spontaneous eye opening. Looking at the column total, we see that Emergency Physician #2 thought that 17 patients opened their eyes to command. So, based on these marginals, we would expect that Physician #1 would classify that 78/116 of these 17 patients as opening their eyes spontaneously: $78/116 \times 17 = 11.4$. We calculate all the expected values in the same way:

**Table 2.3.** Linear weights for four categories

|  |  | Rater #2 | | | |
|---|---|---|---|---|---|
|  |  | Category 1 | Category 2 | Category 3 | Category 4 |
|  | Category 1 | 1 | 2/3 | 1/3 | 0 |
| Rater #1 | Category 2 | 2/3 | 1 | 2/3 | 1/3 |
|  | Category 3 | 1/3 | 2/3 | 1 | 2/3 |
|  | Category 4 | 0 | 1/3 | 2/3 | 1 |

**Expected Numbers in Each Cell Based on the Marginals**

|  |  | Emergency Physician #2 |  |  |  |  |
|---|---|---|---|---|---|---|
|  |  | None | To Pain | To Command | Spontaneous | Total |
|  | None | 2.5 | 1.0 | 2.5 | 11.0 | 17 |
| Emergency | To Pain | 1.0 | 0.4 | 1.0 | 4.5 | 7 |
| Physician #1 | To Command | 2.1 | 0.8 | 2.1 | 9.1 | 14 |
|  | Spontaneous | 11.4 | 4.7 | 11.4 | 50.4 | 78 |
|  | Total | 17 | 7 | 17 | 75 | 116 |

Now we calculate unweighted kappa. The observed number of agreements is:

$11 + 1 + 8 + 68 = 88$.

And the observed % agreement is

$88/116 = 76\%$.

The expected number of (perfect) agreements is

$(2.5 + 0.4 + 2.1 + 50.4) = 55.4$.

And the expected % agreement is

$55.4/116 = 48\%$.

So, (unweighted) kappa is:

$(76\% - 48\%)/(100\% - 48\%) = 0.54$.

Now, we apply the linear weights shown in Table 2.3. Above we saw that the number of observed exact agreements was 88. These get a weight of 1.
   The number of observations one category apart is:

$2 + 2 + 3 + 4 + 3 + 7 = 21$.

These observations get a weight of 2/3.
   The number of observations two categories apart is:

$0 + 0 + 0 + 1 = 1$.

This observation gets a weight of 1/3.
   The disagreements three categories apart, in the upper right and lower left corners of the table, get a weight of 0 and we can ignore them.
   So, we have 88 exact agreements, 21 disagreements 1 category apart, to be weighted by 2/3, and 1 disagreement 2 categories apart to be weighted by 1/3. Our total observed (weighted) number of agreements is:

$88 \times 1 + 21 \times 2/3 + 1 \times 1/3 = 88 + 14.33 = 102.33$.

And observed % agreement (weighted) is

$102.33/116 = 88\%$.

We calculate the expected (weighted) agreement the same way. For unweighted kappa, we calculated the number of expected exact agreements to be 55.4. These get fully weighted.

The expected number of disagreements one category apart is

$$1 + 1 + 9.1 + 1 + 0.8 + 11.4 = 24.3,$$

which will be weighted by 2/3.

The expected number of disagreements two categories apart is:

$$2.5 + 4.5 + 2.1 + 4.7 = 13.8,$$

which will be weighted by 1/3.

So the total weighted expected number of agreements is:

$$55.4 \times 1 + 24.3 \times 2/3 + 13.8 \times 1/3 = 55.4 + 16.2 + 4.6 = 76.2.$$

And expected % weighted agreement is:

$$76.2/116 = 66\%.$$

Weighted observed % agreement: 88%.

Weighted expected % agreement: 66%.

Weighted kappa $= (88\% - 66\%)/(100\% - 66\%) = 0.66$

As is usually the case, the weighted kappa using linear weights (0.66) is higher than the unweighted kappa (0.54).

### Custom weights

Of course, these linear weights are just one way to do it. You may feel like some disagreements are much worse than others.

**Example 2.8**  Gill et al. (see Example 2.7) actually calculated weighted kappa giving half-credit for disagreements differing by only one category and no credit for disagreements differing by two or three categories. Their custom weights are shown below.

**Custom Weights for the Four Eye-Opening Ratings**

|  | None | To Pain | To Command | Spontaneous |
|---|---|---|---|---|
| **None** | 1 | 0.5 | 0 | 0 |
| **To Pain** | 0.5 | 1 | 0.5 | 0 |
| **To Command** | 0 | 0.5 | 1 | 0.5 |
| **Spontaneous** | 0 | 0 | 0.5 | 1 |

In this case, the kappa using custom weights was greater than the unweighted kappa and slightly less than the linear weighted kappa. This makes sense because linear weighted kappa gave more credit for disagreements differing by one category (2/3 vs. 1/2 weight).

Although weighted kappa is generally used for ordinal variables, it can be used for nominal variables as well, if some types of disagreement are more significant than others.

**Example 2.9** In Example 2.6, we could give 70% credit for disagreements where both observers agree the ear drum is abnormal but disagree on whether it is OME versus acute OM, and we could give no credit if one observer thinks the drum is normal and the other does not:

**Custom Weights for the Otoscopy Ratings in Example 2.6**

|  |  | Pediatrician #2 | | |
|---|---|---|---|---|
|  |  | Normal | OME | Acute OM |
|  | **Normal** | 1 | 0 | 0 |
| **Pediatrician #1** | **OME** | 0 | 1 | 0.7 |
|  | **Acute OM** | 0 | 0.7 | 1 |

Whatever weighting scheme we choose, it should be symmetric along the diagonal, so that the answer does not depend on which observer is #1 and which is #2.

Kappa also generalizes to more than two observers, although then it is much easier to use a statistics software package. Note that it is not required that each item be rated by the same raters. For example, there can be three raters, with each item rated by only two of them.

## Quadratic weights

A commonly used alternative to linear weights is quadratic weights. With quadratic weights, the penalty for disagreement at each level, $\frac{i-j}{k-1}$, is squared:

$$\text{Quadratic Weight for Cell at Row i and Column j} = 1 - \left(\frac{i-j}{k-1}\right)^2 \qquad \text{(Eq. 2.3)}$$

Because this penalty $\frac{i-j}{k-1}$ is less than 1, squaring it makes it smaller, and the effect of quadratic weights is to give *more credit* for partial agreement. For example, if there are three categories, the weight for partial agreement is $1 - (1/2)^2 = 0.75$, rather than 0.5; if there are four categories, the weight for being off by one category is $1 - (1/3)^2 = 8/9$, rather than 2/3.

**Example 2.10** Here are the quadratic weights for Example 2.7.

**Quadratic Weights for the Four Eye-Opening Ratings**

|  | None | To Pain | To Command | Spontaneous |
|---|---|---|---|---|
| **None** | 1 | 8/9 | 5/9 | 0 |
| **To Pain** | 8/9 | 1 | 8/9 | 5/9 |
| **To Command** | 5/9 | 8/9 | 1 | 8/9 |
| **Spontaneous** | 0 | 5/9 | 8/9 | 1 |

The quadratic weighted kappa for these data is 0.84. This is higher than the linear weighted kappa of 0.75.

Quadratic weighted kappa will generally be higher (and hence look better) than a linear weighted kappa, because the penalty for anything other than complete disagreement is smaller.

**Table 2.4.** Kappa classifications

| Kappa | Sackett et al. (1991) | Altman (1991) |
|-------|----------------------|---------------|
| 0–0.2 | Slight | Poor |
| 0.2–0.4 | Fair | Fair |
| 0.4–0.6 | Moderate | Moderate |
| 0.6–0.8 | Substantial | Good |
| 0.8–1.0 | Almost Perfect | Very Good |

### What is a good kappa?

Most reviews of kappa have some sort of guideline about what constitutes a good kappa. A couple of sample classifications are shown in Table 2.4.

Comparing kappa values between studies can be misleading. We saw that with two-category kappas, for a given level of observed agreement, kappa depends on both the overall prevalence of the abnormality and whether disagreements are balanced or unbalanced. In our discussion of kappa for three or more categories, several new problems became apparent. It should be clear from Example 2.6 that unweighted kappa can be higher when you collapse the table by combining similar categories. This is generally true of weighted kappa as well. It should also be clear from Example 2.7 that weighted kappa depends on the weights used. Gill et al. (2004) defined the custom weights that they used in their paper on the inter-rater reliability of the Glasgow Coma Scale. In contrast, a widely quoted paper on the inter-rater reliability of the National Institutes of Health Stroke Scale (Meyer et al. 2002) reported weighted kappas without stating whether the weights were linear, quadratic, or custom.

## Reliability of continuous measurements

With continuous variables, just as with categorical and ordinal variables, we are interested in the variability in repeated measurements by the same observer or instrument and in the differences between measurements made by two different observers or instruments.

### Test–retest reliability

The random variability of some continuous measurements is well known. Blood pressures, peak expiratory flows, and grip strengths will vary between measurements done in rapid succession. Because they are easily repeatable, most clinical research studies use the average of several repetitions rather than a single value. We tend to assume that the variability between measurements is random, not systematic, but this may not be the case. For example, if the first grip strength measurement fatigued the subject so that the second measurement was systematically lower, or the patient got better at the peak flow measurement with practice, then we could not assess test–retest reliability because the quantities (grip strength and peak flow) are changed by the measurement process itself.

When the variability can be assumed to be purely random, this random variability can be approximately constant across all magnitudes of the measurement or it can vary (usually increase) with the magnitude of the measurement.

### Within-subject standard deviation and repeatability

The simplest description of a continuous measurement's variability is the within-subject standard deviation, $S_w$ (Bland and Altman 1996a). This requires a dataset of several subjects on whom the measurement was repeated multiple times. You calculate each subject's sample variance according to the following formula:

$$\text{Single Subject Sample Variance} = \frac{(M_1 - M_{avg})^2 + (M_2 - M_{avg})^2 + (M_3 - M_{avg})^2 + \cdots + (M_N - M_{avg})^2}{(N - 1)}$$

(Eq. 2.4)

Where

N is the total number of repeated measurements on a single subject,

$M_1, M_2, M_3 \ldots M_N$ are the repeated measurements on a single subject, and

$M_{avg}$ is the average of all N measurements on a single subject.

Then, you average these sample variances across all the subjects in the sample and take the square root to get $S_w$. When there are only two measurements per subject, the formula for within subject sample variance simplifies to:

Sample Variance for two measurements $= (M_1 - M_2)^2/2$     (Eq. 2.5)[3]

**Example 2.11** Suppose you want to assess the test–retest reliability of a new pocket glucometer. You measure the finger-stick glucose twice on each of ten different subjects:

**Calculation of Within-Subject Standard Deviation on Duplicate Glucose Measurements**

| Specimen | Glucose Measurement (mg/dL) #1 | #2 | Difference | Variance $= (M_1 - M_2)^2/2$ |
|---|---|---|---|---|
| 1 | 80 | 92 | −12 | 72 |
| 2 | 89 | 92 | −3 | 4.5 |
| 3 | 93 | 109 | −16 | 128 |
| 4 | 97 | 106 | −9 | 40.5 |
| 5 | 103 | 87 | 16 | 128 |
| 6 | 107 | 104 | 3 | 4.5 |
| 7 | 100 | 105 | −5 | 12.5 |
| 8 | 112 | 104 | 8 | 32 |
| 9 | 123 | 110 | 13 | 84.5 |
| 10 | 127 | 120 | 7 | 24.5 |

**Average Variance $= 53.1$**

$S_w = 7.3$

---

[3] This may look odd, but you will see it is correct if you substitute $(M_1 + M_2)/2$ for $M_{avg}$ in Eq. 2.5, and do the algebra.

For Subject 1, the difference between the two measurements was $-12$. You square this to get 144, and divide by 2 to get a within-subject variance of 72. Averaging together all ten variances yields 53.1, so the within-subject standard deviation $S_w$ is $\sqrt{53.1}$ or 7.3.[4]

If we assume that the measurement error is distributed in a normal ("Gaussian" or bell-shaped) distribution, then about 95% of our measurements (on a single specimen) will be within 1.96 $S_w$ of the theoretical "true" value for that specimen. In this case, $1.96 \times 7.3 = 14.3$ mg/dL. So about 95% of the glucometer readings will be within about 14 mg/dL of the "true" value. The difference between two measurements on the same subject is expected to be within $(1.96 \times \sqrt{2}) = 2.77 \times S_w$ 95% of the time.[5] In this example, $2.77 \times S_w = 2.77 \times 7.3 = 20.2$. This is called the repeatability. We can expect the difference between two measurements on the same specimen to be less than 20.2 mg/dL 95% of the time.

### Why not use average standard deviation?

Rather than take the square root of the variance for each subject (that subject's standard deviation) and then average those to get $S_w$, we first averaged the variances and then took the square root. We did this to preserve desirable mathematical properties – the same general reason that we use the standard deviation (the square root of the mean square deviation) rather than average deviation. However, because the quantities we are going to average are squared, the effect of outliers (subjects from whom the measurement error was much larger than average) is magnified.

### Why not use the correlation coefficient?

A scatterplot of the data in Example 2.11 looks like Figure 2.2.

You may recall from your basic statistics course that the correlation coefficient measures linear correlation between two measurements, ranging from $-1$ (for perfect inverse correlation) to 1 (for perfect correlation) with a value of 0 if the two variables are independent. For these data, the correlation coefficient is 0.67. Is this a good measure of test-retest reliability? Before you answer, see Example 2.12.

**Example 2.12** Let us replace the last pair of measurements (127, 120) in Example 2.11 with a pair of measurements (300, 600) on a hyperglycemic specimen. This pair of measurements does not show very good reliability. The glucose level of 300 might or

---

[4] If there are more than 2 measurements per subject, and especially if there are different numbers of measurements per subject, it is easiest to get the average within-subject variance by using a statistical package to perform a one way analysis of variance (ANOVA). In the standard one-way ANOVA table, the residual mean square is the within-subject variance (Bland and Altman 1996a).

[5] The variance of the difference between two independent random variables is the sum of their individual variances. Since both measurements have variance equal to the within-specimen variance, the difference between them has variance equal to twice the within-specimen variance and the standard deviation of the difference is $\sqrt{2} \times S_{within}$. If the difference between the measurements is normally distributed, 95% of these differences will be within 1.96 standard deviations of the mean difference, which is 0.

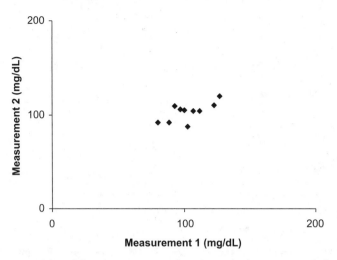

Figure 2.2    Scatterplot of the glucometer readings in Example 2.11. Correlation coefficient = 0.67.

might not prompt a patient using the pocket glucometer to adjust his insulin dose. The glucose level of 600 should prompt him to call his doctor. Here are the new data:

**Duplicate Glucose Measurements from Example 2.11** (except for the last observation)

**Glucose Measurement (mg/dL)**

| Specimen | #1 | #2 | Difference | Variance |
|---|---|---|---|---|
| 1 | 80 | 92 | −12 | 72.0 |
| 2 | 89 | 92 | −3 | 4.5 |
| 3 | 93 | 109 | −16 | 128.0 |
| 4 | 97 | 106 | −9 | 40.5 |
| 5 | 103 | 87 | 16 | 128.0 |
| 6 | 107 | 104 | 3 | 4.5 |
| 7 | 100 | 105 | −5 | 12.5 |
| 8 | 112 | 104 | 8 | 32.0 |
| 9 | 123 | 110 | 13 | 84.5 |
| *10* | *300* | *600* | *−300* | *45000.0* |

Average Variance = 4550.7

$S_w = 67.5$

And the new scatterplot is shown in Figure 2.3.

The correlation coefficient for these data is 0.99. We have added a single pair of measurements that do not even agree with each other very well, and yet the correlation coefficient has gone from 0.67 to 0.99 (almost perfect). Meanwhile, the within-subject standard deviation $S_w$ has increased from 7.3 to 67.5 mg/dL (it has gotten much worse), and the repeatability has increased from 20.2 to 186.9 mg/dL.

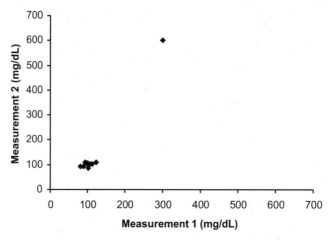

Figure 2.3    Scatterplot of the glucometer readings in Example 2.12. Correlation coefficient = 0.99.

Although it is tempting to use the correlation coefficient between the first and second measurements on each subject, here is why you should not do it (Bland and Altman 1996b):

1. As we just saw, the correlation coefficient is very sensitive to outliers.
2. (Related to 1): The correlation coefficient will automatically be higher if the range of measurements is higher, even though the precision of the measurement stays the same.
3. The correlation coefficient is high for any linear relationship, not just when the first measurement equals the second measurement. If the second measurement is always 300 mg/dL higher or 40% lower than the first measurement, the correlation coefficient is 1, although the measurements do not agree at all.
4. The test of significance for the correlation coefficient uses the absence of relationship as the null hypothesis. This will almost invariably be rejected because of course there is likely to be a relationship between the first and second measurements, even if they do not agree with each other very well.

### Measurement error proportional to magnitude

Sometimes the random error of a measurement is proportional to the magnitude of the measurement. We can visually assess whether error increases with magnitude by graphing the absolute difference between the two measurements versus their average. The glucometer readings from Example 2.11 show no clear trend of error increasing with the magnitude of the measurement, as shown in Figure 2.4.

If the random error of a measurement is proportional to the magnitude of the measurement, we cannot use a single value for the within-subject (or within-specimen) standard deviation, because it increases with the level of the measurement. This would be the case if, for example, a measurement was accurate to ±10%, rather than a certain number of mg/dL. In cases like this, rather than using a single within-subject standard deviation, the variability could be better summarized with the average coefficient of variation (CV), equal to the standard deviation divided by the mean.

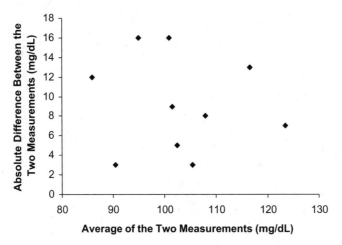

Figure 2.4    Plot of the absolute difference between the two measurements against their average for the data in Example 2.11.

**Example 2.13**  Sometimes the difference between measurements tends to increase as the magnitude of the measurements increases.

**Duplicate Glucose Measurements Illustrating Increasing Error Proportional to the Mean**

| Specimen | Glucose Measurement (mg/dL) #1 | #2 | Difference | Variance | SD | CV |
|---|---|---|---|---|---|---|
| 11 | 93 | 107 | −14 | 98 | 9.9 | 9.9% |
| 12 | 132 | 117 | 15 | 112.5 | 10.6 | 8.5% |
| 13 | 174 | 199 | −25 | 312.5 | 17.7 | 9.5% |
| 14 | 233 | 277 | −44 | 968 | 31.1 | 12.2% |
| 15 | 371 | 332 | 39 | 760.5 | 27.6 | 7.8% |
| 16 | 364 | 421 | −57 | 1624.5 | 40.3 | 10.3% |
| 17 | 465 | 397 | 68 | 2312 | 48.1 | 11.2% |
| 18 | 518 | 446 | 72 | 2592 | 50.9 | 10.6% |
| 19 | 606 | 540 | 66 | 2178 | 46.7 | 8.1% |
| 20 | 682 | 806 | −124 | 7688 | 87.7 | 11.8% |

Again, this is better appreciated by plotting the absolute difference between the two measurements against their average (Figure 2.5).

Note that, in table for this example, the CV remains relatively constant at about 10%.

## Method comparison

In our discussion of test–retest reliability, we assumed that no systematic difference existed between initial and repeat applications of a single test. When we compare two different testing methods (or two different instruments or two different testers), we can make no such assumption. Oral temperatures are usually lower than rectal

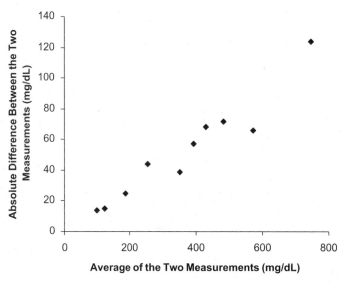

Figure 2.5    Check for error proportional to the mean by plotting the absolute difference between the two measurements against their average. This is done for the data in Example 2.13.

temperatures, abdominal aortic aneurysm diameters are usually lower when assessed by ultrasound than by computed tomography (CT) (Lederle et al. 1995), and mean arterial pressures are usually lower when measured by a finger cuff than by a line in the radial artery (Bos et al. 1996). So, when we are comparing two methods, we need to quantify both systematic bias and random differences between the measurements.

Researchers comparing methods of measurement often present their data by plotting the first method's measurement versus the second method's measurement, and by calculating a regression line and a correlation coefficient. We have seen that the correlation coefficient is not good for assessing measurement agreement.

**Example 2.14**   We compare two methods of measuring bone mineral density (BMD) in children in Figure 2.6: quantitative CT (qCT) and dual-energy x-ray absorptiometry (DXA) (Wren et al. 2005). Both qCT and DXA results are reported as Z scores, equal to the number of standard deviations the measurement is from the mean among normals.[6] We would like to get the same Z score whether we use qCT or DXA.

In the dataset depicted in Figure 2.6, we can replace a pair of measurements showing moderate agreement ($Z_{DXA} = 3$, $Z_{CT} = 2.25$) with a pair of measurements showing *perfect* agreement ($Z_{DXA} = 0$, $Z_{CT} = 0$), and the correlation coefficient decreases from 0.61 to 0.51. The regression line is not particularly informative either, because we want the two methods of measurement to be interchangeable, not just linearly related. Rather than graph the regression line, most of us would prefer the line of identity on which the measurement by the second method *equals* the measurement by the first method (Figure 2.7).

---

[6] If m and s are the mean BMD and standard deviation in the normal population, then $Z = (BMD - m)/s$.

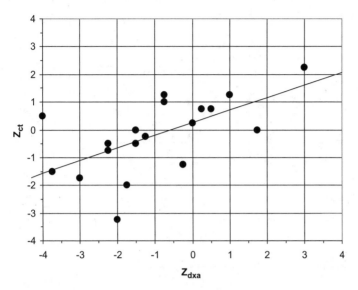

Figure 2.6    Comparison of BMD Z scores obtained by quantitative CT ($Z_{CT}$) and DXA ($Z_{DXA}$) ($r = 0.61$). [Fictional data based on Wren et al. (2005).]

Looking at the points relative to the line of identity in Figure 2.7 reveals that in this dataset, where most of the measurements are negative, qCT gives a higher (less negative) measurement than DXA. This is easier to see by plotting the differences between the measurements versus their average, a so-called Bland–Altman plot(Bland and Altman 1986; Bland and Altman 1999) (Figure 2.8).

The mean difference ($Z_{CT} - Z_{DXA}$) is 0.75, and the standard deviation of the differences is 1.43. The 95% limits of agreement are $0.75 \pm (1.96 \times 1.43)$ or $-2.06$ to 3.56. This means that 95% of the time the difference between the Z scores, as assessed by CT and DXA, will be within this range. A Bland–Altman plot shows the mean difference and the 95% limits of agreement (Figure 2.9).

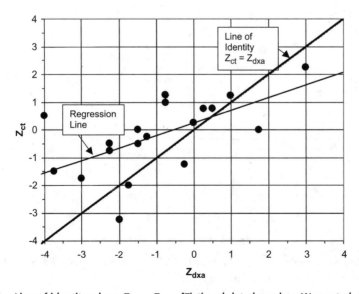

Figure 2.7    Line of identity where $Z_{CT} = Z_{DXA}$. [Fictional data based on Wren et al. (2005).]

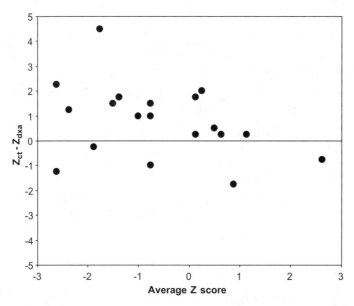

Figure 2.8   Bland–Altman plot showing the difference in BMD Z scores as measured by CT versus DXA.

That BMD Z scores by CT are, on average, higher than by DXA is not a severe problem. After all, we know that rectal temperatures are consistently higher than oral temperatures and can adjust accordingly. However, the large variability in the differences and the resulting wide limits of agreement make it hard to accept the use of these BMD measurements interchangeably.

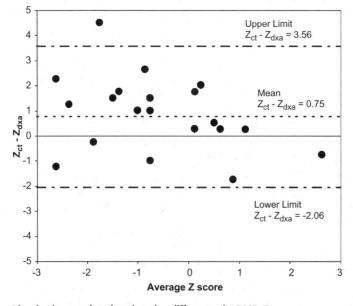

Figure 2.9   Bland–Altman plot showing the difference in BMD Z scores as measured by CT versus DXA with mean difference and 95% limits of agreement.

## Calibration

Method comparison becomes "calibration" when one of the two methods being compared using a plot like Figure 2.9 is considered the gold standard and gives the "true" value of a measurement. For a true calibration problem, the gold standard method should be much more precise than the newer method. In fact, the test–retest variability of the gold standard method should be so much lower that it can be ignored. The x-axis of the plot should then correspond to the measurement by the gold standard method rather than the mean of the two measurements (one by each method). The plot then compares the difference between the new methods versus the gold standard value. For more on calibration, see Krouwer (2008).

## Using studies of reliability from the literature

Suppose we want to evaluate a study of test reliability.[7] First, consider the study subjects. In studies of reliability, there are really two sets of subjects: the patients, who may or may not have the finding, and the examiners. If we want to know whether results are applicable in our own clinical setting, the patients in the study should be representative of those that we or our colleagues are likely to see. Specifically, the way in which we would like them to be representative is that their findings should be as easy or as difficult to discern as those of patients in our own clinical population – neither very subtle nor very obvious findings should be over-represented. Watch for studies in which subjects with ambiguous or borderline results are under-sampled or not included at all. Similarly, consider whether the examiners in the study are representative. How were they selected? Perhaps, because of their interest in a research project on inter-observer variability or their location in a center with a particular interest in the problem, the examiners in the study will perform better than what might be expected elsewhere. But the opposite is also possible: sometimes investigators are motivated to study inter-observer variability in a particular setting because they have the impression that it is poor.

In testing the reliability of two observers on a normal/abnormal rating, it does not make sense to include only subjects rated abnormal by at least one of the two raters. This excludes all the agreements where both raters thought the subject was normal. Nor does it make sense for the second rating to occur only if the first rating is abnormal. This excludes disagreements of type normal/abnormal and only allows type abnormal/normal.

Second, think about the measurements in the study. Were they performed similarly to how such measurements are performed in your clinical setting? Were there optimal conditions, such as a quiet room, good lighting, or special instruments to do the measurements? Is the whole process for making the measurement being studied, or have the authors selected only a single step? For example, a study of inter-rater reliability of interpretation of mammograms, in which two observers read the same

---

[7] As mentioned above, these can also be referred to as studies of test reproducibility.

films, will capture variability only in the interpretation of images, not in how the breast was imaged. This will probably overestimate reliability. On the other hand, cardiologists reading a videotaped echocardiogram might show lower reliability than if they were performing the echocardiogram themselves.

For further discussion of these issues, see Chapter 12 of *Designing Clinical Research* (Newman et al. 2007).

## Summary of key points

1. The methods used to quantify inter- and intra-rater reliability of measurements depend on variable type.
2. For categorical variables, the **observed % agreement** is simply the proportion of the measurements upon which both observers agree exactly.
3. Particularly when observers agree that the prevalence of any of the different categories is high or low, it may be desirable to calculate **kappa** ($\kappa$), an estimate of agreement beyond that expected based on the row and column totals ("marginals") in a table summarizing the results.
4. For ordered categories, kappa can be weighted to allow partial credit for close but not exact agreement. Linear, quadratic, or custom weights can be used.
5. For continuous measurements, the within-subject standard deviation expresses the spread of measurements around the subject's mean.
6. When measurement error increases with the value of the mean (e.g., a measurement is accurate to $\pm 3\%$), the **coefficient of variation**, equal to the within-subject standard deviation divided by the mean, is a better way to express reproducibility.
7. Bland–Altman plots are helpful for comparing methods of measurement; they show the scatter of differences between the methods, whether the difference tends to increase with the magnitude of the measurement, and any systematic difference or bias.

## References

Altman, D. G. (1991). *Practical Statistics for Medical Research*. London, Chapman and Hall.

Bland, J. M., and D. G. Altman (1986). "Statistical methods for assessing agreement between two methods of clinical measurement." *Lancet* **1**(8476): 307–10.

Bland, J. M., and D. G. Altman (1996a). "Measurement error." *Br Med J* **313**(7059): 744.

Bland, J. M., and D. G. Altman (1996b). "Measurement error and correlation coefficients." *Br Med J* **313**(7048): 41–2.

Bland, J. M., and D. G. Altman (1999). "Measuring agreement in method comparison studies." *Stat Methods Med Res* **8**(2): 135–60.

Bos, W. J., J. van Goudoever, et al. (1996). "Reconstruction of brachial artery pressure from noninvasive finger pressure measurements." *Circulation* **94**(8): 1870–5.

Feinstein, A. R., and D. V. Cicchetti (1990). "High agreement but low kappa. I. The problems of two paradoxes." *J Clin Epidemiol* **43**(6): 543–9.

Gill, M. R., D. G. Reiley, et al. (2004). "Interrater reliability of Glasgow Coma Scale scores in the emergency department." *Ann Emerg Med* **43**(2): 215–23.

Krouwer, J. S. (2008). "Why Bland-Altman plots should use X, not (Y + X)/2 when X is a reference method." *Stat Med* **27**(5): 778–80.

Lederle, F. A., S. E. Wilson, et al. (1995). "Variability in measurement of abdominal aortic aneurysms. Abdominal Aortic Aneurysm Detection and Management Veterans Administration Cooperative Study Group." *J Vasc Surg* **21**(6): 945–52.

Meyer, B. C., T. M. Hemmen, et al. (2002). "Modified National Institutes of Health Stroke Scale for use in stroke clinical trials: prospective reliability and validity." *Stroke* **33**(5): 1261–6.

Newman, T. B., W. S. Browner, et al. (2007). "Designing Studies of Medical Tests" in *Designing Clinical Research*. S. B. Hulley, et al. Philadelphia, PA, Lippincott Williams & Wilkins.

Sackett, D., R. Haynes, et al. (1991). *Clinical Epidemiology: A Basic Science for Clinical Medicine*. Boston, Little, Brown and Company.

Wren, T. A., X. Liu, et al. (2005). "Bone densitometry in pediatric populations: discrepancies in the diagnosis of osteoporosis by DXA and CT." *J Pediatr* **146**(6): 776–9.

Yen, K., A. Karpas, et al. (2005). "Interexaminer reliability in physical examination of pediatric patients with abdominal pain." *Arch Pediatr Adolesc Med* **159**(4): 373–6.

## Chapter 2 Problems: reliability and measurement error

1. In a chart review of patients presenting to the emergency department with chest pain (CP), a subgroup of 60 patients had either unstable angina or atypical CP. They were assigned to these 2 diagnoses based on either the primary discharge ICD-9 code or the consensus of 2 chart reviewers (who were blinded to the ICD-9 code). (ICD-9 refers to the 9th revision of the International Classification of Diseases system for coding diagnoses.)

|           |                 | ICD-9 Code |            |    |
|-----------|-----------------|:----------------:|:------------:|:----:|
|           |                 | Unstable Angina | Atypical CP |    |
| Consensus | Unstable Angina | 16               | 3            | 19 |
|           | Atypical CP     | 14               | 27           | 41 |
|           |                 | 30               | 30           | 60 |

a) Based on ICD-9 code, what proportion of the 60-patient sample was assigned to the unstable angina group?

b) Based on the reviewers' consensus, what proportion was assigned to the unstable angina group?

c) What is the observed agreement (concordance rate) between the group assignments based on ICD-9 code versus reviewers' consensus?

d) What is the expected proportion agreement?

e) What is kappa?

f) Are the disagreements balanced or unbalanced? How would this affect your interpretation of a study by these investigators of the prevalence of unstable angina, if the diagnosis was based on ICD-9 codes? (Assume for this problem that the main source of error in diagnosis is the distinction between unstable angina and atypical chest pain.)

2. Yen et al. (2005) compared abdominal exam findings suggestive of appendicitis, such as tenderness to palpation, between pediatric emergency physicians and pediatric surgical residents.

    Assume that the emergency physician and the surgeon each examine the same 10 patients for right lower quadrant tenderness with the following results:

|  |  | Surgeon | | |
|---|---|---|---|---|
|  |  | Tender | Not Tender | Total |
| Emergency | Tender | 3 | 2 | 5 |
| Physician | Not Tender | 2 | 3 | 5 |
|  | Total | 5 | 5 | 10 |

    a) Note that the observed agreement is $3 + 3 = 6/10 = 60\%$. Calculate kappa.
    b) Now, assume that the emergency physician and the surgeon both find a higher prevalence of right lower quadrant tenderness, but still have 60% observed agreement:

|  |  | Surgeon | | |
|---|---|---|---|---|
|  |  | Tender | Not Tender | Total |
| Emergency | Tender | 5 | 2 | 7 |
| Physician | Not Tender | 2 | 1 | 3 |
|  | Total | 7 | 3 | 10 |

    Calculate kappa.
    c) Compare the values of kappa for the tables in part (a) and part (b). The observed agreement was 60% in both cases; why is kappa different?
    d) Now, assume that the surgeon has a much higher threshold than the emergency physician for calling tenderness (e.g., the child has to scream and cry rather than just wince). This is a source of systematic disagreement. Results follow:

|  |  | Surgeon | | |
|---|---|---|---|---|
|  |  | Tender | Not Tender | Total |
| Emergency | Tender | 3 | 4 | 7 |
| Physician | Not Tender | 0 | 3 | 3 |
|  | Total | 3 | 7 | 10 |

    Note that the observed agreement is still 6/10 or 60% and calculate kappa.
    e) If you answered (a), (b), and (d) correctly, you found that the highest value of kappa occurred in (d) when disagreements were unbalanced. Why?

3. Make a $2 \times 2$ table (2 observers rating a sample of patients as either positive or negative for a finding) where the observed agreement is less than 50%, but kappa is nonetheless more than 0.

4. A brave group of investigators (Sinal et al. 1997) examined inter-rater reliability for diagnosing sexual abuse in prepubertal girls. Experienced clinicians (N = 7) rated sets of culposcopic photographs on a 5-point scale (1, normal; 2, nonspecific findings; 3, suspicious for abuse; 4, suggestive of penetration; 5, clear evidence of penetration).

   a) The published unweighted kappa in this study was 0.20; the published weighted kappa (using quadratic weights) was 0.62. Why do you think there is a big difference? Which is preferable?

   b) The data collection form for the study included a sixth category: "unable to interpret." Most of the kappa values published for the study were based on the subset of 77 (55%) of 139 sets of photographs that were "interpretable" by all 7 clinicians.

      i. Did the exclusion of this group probably increase or decrease kappa?

      ii. How else could they have handled that sixth "unable to interpret" category?

   c) The practitioners who participated in this study were all trained in evaluating suspected sexual abuse, with a minimum experience of 50 previous cases (6 of 7 had seen more than 100 previous cases). How does this affect the generalizability of the results and your conclusions?

   d) The authors actually assessed inter-observer agreement in two groups of clinicians, both with and without blinding them to the patients' histories. Results are shown below:

   **(Unweighted) Kappa Values for Interpretation of Culposcopic Photos on a 5-Point Scale**

   |         | Blinded (N = 456)[a] | Provided History (N = 510)[a] |
   |---------|----------------------|-------------------------------|
   | Group 1 | 0.22                 | 0.11                          |
   | Group 2 | 0.31                 | 0.15                          |

   [a] These N values indicate the number of pairwise comparisons in which both clinicians considered the photograph to be interpretable.

   What are some possible explanations for the higher kappa values when observers were blinded to the history?

5. In the chapter, we provided an example of the Eye Opening portion of the Glasgow Coma Scale (GCS). The full GCS is calculated as the sum of scores in three areas, as shown below:

   | Eye Opening    | Verbal Activity     | Motor Activity       |
   |----------------|---------------------|----------------------|
   |                |                     | 6 Obeys commands     |
   |                | 5 Oriented          | 5 Localizes pain     |
   | 4 Spontaneous  | 4 Confused          | 4 Withdraws to pain  |
   | 3 To command   | 3 Inappropriate     | 3 Flexion to pain    |
   | 2 To pain      | 2 Incomprehensible  | 2 Extension to pain  |
   | 1 None         | 1 None              | 1 None               |

In the study by Gill et al. (2004), two Emergency Department attending physicians independently assessed the scores within 5 minutes of each other. For this problem, we will now focus on the Verbal Activity score. These were their results:

**Verbal Activity**

|  |  | Second Measure (within 5 minutes) |  |  |  |  |  |
|---|---|---|---|---|---|---|---|
|  |  | 1 | 2 | 3 | 4 | 5 | Total |
| First | 1 | 30 | 5 | 2 | 4 | 0 | 41 |
| Measure | 2 | 2 | 4 | 3 | 4 | 1 | 14 |
|  | 3 | 0 | 0 | 1 | 1 | 0 | 2 |
|  | 4 | 2 | 5 | 6 | 28 | 3 | 44 |
|  | 5 | 1 | 1 | 0 | 12 | 1 | 15 |
|  | Total | 35 | 15 | 12 | 49 | 5 | 116 |

a) Calculate observed % agreement, expected % agreement, and unweighted kappa. Do you get the same answer as the authors? [See the table in part (b).]

b) Here is an excerpt from Table 2 of the paper:

Measures of inter-rater reliability between paired ratings

| Measure | Verbal[a] |
|---|---|
| Agreement (%) | 55 |
| Unweighted kappa | 0.37 |
| Weighted kappa[b] | 0.48 |

[a] A subset analysis of this measure in the subset of non-intubated patients (n = 98) yielded slightly less reliable results: percentage agreement 47%; kappa = 0.24 ("fair").

[b] Exact matches weighted 1.0, misses of 1 point weighted 0.5, and misses of $\geq 2$ points weighted as 0.

Note that 18 of the 116 patients were intubated (had breathing tubes in their tracheas) at the time that the GCS was assessed. A verbal score cannot be assessed in an intubated patient, so all 18 intubated patients were assigned Verbal scores of "1" by both observers. As per the "a" footnote, the authors performed a subset analysis excluding these 18 patients.

Modify the 5 × 5 results table in part (a) for the exclusion of intubated patients, calculate kappa for the modified results, and again compare with the results reported by the authors.

c) Should the kappa calculated for the subset of 98 nonintubated patients (excluding the 18 intubated patients) be higher or lower than the kappa for all 116 patients? Explain.

d) The authors also calculated weighted kappa. As you see from the **(b)** note in Table 2 from that paper:

"Exact matches weighted 1.0, misses of 1 point weighted 0.5, and misses of $\geq 2$ points weighted as 0."

Create the table of weights that the authors used and calculate weighted kappa for the table in part (a).

e) The "Limitations" section includes the following:

"Because our paired measures could occur up to 5 minutes apart, it is possible that some of our observed differences represent actual patient changes in function over time rather than inter-rater variation."

This may be an important limitation. In Emergency Department patients with altered mentation, mental status does change (either deteriorates or improves) rapidly, especially just after arrival. These patients were all evaluated shortly after arrival. What study design changes could the investigators have made both to address this limitation and to estimate its importance?

6. One of the accepted operative indications for abdominal aortic aneurysm (AAA) repair is maximal aneurysm diameter larger than 5.0 to 5.5 cm (50 to 55 mm).

Sprouse et al. (2003) compared the maximal diameter of 334 AAAs as measured by CT ($CT^{max}$) and as measured by ultrasound ($US^{max}$). Figure 2 from the paper is reprinted below.

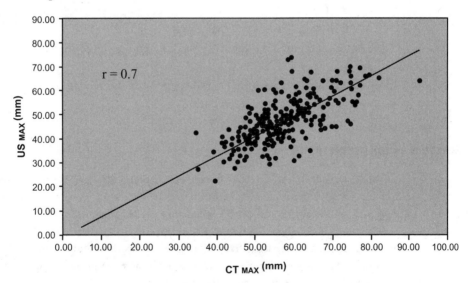

Correlation between $CT^{max}$ and $US^{max}$. From Sprouse et al. (2003). Used with permission.

a) Do US measurements of AAA diameter tend to be higher than CT measurements, or lower?

b) In the discussion of the results, the authors write:

"Although the difference between $CT^{max}$ and $US^{max}$ was statistically significant, the correlation (Fig. 2) between $CT^{max}$ and $US^{max}$ in all groups was good (correlation coefficient, 0.705)."

If the goal is to determine whether clinicians can use CT$^{max}$ and US$^{max}$ interchangeably in the management of patients with AAA, what does this "good" correlation coefficient mean?

c)  Here is Figure 3 from the same article:

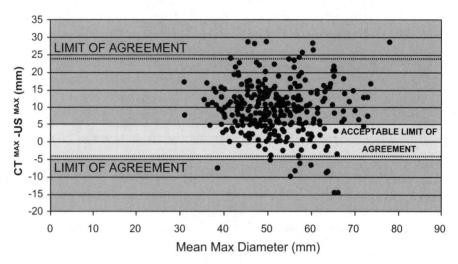

Limits of agreement (broken lines) between CT$^{max}$ and US$^{max}$ ($-4.5$ to $23.6$ mm) compared with clinically acceptable limits of agreement (highlighted area) between CT$^{max}$ and US$^{max}$ ($-5.0$ to $5.0$ mm). From Sprouse et al. (2003). Used with permission.

What is the name of this type of graph?

d)  Based on Figure 3, does US or CT tend to give higher AAA diameter measurements?

e)  Can CT and US assessment of AAA be used interchangeably for purposes of deciding on operative intervention?

## References for problem set

Gill, M. R., D. G. Reiley, et al. (2004). "Interrater reliability of Glasgow Coma Scale scores in the emergency department." *Ann Emerg Med* **43**(2): 215–23.

Sinal, S. H., M. R. Lawless, et al. (1997). "Clinician agreement on physical findings in child sexual abuse cases." *Arch Pediatr Adolesc Med* **151**(5): 497–501.

Sprouse, L. R., 2nd, G. H. Meier, 3rd, et al. (2003). "Comparison of abdominal aortic aneurysm diameter measurements obtained with ultrasound and computed tomography: Is there a difference?" *J Vasc Surg* **38**(3): 466–71; discussion 471–2.

Yen, K., A. Karpas, et al. (2005). "Interexaminer reliability in physical examination of pediatric patients with abdominal pain." *Arch Pediatr Adolesc Med* **159**(4): 373–6.

# Dichotomous tests

## Introduction

In this chapter and the next, we move from assessing test reliability (reproducibility) to assessing accuracy. We are no longer comparing repeated administrations of an imperfect test or comparing one imperfect test with another; we are comparing the test result to the patient's true disease state (D+ or D−) in order to quantify how often the test gives the right answer. This requires that we have a "gold standard" (also known as "reference standard") against which to compare our test. In this chapter, we introduce these concepts with dichotomous tests. In Chapter 4, we extend the discussion to multilevel and continuous tests.

## Sensitivity, specificity, prevalence, predictive value, and accuracy

We will review the definitions of sensitivity, specificity, prevalence, predictive value and accuracy using as an example the evaluation of a rapid bedside test for influenza virus reported by Poehling et al. (2002). Simplifying somewhat, the study compared results of a rapid bedside test for influenza called QuickVue with the true influenza status in children hospitalized with fever or respiratory symptoms. The authors used as a gold standard for diagnosing influenza either a positive viral culture or two positive polymerase chain reaction tests. We present the data using just the polymerase chain reaction test results as the gold standard.[1] The results were as shown in Table 3.1.

"Sensitivity" is the probability that a patient with the disease will have a positive test. In this case, there were eighteen patients with influenza, of whom fourteen had a positive test, so the sensitivity was $14/18 = 78\%$. A mnemonic for sensitivity is PID, which stands for "Positive In Disease." (This is easy to remember because the other PID, Pelvic Inflammatory Disease, is a problem that requires clinician sensitivity.) A

---

[1] Although the authors' gold standard may have been more appropriate, using it resulted (by coincidence) in the number of false positives exactly equalling the number of false negatives, which is potentially confusing.

**Table 3.1.** Results of "QuickVue" influenza test in a 2 × 2 table

|        | Flu+ | Flu− | Total |
|--------|------|------|-------|
| Test+  | 14   | 5    | **19**    |
| Test−  | 4    | 210  | **214**   |
| **Total**  | **18**   | **215**  | **233**   |

perfectly sensitive test (sensitivity = 100%) will never give a false negative (never be negative in disease), so a "perfectly **Sen**sitive test, when **N**egative, rules **OUT** disease" (mnemonic, SnNOUT). An example would be the highly sensitive urine pregnancy test in a young woman with abdominal pain, where the disease in question is ectopic pregnancy. A negative urine pregnancy test rules out ectopic pregnancy.

"Specificity" is the probability that a patient without the disease will have a negative test. In our example above, there were 215 patients without the disease, of whom 210 had a negative test, so the specificity was 210/215 = 98%. A mnemonic for specificity is NIH for "Negative In Health." (Remember this by recalling that the other NIH, the National Institutes of Health, are very specific in their requirements on grant applications.) A perfectly specific test (specificity = 100%) will never give a false positive (never be positive in health), so a "perfectly **S**pecific test, when **P**ositive, rules disease **IN** (SpPIN). An example of this would be "pathognomonic" findings, such as visualization of head lice for that infestation or gram-negative diplococci on gram stain of the cerebrospinal fluid for meningococcal meningitis. These findings are highly specific; they never or almost never occur in patients without the disease, so their presence rules the disease in. Note that, although "NIH" is a helpful way to remember specificity, we want the test not just to be "negative in health," we want it to be negative in everything that is not the disease being tested for, including other diseases that may mimic it.

"Prevalence" is the proportion of patients in the at-risk population who *have* the disease *at one point in time*. It should not be confused with "incidence," which is the proportion who *get* the disease *over a period of time*. In Table 3.1, there were 233 children hospitalized for fever or respiratory symptoms, of whom 18 had the flu. In this population, the prevalence of flu was 18/233 or 7.7%.

"Positive predictive value" is the probability that a patient with a positive test has the disease. In Table 3.1, there are nineteen patients with a positive test, of whom fourteen had the disease, so the positive predictive value was 14/19 = 74%. This means that, in a population like this one (hospitalized children with fever or respiratory symptoms), about three out of four patients with a positive bedside test will have the flu.

"Negative predictive value" is the probability that a patient with a negative test does not have the disease. In Table 3.1, there were 214 patients with a negative test, of whom 210 did not have the flu, so the negative predictive value was 210/214 = 98%. This means that, in a population such as this one, the probability that a patient with a negative bedside test does not have the flu is about 98%.[2] Another way to say this is: the probability that a patient with a negative test *does* have the flu is about $100\% - 98\% = 2\%$.

The negative predictive value of 98% is not as good as it sounds. The probability of flu before obtaining the test result, the pre-test probability, was already only 7.7%, so the probability that a patient in this study did not have the flu was already $100\% - 7.7\% = 92.3\%$ before the test was done. Negative predictive values will always be high when the pre-test probability of disease is low.

"Accuracy" has both general and more precise definitions. We have been using the term "accuracy" in a general way to refer to how closely the test result agrees with the true disease state as determined by the gold standard. The term accuracy also refers to a specific numerical quantity: the percent of all results that are correct. In other words, accuracy is the sum of true positives and true negatives, divided by the total number tested. Table 3.1 shows 14 true positives and 210 true negatives out of 233 tested. The accuracy is therefore $(14 + 210)/233 = 96.1\%$.

Accuracy can be understood as a prevalence-weighted average of sensitivity and specificity:

$$\text{Accuracy} = \text{Prevalence} \times \text{Sensitivity} + (1 - \text{Prevalence}) \times \text{Specificity}.$$

Although completeness requires that we provide this numerical definition of accuracy, it is not a particularly useful quantity. Because of the weighting by prevalence, for all but very common diseases, accuracy is mostly determined by specificity. Thus, a test for a rare disease can have extremely high accuracy just by always coming out negative.

## Importance of the sampling scheme

It is not always possible to calculate prevalence and positive and negative predictive values from a $2 \times 2$ table as we did above. What if this study had sampled children with and without flu separately (a "case-control" sampling scheme) with one non-flu control for each of the 18 patients with the flu, as in Table 3.2?

**Table 3.2.** Sample $2 \times 2$ table for the flu test when subjects with and without flu are sampled separately, leading to meaningless "prevalence" of 50%

|        | Flu+ | Flu− | Total |
|--------|------|------|-------|
| Test+  | 14   | 1    | 15    |
| Test−  | 4    | 17   | 21    |
| Total  | 18   | 18   | 36    |

---

[2] It is just a coincidence that the negative predictive value 210/215 and the specificity 210/214 both round to 98%. As we shall see, the probability that a patient without the disease will have a negative test (specificity) is *not* the same as the probability that a patient with a negative test does not have the disease (negative predictive value).

## Box 3.1: Dichotomous tests: definitions

|  | Disease+ | Disease− | Total |
|---|---|---|---|
| Test + | a<br>True Positives | b<br>False Positives | a + b<br>Total Positives |
| Test− | c<br>False Negatives | d<br>True Negatives | c + d<br>Total Negatives |
| Total | a + c<br>Total With Disease | b + d<br>Total Without Disease | a + b + c + d<br>Total N |

**Sensitivity:** the probability that the test will be positive in someone with the disease: $\dfrac{a}{a+c}$

> Mnemonics: PID = Positive In Disease; SnNOUT = Sensitive tests, when Negative, rule OUT the disease

**Specificity:** the probability that the test will be negative in someone who does not have the disease: $\dfrac{d}{b+d}$

> Mnemonics: NIH = Negative In Health; SpPIN = Specific tests, when Positive, rule IN a disease

The following four parameters can be calculated from a 2 × 2 table only if there was cross-sectional sampling:

**Prevalence:** the probability of disease in the entire population: $\dfrac{a+c}{a+b+c+d}$.

**Positive Predictive Value:** the probability that a person with a positive test has the disease: $\dfrac{a}{a+b}$.

**Negative Predictive Value:** the probability that a person with a negative test does NOT have the disease: $\dfrac{d}{c+d}$.

**Accuracy:** the proportion of those tested in which the test gives the correct answer: $\dfrac{a+d}{a+b+c+d}$.

We could still calculate the sensitivity as 14/18 = 78% and would estimate specificity as 17/18 = 94%, but calculating the prevalence as 18/36 = 50% is meaningless. The 50% proportion was determined by the investigators when they decided to have one non-flu control for each flu patient; it does not represent the proportion of the at-risk population with the disease. When patients are sampled in this case-control fashion, we cannot estimate prevalence or positive or negative predictive value – both of which depend on prevalence.[3] Calculating prevalence, positive predictive value, and negative predictive value from a 2 × 2 table requires sampling the D+ and D− patients together from a whole population, rather than sampling separately by disease status. This is called "cross-sectional" (as opposed to "case-control") sampling.

---

[3] "Accuracy" also depends on prevalence, but as mentioned above, it is not a useful quantity.

> **Box 3.2: Brief digression: the "|" symbol**
>
> The "|" symbol is used to represent a conditional probability. It is read "given." The expression P(A|B) is read "the probability of A given B" and means the probability of A being true (or occurring) if B is known to be true (or to occur). Here are some examples:
>
> P(Headache|Brain tumor) = Probability of headache given that the patient has a brain tumor = 0.7.
>
> P(Brain tumor|Headache) = Probability of a brain tumor given that the patient has a headache = 0.001.
>
> Note, as illustrated above, P(A|B) will generally be quite different from P(B|A).
>
> Using the "|" symbol,
>
> Sensitivity = P(+|D+) = Probability of a positive test given disease.
>
> Specificity = P(−|D−) = Probability of a negative test given no disease.
>
> Positive Predictive Value = P(D+|+) = Probability of disease given a positive test.
>
> Negative Predictive Value = P(D−|−) = Probability of no disease given a negative test.

## Combining information from the test with information about the patient

We can express a main idea of this book as:

What you thought before + New information = What you think now

This applies generally, but with regard to diagnostic testing, "what you thought before" is also known as the prior (or pre-test) probability of disease. This is the probability that the patient had the disease before the test result was known. For screening tests, this is often just the prevalence of disease. For diagnostic tests, it will depend on the patient's signs and symptoms and other test results, and on how much these suggest the disease in question.

"What you think now" is also known as the posterior (or post-test) probability of disease. Now that you know the test result, what is your revised estimate of the probability of disease? In the case of a positive dichotomous test, this is the same as positive predictive value. What about the posterior probability of disease after a negative test? This can be confusing. It is the probability that a patient with a negative test *has* the disease. Hence, it is 1 − Negative Predictive Value. (The negative predictive value is the probability that a patient with a negative test *does not have* the disease.) We will spend a fair amount of time in this and the next chapter discussing how to use the result of a diagnostic test to update the prior probability and obtain the posterior probability of disease. The first method that we will discuss is the "2 × 2 Table Method"; the second uses likelihood ratios.

## 2 × 2 table method for updating prior probability

This method uses the sensitivity and specificity of a test to fill in the 2 × 2 table that would result if the test were applied to an entire population with a given prior probability of disease. Thus, we assume either that the entire population is studied or that a random sample is taken, so that the proportions in the "Disease" and "No Disease" columns are determined by the prior probability of disease, $P(D+)$. As mentioned above, this is referred to as cross-sectional sampling, because subjects are sampled according to their frequency in the population, not separately based on either disease status or test result.

The formula for posterior probability after a positive test is:

$$\frac{\text{Sensitivity} \times \text{Prior Probability}}{\text{Sensitivity} \times \text{Prior Probability} + (1 - \text{Specificity}) \times (1 - \text{Prior Probability})}$$

To understand what is going on, it helps to fill the numbers into a $2 \times 2$ table, as shown in a step-by-step "cookbook" fashion in Example 3.1.

**Example 3.1**   $2 \times 2$ Table Method Instructions for Screening Mammography Example

One of the clinical scenarios in Chapter 1 involved a 45-year-old woman who asks about screening mammography. If this woman gets a mammogram and it is positive, what is the probability that she actually has breast cancer? Based on Kerlikowske et al. (1996a, 1996b), the prevalence of undetected invasive breast cancer in previously unscreened women at age 45 is about 2.8/1000, that is, 0.28%. The sensitivity of mammography is about 75% and the specificity about 93%. Here are the steps to get her posterior probability of breast cancer:

1. Make a $2 \times 2$ table, with *"Disease"* and *"No Disease"* on top and *"Test+"* and *"Test−"* on the left, like the one below.

**Blank $2 \times 2$ Table to Use for Calculating Posterior Probability**

|         | Disease | No Disease | Total |
|---------|---------|------------|-------|
| Test +  |         |            |       |
| Test−   |         |            |       |
| **Total** |       |            |       |

2. Put a large, round number below and to the right of the table for your total N. We'll use 10,000.
3. Multiply that number by the prior probability (prevalence) of disease to get the left column total, the number with disease or $(a + c)$. In this case, it is $2.8/1000 \times 10,000 = 28$.
4. Subtract the left column total from the total N to get the total number without disease $(b + d)$. In this case, it is $10,000 - 28 = 9972$.
5. Multiply the "total with disease" $(a + c)$ by the sensitivity, $a/(a + c)$ to get the number of true positives $(a)$; this goes in the upper left corner. In this case, it is $28 \times 0.75 = 21$.
6. Subtract this number $(a)$ from the "total with disease" $(a + c)$ to get the false negatives $(c)$. In this case, it is $28 - 21 = 7$.
7. Multiply the "number without disease" $(b + d)$ by the specificity, $d/(b + d)$, to get the number of true negatives $(d)$. Here, it is $9972 \times 0.93 = 9274$.

8. Subtract this number from the "total without disease" (b + d) to get the false positives (b). In this case, $9972 - 9274 = 698$.

9. Calculate the row totals. For the top row, $21 + 698 = 719$. For the bottom row, $7 + 9274 = 9281$.

   The completed table is shown below.

**Completed 2 × 2 Table to Use for Calculating Posterior Probability**

|  | Breast (Cancer) | No Breast Cancer | Total |
|---|---|---|---|
| **Mammogram (+)** | 21 | 698 | 719 |
| **Mammogram (−)** | 7 | 9274 | 9281 |
| **Total** | 28 | 9972 | 10,000 |

10. Now you can get posterior probability from the table by reading across in the appropriate row and dividing the number with disease by the total number in the row with that result. So the posterior probability if the mammogram is positive (positive predictive value) = $21/719 = 2.9\%$, and our 45-year-old woman with a positive mammogram has only about a 2.9% chance of breast cancer!

   If her mammogram is negative, the posterior probability (1 − Negative Predictive Value) is $7/9281 = 0.075\%$, and the negative predictive value is $1 - 0.075\% = 99.925\%$. This negative predictive value is very high. However, this is due more to the very low prior probability than to the sensitivity of the test, which was only 75%.

## Likelihood ratios for dichotomous tests

One way to think of the likelihood ratio is as a way of quantifying how much a given test result changes the probability of disease in your patient. More exactly, it is the factor by which the odds of disease either increase or decrease as a result of your test. (Note the distinction between odds and probability below). There are two big advantages to using likelihood ratios to calculate posterior probability. First, as discussed in the next chapter, unlike sensitivity and specificity, likelihood ratios work for nondichotomous tests. Second, they simplify the process of estimating posterior probability.

You have seen that it is possible to get posterior probability from sensitivity, specificity, prior probability, and the test result by filling in a 2 × 2 table. You have also seen that it is kind of a pain. We would really love to just multiply the prior probability by some constant derived from a test result to get the posterior probability. For instance, wouldn't it be nice to be able to say that a positive mammogram increases the probability of breast cancer about tenfold, or that a white blood cell count of more than 15,000 triples the probability of bacteremia?

But there is a problem with this: probabilities cannot exceed one. So if the prior probability of breast cancer is greater than 10%, there is no way you can multiply it by ten. If the prior probability of bacteremia is more than one-third, there is no way

**Box 3.3: Avoiding a common error: be clear on the denominator of "False Positives" and "False Negatives"!**

A common source of confusion arises from the inconsistent use of terms like "False-Positive Rate" and "False-Negative Rate." The numerators of these terms are clear – in 2 × 2 tables like the ones above, they correspond to cells b and c, respectively. The trouble is that the denominator is not used consistently. For example, the False-Negative Rate is generally defined as (1 − Sensitivity), i.e., the denominator is (a + c). But sometimes the term is used when the denominator is (c + d) or even (a + b + c + d).

Here's an example of how this error can get us into trouble. We have often heard the following rationale for requiring a urine culture to rule out a urinary tract infection (UTI), even when the urinalysis (UA) is negative:

1. The sensitivity of the UA for a UTI is about 80%.
2. Therefore, the false-negative rate is 20%.
3. Therefore, after a negative UA, there is a 20% chance that it's a false negative and that a UTI will be missed.
4. The 20% chance of missing a UTI is too high; therefore, always culture, even if the UA is negative.

Do you see what has happened here? The decision to culture should be based on the posterior probability of UTI after the UA (which is the prior probability before the culture). We do want to know the chance that a negative UA represents a false negative, so it seems like the false-negative rate should be relevant. But the false-negative rate we want is (1 − Negative Predictive Value), not (1 − Sensitivity). In the example above, in Statement 2, we began with a false-negative rate that was (1 − Sensitivity), and then in Statement 3, we switched to (1 − Negative Predictive Value). But we can't know negative predictive value just from the sensitivity; it will depend on the prior probability of UTI (and the specificity of the test) as well.

This is illustrated below for two different prior probabilities of UTI in a 2-month-old boy. In the high-risk scenario, the baby is uncircumcised, has a high (39.3°C) fever, and a UTI risk of about 40%. In the low-risk scenario, the baby is circumcised, has a lower (38.3°C) fever, and a UTI risk of only ~2% (Newman et al. 2002). The sensitivity of the UA is assumed to be 80% and the specificity 85%.

| High-Risk Boy: Prior = 40% | | | | Low Risk-Boy: Prior = 2% | | |
| --- | --- | --- | --- | --- | --- | --- |
| | UTI | No UTI | Total | | UTI | No UTI | Total |
| UA+ | 320 | 90 | 410 | UA+ | 16 | 147 | 163 |
| UA− | 80 | 510 | 590 | UA− | 4 | 833 | 837 |
| Total | 400 | 600 | 1000 | Total | 20 | 980 | 1000 |
| Posterior probability after negative UA = 80/590 = 13.5% | | | | Posterior probability after negative UA = 4/837 = 0.4% | | | |

For the high-risk boy, the posterior probability after a negative UA is still 13.5%, perhaps justifying a urine culture. In the low-risk boy, however, the posterior probability is down to 0.4%, meaning that 250 urine cultures would need to be done on such infants for each 1 expected to be positive.

There are many similar examples of this problem, where Test A is not felt to be sufficiently sensitive to rule out the disease, so if it is negative, we are taught that Test B needs to be done. This only makes sense if Test A is never done when the prior probability is low.

**Box 3.4: Understanding odds and probability using pizzas**

It might help to visualize a delicious but insufficient pizza to be completely divided between you and a hungry friend when you are on-call together. If your portion is half as big as his, it follows that your portion is one-third of the pizza. Expressing the ratio of the size of your portion to the size of his is like odds; expressing your portion as a fraction of the total is like probability. If you get confused about probability and odds, just draw a pizza!

**Call night #1:** Your portion is half as big as his. What percent of the pizza do you eat?

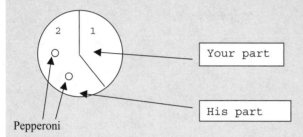

Pepperoni

Answer: 1/3 of the pizza (if odds = 1:2, probability = 1/3).

**Call night #2:** You eat 10% of the pizza. What is the ratio of the size of your portion to the size of your friend's portion?

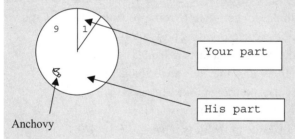

Anchovy

Answer: Ratio of the size of your portion to the size of her portion, 1:9 (if probability = 10%, odds = 1:9).

you can triple it. To get around this problem, we switch from probability to odds. Then we will be able to say:

Prior Odds × Likelihood Ratio = Posterior odds

## Necessary digression: a crash course in odds and probability

This topic trips up a lot of people, but it really is not that hard. "Odds" are just a probability (P) expressed as a ratio to (1 − P); in other words, the probability that something *will* happen (or already exists) divided by the probability that it *won't* happen (or does not already exist). For our current purposes, we are mostly interested in the odds for diagnosing diseases, so we are interested in:

$$\frac{\text{Probability of having the disease}}{\text{Probability of } not \text{ having the disease}}$$

If your only previous experience with odds comes from gambling, do not get confused – in gambling they use betting odds, which are based on the odds of *not*

**Box 3.5: Practice with odds and probabilities**

Convert the following probabilities to odds:

a)      0.01
b)      0.25
c)      3/8
d)      7/11
e)      0.99

Convert the following odds to probabilities:

a)      0.01
b)      1:4
c)      0.5
d)      4:3
e)      10

winning. That is, if the tote board shows a horse at 2:1, the odds of the horse winning are 1:2 (or a little less to allow a profit for the track).

We find it helpful always to express odds with a colon, like a:b. However, mathematically, odds are ratios, so 4:1 is the same as 4/1 or 4, and 1:5 is 1/5 or 0.2.

Here are the formulas for converting from probability to odds and vice versa:

If probability is P, the corresponding odds are $P/(1 - P)$.

- If the probability is 0.5, the odds are 0.5:0.5 = 1:1.
- If the probability is 0.75, the odds are 0.75:0.25 = 3:1.

If odds are a:b, the corresponding probability is $a/(a + b)$.

- If the odds are 1:9, the probability is $1/(1 + 9) = 1/10$.
- If the odds are 4:3, the probability is $4/(4 + 3) = 4/7$.

If the odds are already expressed as a single number (e.g., 0.5 or 2), then the formula simplifies to: Probability = Odds/(Odds + 1) because the "b" value of the a:b way of writing odds is implicitly equal to 1.

The only way to learn this is just to do it. Box 3.5 has some problems to practice on your own right now. (The answers are in Appendix 3.4.)

One thing you probably noticed in these examples (and could also infer from the formulas) is that, when probabilities are small, they are almost the same as odds. Another thing you notice is that *odds are always higher than probabilities* (except when both are zero). Knowing this may help you catch errors. Finally, probabilities cannot exceed one, whereas odds can range from zero to infinity.

The last thing you will need to know about odds is that, because they are just ratios, when you want to multiply odds by something, you multiply only the numerator (on the left side of the colon). So if you multiply odds of 3:1 by 2, you get 6:1. If you multiply odds of 1:8 by 0.4, you get odds of $(0.4 \times 1):8 = 0.4/8 = 0.05$ or 5:100.

**Table 3.3.** $2 \times 2$ table for likelihood ratio derivation

|  | Disease+ | Disease− | Total |
|---|---|---|---|
| Test+ | a | b | a + b |
|  | True Positives | False Positives | Total Positives |
| Test− | c | d | c + d |
|  | False Negatives | True Negatives | Total Negatives |
| Total | a + c | b + d | a + b + c + d |
|  | Total With Disease | Total Without Disease | Total N |

## Deriving likelihood ratios ("lite" version)

Suppose we want to find something by which we can multiply the prior odds of disease in order to get the posterior odds. What would that something have to be?

Recall the basic $2 \times 2$ table and assume we study an entire population or use cross-sectional sampling, so that the prior probability of disease is $(a + c)/N$ (Table 3.3).

What, in terms of a, b, c, and d, are the prior odds of disease? The prior odds are just the probability of having disease divided by the probability of *not* having disease, based on knowledge we have before we do the test. So

$$\text{prior odds} = \frac{P(\text{disease})}{P(\text{no disease})} = \frac{\text{Total with disease/Total N}}{\text{Total without disease/Total N}}$$

$$= \frac{(a + c)/N}{(b + d)/N} = \frac{(a + c)}{(b + d)}$$

Now, if the test is positive, what are the posterior odds of disease? We want to calculate the odds of disease as above, except now use information we have derived from the test. Because the test is positive, we can focus on just the upper (positive test) row of the $2 \times 2$ table. The probability of having disease is now the same as the posterior probability: True Positives/All Positives or $a/(a + b)$. The probability of not having disease if the test is positive is: False Positives/All Positives or $b/(a + b)$. So the posterior odds of disease if the test is positive are:

$$\frac{P(\text{Disease}|\text{Test}+)}{P(\text{No Disease}|\text{Test}+)} = \frac{\text{True Positive/Total Positive}}{\text{False Positive/Total Positive}} = \frac{a/(a + b)}{b/(a + b)} = \frac{a}{b}$$

So now the question is: by what could we multiply the prior odds $(a + c)/(b + d)$ in order to get the posterior odds $(a/b)$?

$$\frac{a + c}{b + d} \times ? = \frac{a}{b}$$

The answer is:

$$\frac{a + c}{b + d} \times \frac{a/(a + c)}{b/(b + d)} = \frac{a}{b}$$

So,

$$? = \frac{a/(a+c)}{b/(b+d)}$$

This must be the likelihood ratio (LR) we have been searching for![4]

But look more closely at the formula for the LR that we just derived – some of it should look familiar. Remember what $a/(a+c)$ is? That's right, sensitivity! And $b/(b+d)$ is (1 − Specificity). So the LR for a positive dichotomous test is just Sensitivity/(1 − Specificity).

You do not need to derive this every time you want to know what an LR is, although you could. Instead, just remember this one formula:

$$\text{Likelihood ratio (result)} = \frac{P(\text{result}|\text{disease})}{P(\text{result}|\text{no disease})}.$$

Stated in words, this says that the likelihood ratio for a test result is the probability of obtaining this test result in those *with* the disease divided by the probability of obtaining this result in those *without* the disease. This formula is a good one to memorize, because, as we will see in Chapter 4, it works for all tests, not just dichotomous ones. The numerator refers to patients *with* the disease, and the denominator refers to patients *without* the disease. One way to remember it is WOWO, which is short for "With Over WithOut."[5] Each possible test result has an LR. For dichotomous tests, there are two possible results and therefore two LRs: LR(+), the LR of a positive result, and LR(−), the LR of a negative result.

To derive the formula for the LR for a negative result, you might first find it helpful to go back to the 2 × 2 table and retrace the steps we took to get the LR for a positive result, but instead use the cell values for the negative test, which appear in the lower row of the 2 × 2 table. If you do this, at the end you should have derived for the "?" factor the formula $\dfrac{c/(a+c)}{d/(d+b)}$. If you think about what other ways we have to express this, you should come up with

$$\text{Likelihood ratio}(-) = \frac{P(-|\text{disease})}{P(-|\text{no disease})} = \frac{1 - \text{Sensitivity}}{\text{Specificity}}$$

or the likelihood of a negative result in patients with the disease divided by the likelihood of a negative result in patients without the disease.

---

[4] In case you are wondering why we call this the "lite" derivation, it is because the formula for the LR works even when sensitivity and specificity come from a study that does not have cross-sectional sampling, but this derivation would not work in such a study.

[5] Thanks to Dr. Warren Browner for this mnemonic.

**Example 3.2**  Using LRs to Calculate Posterior Probability

Let us return to Example 3.1, where the prevalence (prior probability) of breast cancer was 0.28%, the sensitivity of the mammogram was 75%, and the specificity was 93%. The LR for a positive mammogram would then be [Sensitivity/$(1 - \text{Specificity})$] $= 0.75/0.07 = 10.7$. Since odds and probabilities are almost the same when probabilities are low, let us first try a short cut: simply multiply the prior probability by the LR:

$$0.0028 \times 10.7 = 0.030 = 3\%$$

This is close to the 2.9% we calculated with the $2 \times 2$ table method used before. However, if the prior probability and/or the LR are higher, this shortcut will not work. For example, in a 65-year-old woman (prior probability $\approx 1.5\%$) with a mammogram "suspicious for malignancy" (LR $\approx 100$), we would get [$0.015 \times 100$] $= 1.5$, which doesn't make any sense as a posterior probability, because it is greater than one. In general, if the product of the prior probability and likelihood ratio is more than about 10%, we have to convert to odds and back again. For the example above, the steps are:

1. Convert prior probability (P) to prior odds [$P/(1 - P)$] $= 0.015/(1 - 0.015) = 0.0152$.
2. Find the LR for the patient's test result (r): $\text{LR}(r) = \dfrac{P(r|D+)}{P(r|D-)} = 100$.
3. Multiply prior odds by the LR of the test result: $0.0152 \times 100 = 1.52$.
4. Convert posterior odds back to probability $\left( P = \dfrac{\text{odds}}{1 + \text{odds}} \right)$:

$$P = 1.52/(1 + 1.52) = 1.52/2.52 = 0.60.$$

So if the *prior* probability of breast cancer was 1.5%, a mammogram "suspicious for malignancy" would raise the *posterior* probability to about 60%.

## Using the LR slide rule

Although LRs make calculation of posterior probability a little easier than the $2 \times 2$ table method, it still is rather burdensome, especially if the probabilities are too high to skip the conversion from probability to odds and back. An alternative is to use an LR slide rule, which not only provides an answer, but is also useful for visualizing the process of going from prior to posterior probability. It uses a probability scale that is spread out so that distances on it are proportional to the logarithm of the prior odds. We review logarithms in Appendix 4.1. A cutout version of the LR slide rule is included with this book. To use the slide rule to calculate posterior probability from prior probability and LR:

1. Line up the 1 on the LR portion (sliding insert) with the prior probability on the probability (lower) portion.
2. Find the LR of the test result on the LR (top) half and read off the posterior probability just below.

We will see how the LR slide rule can help us understand testing thresholds.

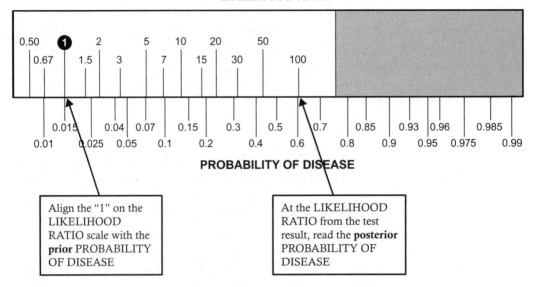

**LIKELIHOOD RATIO**

Align the "1" on the LIKELIHOOD RATIO scale with the **prior** PROBABILITY OF DISEASE

At the LIKELIHOOD RATIO from the test result, read the **posterior** PROBABILITY OF DISEASE

This example shows the position if the prior probability is 0.015 and the likelihood ratio is 100. The posterior probability is about 0.6.

Figure 3.1     LR slide rule

## Treatment and testing thresholds

Recall that in Chapter 1 we said that a good reason to do a diagnostic test is to help you make a decision about administering or withholding treatment. There are two main factors that limit the usefulness of tests:

1. They sometimes give wrong answers.
2. They have a "cost," which includes the financial cost as well as the risks, discomfort, and complications that arise from testing.

Even a costless test has limited usefulness if it is not very accurate, and even a 100% accurate test has limited usefulness if it is very costly. In the following sections, we will show how test inaccuracy and costs narrow the range of prior probabilities for which the expected benefits justify performing the test. Readers interested in a more in-depth discussion should read about decision analysis (Sox 1986; Sox et al. 1988; Detsky et al. 1997a, 1997b; Krahn et al. 1997; Naglie et al. 1997; Naimark et al. 1997).

As an example, we will consider the question of whether to use a rapid bedside test, such as the QuickVue test discussed earlier in this chapter, to guide antiviral treatment for the flu. An antiviral medication, such as oseltamivir, reduces the duration of flu symptoms by about 1 day.

### Quantifying costs and benefits

In order to calculate the range of prior probabilities for which the expected benefits justify testing, we need to quantify three things:

1. *How bad is it to treat someone who does not have the disease?* This quantity is generally denoted "C" (for cost) (Sox et al. 1988; Hilden and Glasziou 1996). C

is the cost[6] of (unnecessarily) treating someone without the disease. In the flu example, we will take the cost of this unnecessary treatment as just the monetary cost of the antiviral medication, about $60.

2. *How bad is it to fail to treat someone who has the disease?* This quantity is generally denoted "B" (Sox et al. 1988; Hilden and Glasziou 1996). You can think of B as the cost of failing to achieve the **B**enefit of treatment. For example, if the value we assign to patients with the flu feeling better 1 day sooner is $160, but the medication costs $60, the net benefit of treatment is $160 - 60 = 100$, so we can think of that missed opportunity to get the $100 benefit of treatment as the net cost of not treating someone with the flu.

3. *What is the cost of the test?* This cost includes the cost of the time, reagents, etc. to do the test, as well as the cost of complications or discomfort from doing the test itself (including assigning a dollar value to any pain and suffering involved). We will denote this test cost as "T."

A note about the term "cost": Some of our colleagues have objected to using the term "cost," because readers might construe it to refer only to monetary costs. Our various "costs" include all harm, pain, suffering, time, and money associated with 1) treating someone unnecessarily, 2) failing to treat someone who needs treatment, and 3) performing the diagnostic test.

### The treatment threshold

First introduced by Pauker and Kassirer (Pauker and Kassirer 1975), the "treatment threshold probability," $P_{TT,}$ is the (posterior) probability of disease at which the expected costs of the two types of mistakes we can make (treating people without the disease and not treating people with the disease) are balanced. By expected costs, we mean we multiply the cost of these mistakes (C and B) by their probability of occurring. For example, the expected cost of not treating is P (the probability of disease) $\times$ B. This is because the probability that not treating is the wrong decision is the probability that the person has the disease, or P, and the cost of that wrong decision is B. This makes sense: if $P = 0$, then not treating will not be a mistake, and the cost will be zero. On the other hand, if $P = 1$, the person has the disease, and the cost of not treating is $1 \times B = B$. If $P = 0.5$, then half the time the cost will be zero, and half the time the cost will be B, so the expected cost is $0.5 \times B$. We can graph this expected cost of not treating as a function of the probability of disease: $P \times B$ is the equation for a straight line with slope B and intercept 0, as shown in Figure 3.2

Similarly, the expected cost of treating is $(1 - P) \times C$. The probability that treating is the wrong decision is the probability that the person does not have the disease $(1 - P)$, and the cost of treating someone who does not have the disease is C. Because $(1 - P) \times C = C - C \times P$, the expected cost of treating is a straight line,

---

[6] What we refer to as "cost" might more strictly be termed "regret," the difference in outcome between the action we took and the best action we could, in retrospect, have taken. (See Hilden and Glasziou 1996. ) The regret associated with treating a patient who turns out to have the disease is zero, since it was the best action we could have taken. Similarly, the regret associated with not treating an individual who turns out not to have the disease is also zero.

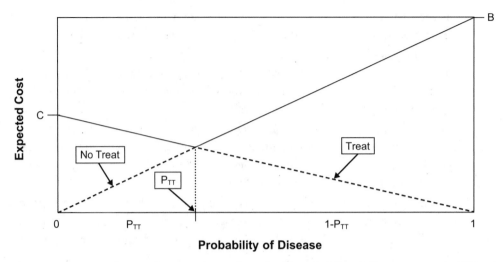

**Probability of Disease**

Figure 3.2    Expected costs of not treating and treating by probability of disease. For probabilities from 0 to $P_{TT}$, "No Treat" has the lowest expected cost. For probabilities from $P_{TT}$ to 1, "Treat" has the lowest expected cost.

with intercept C and slope $-C$. The place where these two lines cross is the treatment threshold, the probability of disease, $P_{TT}$, at which the expected costs of not treating and treating are equal (Fig. 3.2). Put mathematically, $P_{TT}$ is the probability of disease at which:

$$P_{TT} \times B = (1 - P_{TT}) \times C$$

And therefore, the treatment threshold odds are given by:

$$\frac{P_{TT}}{(1 - P_{TT})} = \frac{C}{B}$$

and the threshold probability is

$$P_{TT} = \frac{C}{(C + B)}$$

Stop here to convince yourself that this formula makes sense. If treating someone who does not have the disease is half as bad as failing to treat someone who does have the disease, we should be willing to treat two people without disease to avoid failing to treat one person who has it, and the threshold probability $P_{TT}$ should be 1/3. Using the formula above, if $B = 2 \times C$, then we get $P_{TT} = C/(C + 2C) = C/3C = 1/3$. Similarly, if the two types of mistakes are equally bad, $C = B$, and $P_{TT}$ should be 0.5.

Finally, look at the graph in Figure 3.2 and visualize what happens as C gets closer to zero. Can you see how the treatment threshold, $P_{TT}$, slides down the "no treat" line, approaching zero? This makes sense: if the cost of treating people without disease is low relative to the benefit of treating someone who has it, you will want to treat even when the probability of disease is low. Similarly, imagine what happens when C goes up in relation to B. The treatment threshold, $P_{TT}$, will move to the right.

As did Pauker and Kassirer (Pauker and Kassirer 1980), we now extend the threshold calculation to the case where a dichotomous diagnostic test is available. There

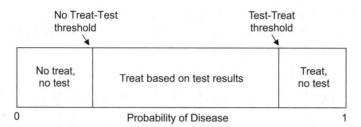

Figure 3.3    The no treat–test and test–treat probability thresholds, between which the test can affect treatment decisions.

are now two threshold probabilities: the "no treat–test threshold" and the "test–treat threshold."

## Testing thresholds for an imperfect but costless test

We will first assume that the test itself has absolutely no monetary cost or risks to the patient. Even if a test is very inexpensive or free, if it isn't perfect, there are some situations in which testing is not indicated because it cannot change the treatment decision. If a dichotomous test has less than perfect specificity (i.e., false positives are possible) and the treatment has some risks (i.e., $C > 0$), there will be some low prior probability below which you would not want to treat even if the test were positive. This is because the low prior probability keeps the posterior probability low, so that the false positives would overwhelm the true positives and there would be too many people treated unnecessarily. That defines a lower testing threshold, the No Treat–Test threshold, below which there is no point performing the test. For a dichotomous test, this lower threshold is related to the LR for a positive result.

At the other end of the spectrum, if the test has less than perfect sensitivity (i.e., false negatives are possible) and the treatment has some benefits (i.e., $B > 0$), there will be some high prior probability above which you would want to treat even if the test were negative. This is because the high prior probability keeps the posterior probability high, so that false negatives would overwhelm the true negatives and testing would lead to too many failures to treat patients with the disease. That defines a higher testing threshold, the Test–Treat threshold, above which one should just treat, rather than do the test. This higher threshold is related to the LR of a negative result for a dichotomous test.

Between these two testing thresholds, there is a zone in which the results of the test have the potential to affect your decision to treat (Fig. 3.3).

**Example 3.3**  In patients with the flu, we quantified the net benefit of antiviral treatment at $100 and the cost of unnecessary treatment at $60. Then, our treatment threshold should be $C/(C + B) = 60/160 = 37.5\%$. That is, after we do our rapid bedside antigen test, if the probability of influenza is greater than 37.5%, we will treat the patient. We will assume that the sensitivity of the rapid antigen test is 75% and specificity is 95%. (These are close to, but slightly worse than, the estimates from Table 3.1.) What are our testing thresholds in this case – that is, for what range of prior probabilities of influenza should the results of the bedside test affect the decision to treat? (For now, we are assuming that the test is free and harmless to the patient.) Here are the steps to follow:

1. Calculate LRs for positive and negative test results:

$$LR(+) = Sensitivity/(1 - Specificity) = 0.75/(1 - 0.95) = 0.75/0.05 = 15$$

$$LR(-) = (1 - Sensitivity)/Specificity = (1 - 0.75)/0.95 = 0.25/0.95 = 0.26$$

2. Convert the treatment threshold of 0.375 to odds:

$$odds = P/(1 - P) = 0.375/(1 - .375) = 0.6$$

3. Divide $LR(+)$ and $LR(-)$ into treatment threshold to get the prior odds for the testing thresholds:

(since posterior odds = prior odds × LR, then posterior odds/LR = prior odds)

$$Posterior\ odds/LR(+) = (0.6/15) = 0.04 (for\ positive\ test)$$

$$Posterior\ odds/LR(-) = 2.28 (for\ negative\ test)$$

4. Convert each of these prior odds (for testing thresholds) back to a prior probability $P = odds/(1 + odds)$:

$$P = 0.04/1.04 = 0.04\ (for\ positive\ test)$$

$$P = 2.28/3.28 = 0.70\ (for\ negative\ test)$$

5. Interpret the result:
   - If the prior probability of influenza is <4% (the no treat–test threshold), then even if the rapid antigen test is positive, the post-test probability will still be below 37.5% (the treatment threshold), and you would not treat the patient.
   - If the prior probability is >70% (the test–treat threshold), then even if the antigen test is negative, the post-test probability will be above 37.5%, and you would treat the patient in spite of the negative test result.
   - If the prior probability is between 4% and 70%, the test *may* be indicated, because it at least has the potential to affect management.

So far, we have not considered costs or risks of the test (as opposed to those of the treatment). When these are factored in as well, the testing range will be narrower.

### Visualizing testing thresholds

The LR slide rule's log(odds) scale provides a nice way of visualizing testing thresholds when the accuracy of a test (rather than its costs or risks) is the main thing that limits its usefulness. In the flu example (Example 3.3), the positive and negative LRs of the bedside antigen test can be visualized as arrows. If they are placed with their points on the treatment threshold, their origins will define the testing thresholds as in Figure 3.4.

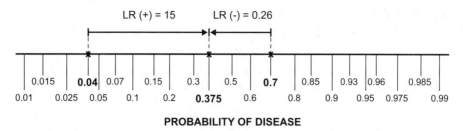

**Figure 3.4**    LR slide rule arrows demonstrate the concept of test and treatment thresholds.

If the prior probability of influenza is less than about 0.04, even if the test is positive, the posterior probability will remain below 0.375, and we shouldn't treat. Similarly, if the prior probability is more than 0.7, even if the test is negative, the posterior probability will remain high enough to treat. These are the same numbers we got algebraically in Example 3.3.

You can also visualize the testing threshold using an X-shaped graph like Figure 3.2. In this case, we draw a line for the expected cost of testing and treating according to the result of the test. When the probability of disease is zero, the expected cost is C × (1 − Specificity). This is the cost of unnecessary treatment (C) times the probability that the test will be falsely positive in patients without the disease. Similarly, when the probability of disease is 1, the expected cost is B × (1 − Sensitivity). This is the cost (B) of failing to treat times the probability that the test will be falsely negative. If we connect these two points with a straight line, we can see that, at very low and very high probabilities of disease, "No Treat" and "Treat" have lower expected costs than "Test," because testing too often leads to wrong answers (Fig. 3.5).

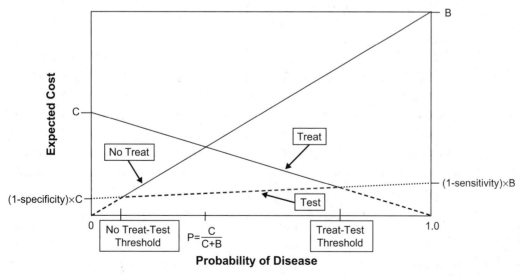

**Figure 3.5**    The expected cost of the "Test" option is higher than the cost of "No Treat" below the No Treat–Test threshold, and higher than the cost of "Treat" above the Test–Treat threshold.

### Testing thresholds for a perfect but risky or expensive test

In the preceding discussion, we showed that, when tests are imperfect, there are some prior probabilities for which the test is not worth doing because the results do not have the potential to affect management. But some tests, with close to 100% sensitivity or specificity, *do* have the potential to change management, even when the prior probability of disease is very close to zero or one. However, because there are risks and costs to tests themselves, even a nearly perfect test may not be worth doing in some patients. Even though it has the potential to change management in some clinical situations, the probability of it doing so is too small to justify the cost of the test. To explore this issue, we now assume that the test is perfect (Sensitivity = Specificity = 100%), but that it has some "cost." Keep in mind that "cost" could represent monetary cost, which is easy to quantify, or risks to the patient (such as pain and loss of privacy), which are harder to quantify. In this situation, there are still two threshold probabilities: 1) the No Treat–Test threshold, where the expected benefits of identifying and treating D+ individuals first justify the testing costs; and 2) the Test–Treat threshold, where the expected savings from identifying and not treating D– individuals no longer justify the testing costs.

If the bedside test for influenza were perfect and the prior probability of influenza were 5%, we would have to test twenty patients to identify one case of the flu. If the prior probability were 10%, we would have to test ten patients to identify one case. For a perfectly sensitive test, the number needed to test to identify one D+ individual is simply $1/P(D+)$, where $P(D+)$ is the prior probability of disease.

To find the No Treat–Test threshold probability, we need to ask how many individuals we are willing to test to identify one D+ individual.

We have already utilized B, the cost of not treating a D+ individual, which we can also think of as the net benefit of treating someone with the disease, and C, the cost of unnecessarily treating a D– individual; now we utilize T, the cost of the test. For a perfect test, the No Treat–Test threshold probability is T/B. (This means we have to assign a dollar benefit to treating people with disease so that T and B can be measured in the same units.)

Assume that the perfect bedside flu testing kits cost $10 each (T = $10). If B = $100 after subtracting the cost of the drug, then T/B = $10/$100 = 10%. This makes sense: for every ten patients we test, on average one will have the flu and be treated, which is worth $100, but the cost of testing those ten people is also 10 × $10 = $100. The costs of testing and benefits of treating are equal, and we break even. If the prior probability of flu is less than 10%, on average we will have to test more than ten people (and hence spend more than $100) for each one who tests positive and gets the treatment; hence the average costs of testing would exceed the benefits.

To understand the test–treat threshold probability, we reverse the logic. We again assume that C, the cost of treating someone without the flu, is just the $60 cost of the medication. Start by assuming that the probability of influenza is 100%. There is no point in testing to identify D– individuals because there aren't any, so we would just treat without testing. As the probability of flu decreases from 100%, it eventually reaches a point where the $60 treatment cost we save by identifying a D– individual

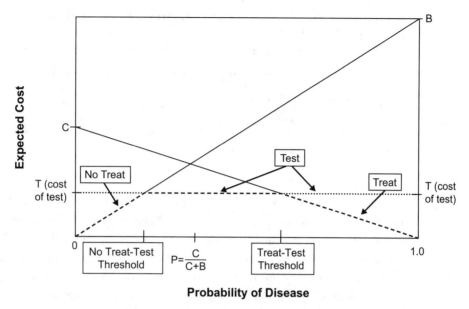

Figure 3.6    "No Treat–Test" and "Test–Treat" thresholds for a perfect but costly test.

justifies the cost of testing to identify that individual. This occurs when the probability of not having the disease is T/C, corresponding to a probability of having the disease of (1 − T/C), the Test–Treat threshold. This makes sense, too. When the probability of nondisease is 1/6, the number needed to test to identify one patient without the disease is six. We test six patients at a testing cost of $10 each in order to save $60 on the one without disease, and hence we come out even. We have to convert this 1/6 probability of nondisease to a probability of disease by subtracting from 100%, so the test–treat threshold probability of disease is 1 − 1/6 = 5/6 = 83.3%.

You can easily visualize testing thresholds for a perfect but costly test by drawing a horizontal line at expected cost = T for the testing option (Fig. 3.6).

### Testing thresholds for an imperfect and costly test

Using the same parameters, C = $60, B = $100, T = $10 (or $0), Sensitivity = 0.75 (or 1.0), and Specificity = 0.95 (or 1.0), Table 3.4 gives the testing thresholds assuming the test is 1) imperfect and costless, 2) perfect and costly, and 3) imperfect and costly. For interested readers, the formulas for the testing thresholds of an imperfect and costly test are given in Appendix 3.2. The graph showing expected costs would be the same as Figure 3.5, except that the testing line would be displaced upward by an amount equal to the testing cost (T).

In order to do these calculations, we have to express misclassification costs (B and C) and testing costs in common units. It is usually difficult to reduce the costs and risks of testing, as well as failing to treat someone with disease or treating someone without the disease, to units such as dollars. We present the algebra and formulas here, not because we want you to use them clinically, but because we want you to understand them and want to show that the theory here is actually quite simple.

**Table 3.4.** Thresholds for a flu test, taking into account accuracy, cost, and both

| Test characteristics | No treat–test threshold | Test–treat threshold |
|---|---|---|
| Imperfect[a] but costless | 0.04 | 0.70 |
| Perfect but costly[b] | 0.10 | 0.67 |
| Imperfect and costly | 0.17 | 0.57 |

[a] Sensitivity = 0.75; Specificity = 0.95.
[b] T = $10.

Testing thresholds exist both because the test is imperfect (and might lead to too many misclassifications) and because the test has costs and risks that might outweigh the benefits of the additional information. Sometimes, especially when the test is expensive and risky but accurate, the testing costs so outweigh the misclassification risks that you can ignore the misclassification risks. Would you do the test if it were perfect? If the answer is "no," then the risks and costs of the test, not the misclassification risks, are driving your decision. We don't do lumbar punctures on well-looking febrile infants. This is not so much because we are worried about false positives, but because the low probability of a positive does not justify the discomfort, risk, and expense of the test. Would you do the test if it were free of discomfort, risks, and costs? If the answer is "no," then the misclassification risks, not the costs and risks of the test itself, are driving your decision. This is one reason we don't perform screening mammography on 30-year-old women. The false positives would vastly overwhelm the true positives and cause an enormous burden of stress and ultimately unnecessary follow-up testing.

## Summary of key points

1. The accuracy of dichotomous tests can be summarized by the proportion in whom the test gives the right answer in five groups of patients:
   - those with disease (sensitivity),
   - those without the disease (specificity),
   - those who test positive (positive predictive value),
   - those who test negative (negative predictive value), and
   - the entire population tested (accuracy).
2. Although sensitivity and specificity are more useful for evaluating tests, clinicians evaluating patients will more often want to know the posterior probability of disease given a particular test result.
3. Posterior probability can be calculated by using the sensitivity and specificity of the test and the prior probability of disease. This can be done by using the 2 × 2 table method or by converting probabilities to odds and using the LR of the test result (defined as P(Result|Disease)/P(Result|No disease)).
4. The treatment threshold ($P_{TT}$) is the posterior probability of disease at which the expected cost of treating those without disease equals the expected cost of not treating those with the disease. The formula for this is: $P_{TT} = C/(C + B)$.

5. If a test is less than perfectly accurate or has costs or risks, it does not make sense to use it on patients with very low probabilities of disease – probabilities below the "No Treat–Test" threshold.
6. Similarly, sometimes the probability of disease is so high that it makes sense to skip the test and proceed directly to treatment. This occurs when the probability is greater than the "Test–Treat" threshold.
7. Both the "No Treat–Test" and "Test–Treat" thresholds can be visualized graphically or calculated algebraically if the cost of treating someone without the disease (C), the cost of failing to treat someone with the disease (B), and the cost of the test (T) can all be estimated on the same scale.

## Appendix 3.1: General summary of definitions and formulas for dichotomous tests

|         | Disease | No Disease | Totals            |
| ------- | ------- | ---------- | ----------------- |
| **Test+** | a       | b          | a + b             |
| **Test−** | c       | d          | c + d             |
| **Totals** | a + c   | b + d      | N = (a + b + c + d) |

$$\text{Sensitivity} = a/(a + c) \qquad \text{Specificity} = d/(b + d)$$
$$= P(+|D+) \qquad\qquad = P(-|D-)$$
$$1 - \text{Sensitivity} = P(-|D+) \qquad 1 - \text{Specificity} = P(+|D-)$$

If sampling is cross-sectional (i.e., diseased and nondiseased are not sampled separately), then:

Prevalence = prior probability = $(a + c)/N$

Positive Predictive Value (PPV) = Posterior probability if test + = $a/(a + b)$

Negative Predictive Value (NPV) = 1 − Posterior probability if test − = $d/(c + d)$

For tests with dichotomous results:

$$LR(+) = P(+|D+)/P(+|D-) = \text{sensitivity}/(1 - \text{specificity})$$
$$LR(-) = P(-|D+)/P(-|D-) = (1 - \text{sensitivity})/\text{specificity}$$

Probability = $P = \text{odds}/(1 + \text{odds})$;

Odds = $P/(1 - P)$ or

If odds = $a/b$, probability = $a/(a + b)$

Prior odds × LR = posterior odds     (ALWAYS TRUE!)

## Appendix 3.2: Rigorous derivation of likelihood ratios

Here is a real derivation – it is not that hard!

First, you need to accept some basic theorems of probability:

1. $P(A \text{ and } B) = P(B \text{ and } A)$
2. $P(A \text{ and } B) = P(A|B)P(B)$. This just says the probability of both A and B is the probability of B times the probability of A *given* B.

From 1 and 2 (which both seem self-evident), it is easy to prove Bayes's theorem:

3. $P(A|B)P(B) = P(A \text{ and } B) = P(B \text{ and } A) = P(B|A)P(A)$. Therefore, $P(A|B) = P(B|A)P(A)/P(B)$, which is how Bayes's theorem is generally written. Now by Bayes's theorem (where r = a specific test result):

4. Posterior probability $= P(D+|r) = P(r|D+)P(D+)/P(r)$

5. $1 -$ Posterior probability $= P(D-|r) = P(r|D-)P(D-)/P(r)$

Dividing 4 by 5 gives:

6. $$\frac{P(D + |r)}{P(D - |r)} = \frac{P(r|D+)}{P(r|D-)} \times \frac{P(D+)}{P(D-)}$$
Posterior odds $=$ LR(r) $\times$ Prior odds

Note that this derivation applies regardless of the form the result takes (dichotomous, continuous, etc.) and requires no assumptions other than the probability theorems we started with.

## Appendix 3.3: Formulas for testing thresholds for dichotomous tests

B $=$ Net Benefit of Treating a D+ individual

C $=$ Cost of Unnecessarily Treating a D−individual

C/B $=$ Treatment Threshold Odds

T $=$ Cost of Test

### 3.3a: For an imperfect but costless test:

No Treat-Test Threshold Odds $= \dfrac{C/B}{LR(+)}$

$= \dfrac{(C)P(+|D-)}{(B)P(+|D+)}$

No Treat-Test Threshold Prob $= \dfrac{(C)P(+|D-)}{(B)P(+|D+) + (C)P(+|D-)}$

Test-Treat Threshold Odds $= \dfrac{C/B}{LR(-)}$

$= \dfrac{(C)P(-|D-)}{(B)P(-|D+)}$

Test-Treat Threshold Prob $= \dfrac{(C)P(-|D-)}{(B)P(-|D+) + (C)P(-|D-)}$

**Example:** Imperfect but costless test for influenza

B $=$ Net Benefit of Antiviral Treatment $=$ \$100

C $=$ Net Cost of Antiviral Treatment $=$ \$60

Sensitivity $= P(+|D+) = 0.75$; $1 -$ Sensitivity $= P(-|D+) = 0.25$

Specificity $= P(-|D-) = 0.95$; $1 -$ Specificity $= P(+|D-) = 0.05$

No Treat-Test Threshold Prob $= \dfrac{(C)P(+|D-)}{(B)P(+|D+) + (C)P(+|D-)}$

$= \dfrac{(60)0.05}{(100)0.75 + (60)0.05}$

$= 0.04$

$$\text{Test-Treat Threshold Prob} = \frac{(C)P(-|D-)}{(B)P(-|D+) + (C)P(-|D-)}$$

$$= \frac{(60)0.95}{(100)0.25 + (60)0.95}$$

$$= 0.70$$

### 3.3b: For a perfect but costly test:

No Treat-Test Threshold Probability $= T/B$
Test-Treat Threshold Probability $= 1 - T/C$

**Example:** Perfect but costly test for influenza

B = Net Benefit of Antiviral Treatment = \$100
C = Antiviral Treatment Cost = \$60
T = Cost of the Perfect Bedside Test = \$10

No Treat-Test Threshold Probability $= T/B = \$10/\$100 = 0.10$
Test-Treat Threshold Probability $= 1 - T/C = 100\% - \$10/\$60 = 0.833$

### 3.3c: For an imperfect and costly test:

$$\text{No Treat-Test Threshold Odds} = \frac{(C)P(+|D-) + T}{(B)P(+|D+) - T}$$

$$\text{No Treat-Test Threshold Prob} = \frac{(C)P(+|D-) + T}{(B)P(+|D+) + (C)P(+|D-)}$$

$$\text{Test-Treat Threshold Odds} = \frac{(C)P(-|D-) - T}{(B)P(-|D+) + T}$$

$$\text{Test-Treat Threshold Prob} = \frac{(C)P(-|D-) - T}{(B)P(-|D+) + (C)P(-|D-)}$$

**Example:** Imperfect and costly test for influenza

B = Net Benefit of Antiviral Treatment = \$100

C = Antiviral Treatment Cost = \$60

T = Cost of Test = \$10

Sensitivity $= P(+|D+) = 0.75; 1 - \text{Sensitivity} = P(-|D+) = 0.25$
Specificity $= P(-|D-) = 0.95; 1 - \text{Specificity} = P(+|D-) = 0.05$

$$\text{No Treat-Test Threshold Prob} = \frac{(C)P(+|D-) + T}{(B)P(+|D+) + (C)P(+|D-)}$$

$$= \frac{(60)0.05 + 10}{(100)0.75 + (60)0.05}$$

$$= 0.167$$

$$\text{Test-Treat Threshold Prob} = \frac{(C)P(-|D-) - T}{(B)P(-|D+) + (C)P(-|D-)}$$

$$= \frac{(60)0.95 - 10}{(100)0.25 + (60)0.95}$$

$$= 0.573$$

## Appendix 3.4: Answers to odds/probability conversions in Box 3.5

If probability is P, Odds are $P/(1 - P)$

|     | Probability | Odds |
|-----|-------------|------|
| a.  | .01         | 1/99 |
| b.  | .25         | 1/3  |
| c.  | 3/8         | 3/5  |
| d   | 7/11        | 7/4  |
| e.  | .99         | 99   |

If odds are $a/b$, probability is $a/(a + b)$.

|     | Odds | Probability     |
|-----|------|-----------------|
| a.  | .01  | 1/101           |
| b.  | 1:4  | 1/5             |
| c.  | .5   | $.5/1.5 = 1/3$  |
| d.  | 4:3  | 4/7             |
| e.  | 10   | 10/11           |

## References

Detsky, A. S., G. Naglie, et al. (1997a). "Primer on medical decision analysis: Part 1. Getting started." *Med Decis Making* **17**(2): 123–5.

Detsky, A. S., G. Naglie, et al. (1997b). "Primer on medical decision analysis: Part 2. Building a tree." *Med Decis Making* **17**(2): 126–35.

Hilden, J., and P. Glasziou (1996). "Regret graphs, diagnostic uncertainty and Youden's Index." *Stat Med* **15**(10): 969–86.

Kerlikowske, K., D. Grady, et al. (1996a). "Effect of age, breast density, and family history on the sensitivity of first screening mammography." *JAMA* **276**(1): 33–8.

Kerlikowske, K., D. Grady, et al. (1996b). "Likelihood ratios for modern screening mammography. Risk of breast cancer based on age and mammographic interpretation." *JAMA* **276**(1): 39–43.

Krahn, M. D., G. Naglie, et al. (1997). "Primer on medical decision analysis: Part 4. Analyzing the model and interpreting the results." *Med Decis Making* **17**(2): 142–51.

Naglie, G., M. D. Krahn, et al. (1997). "Primer on medical decision analysis: Part 3. Estimating probabilities and utilities." *Med Decis Making* **17**(2): 136–41.

Naimark, D., M. D. Krahn, et al. (1997). "Primer on medical decision analysis: Part 5. Working with Markov processes." *Med Decis Making* **17**(2): 152–9.

Newman, T. B., J. A. Bernzweig, et al. (2002). "Urine testing and urinary tract infections in febrile infants seen in office settings: the Pediatric Research in Office Settings' Febrile Infant Study." *Arch Pediatr Adolesc Med* **156**(1): 44–54.

Pauker, S. G., and J. P. Kassirer (1975). "Therapeutic decision making: A cost-benefit analysis." *N Engl J Med* **293**(5): 229–34.

Pauker, S. G., and J. P. Kassirer (1980). "The threshold approach to clinical decision making." *N Engl J Med* **302**(20): 1109–17.

Poehling, K. A., M. R. Griffin, et al. (2002). "Bedside diagnosis of influenzavirus infections in hospitalized children." *Pediatrics* **110**(1 Pt 1): 83–8.

Sox, H. C., Jr. (1986). "Probability theory in the use of diagnostic tests. An introduction to critical study of the literature." *Ann Intern Med* **104**(1): 60–6.

Sox, H. C., M. A. Blatt, et al. (1988). *Medical Decision Making*. Boston, Butterworths.

## Chapter 3 Problems: dichotomous tests

1. You are informed by your doctor that you have tested positive for Grunder-schnauzer disease. You may ask one question to help you figure out whether you really have it. What do you want to know (choices are sensitivity, specificity, prevalence, predictive value, etc.)?

2. Consider the following excerpt from an abstract about a test for Cat Scratch Disease (Zangwill et al. 1993):

**ABSTRACT**

METHODS. We conducted a physician survey to identify cases of cat scratch disease occurring over a 13-month period in cat owners in Connecticut. We interviewed both the patients (or their parents) and controls matched for age who owned cats. Serum from the patients was tested for antibodies to Rochalimaea henselae with a new, indirect fluorescent-antibody test.

RESULTS. . . . . Of 45 patients [cases], 38 had serum samples with titers of 1:64 or higher for antibody to R. henselae, as compared with 4 of 112 samples from controls (P < 0.001). *The positive predictive value of the serologic test was 91 percent* [italics added] . . .

   a) Make a 2 × 2 table that summarizes the results.

   b) Is the authors' calculation of predictive value (91%) correct?

3. A "rapid strep" test for Group A streptococcal throat infection that used an optical immunoassay (OIA) was reported to have about 91% sensitivity and 95% specificity compared with culture (Roddey et al. 1995). The authors concluded that because "approximately 9% of cultures positive for group A Strep . . . would have been missed by the OIA, we believe that a throat culture should be processed in the case of a negative OIA result." Do you agree? How could you improve on this conclusion?

4. Haydel et al. (2000) studied the usefulness of various clinical findings to predict a positive head CT scan in patients with minor head trauma and a possible loss of consciousness. The head CT scan was not the diagnostic test being evaluated; a positive head scan was the "disease," and the clinical findings were the "tests." They reported their results in the table below. (Footnotes are from the original table.)

Association between selected clinical findings and CT results in 520 patients with minor head injury

| Finding[a] | Total (N = 520) | Positive CT scan (N = 36) no. (%) | Negative CT scan (N = 484) | P value[b] | Likelihood ratio[c] |
|---|---|---|---|---|---|
| Short-term memory deficits | 9 (2) | 5 (14) | 4 (1) | <0.001 | 15.0 |
| Drug or alcohol intoxication | 180 (35) | 22 (61) | 158 (33) | 0.001 | 11.0 |
| Headache | 123 (24) | 12 (33) | 111 (23) | 0.16 | 2.0 |

[a] Some patients had more than one finding.
[b] P values were determined by $\chi^2$ analysis.
[c] The LR indicates the likelihood of a positive CT scan in patients with the finding in question as compared with the likelihood in patients without the finding.

a) Consider the second row of the table, which includes data relating drug or alcohol intoxication to the CT scan results. Calculate the LR for this finding.

b) The authors' definition of LR in footnote **c** is actually a prevalence ratio (like a risk ratio): the probability of disease in those with the finding divided by the probability in those without the finding. For that same row of the table, calculate the prevalence ratio.

c) You have a patient with minor head trauma similar to those in the Haydel et al. study, whose prior probability of a positive CT scan you estimate at about 10% before you find out about drug or alcohol intoxication. If your history reveals drug or alcohol intoxication, what is your estimate of the probability that his CT scan will be positive?

5. A study (Gaitan-Cepeda et al. 2005) of people with HIV/AIDS undergoing highly active antiretroviral therapy (HAART) found that the probability of immune failure in the presence of oral candidiasis was 91%.

a) View the exam for oral candidiasis as a test for immune failure. Which of the test characteristics defined in this chapter does the 91% figure represent?

b) Here are the results of the study's cross-sectional sample of patients with HIV/AIDS on HAART:

| | | **Immune Failure** | | |
|---|---|---|---|---|
| | | **Yes** | **No** | **Total** |
| **Oral** | Yes | 31 | 3 | **34** |
| **Candidiasis** | No | 75 | 37 | 112 |
| **Total** | | **106** | **40** | **146** |

i. What was the prevalence of immune failure in this sample?

ii. What was the probability of immune failure in the absence of oral candidiasis?

iii. What would you call this number?

iv. Calculate the sensitivity of oral candidiasis for immune failure.

v. Calculate the specificity.

c) Do you agree with the authors that oral candidiasis is a good marker for immune failure in patients on HAART?

6. You have a patient with pharyngitis (a sore throat) whom you consider treating with penicillin.

Assume:

i. The drug cost of a course of penicillin to treat acute Group A streptococcal throat infection ("strep throat") is $23 (www.drugstore.com, Penicillin VK 500 mg #30, 9/23/08), and the expected cost in patient inconvenience, risk of adverse or allergic reactions, and contribution to antibiotic resistance is another $17. So, the total expected treatment cost is $40.

ii. Treating someone who really has strep throat (and not some other pharyngitis) decreases symptom severity, length of illness, transmission to others and the (already minute) risk of rheumatic fever. The value of this averages about $100, but since the cost of treatment is $40, the net benefit of treating someone with strep throat is $60. This can also be viewed as the net cost of failing to treat someone with strep throat. Penicillin will not help the patient if the sore throat is caused by something other than Group A strep.

a) Draw a graph like figure 3.2, labeling the axes, lines and intercepts.

b) At what probability of strep throat should you treat with penicillin? Show the point on the graph.

c) If a rapid strep test were 90% sensitive and 91% specific, for what range of prior probabilities would it have the potential to affect management? (Ignore the cost of the test.) Do this calculation using likelihood ratios, then draw a line for "testing" on the graph.

d) Now assume that the perfect "rapid strep" test for Group A streptococcal throat infection has been developed. The test causes negligible discomfort and results are available nearly instantaneously, but the test costs $30. When does it make sense to use this test? Draw a line for testing on the graph and explain.

e) Extra credit: Imagine you have a patient with a particularly severe sore throat. For her, you estimate the net benefit of treatment to be $160 rather than $60. Redraw the graph from part d and explain how your answer would change, if at all. (The algebra is optional – focus on the concept.)

## References for problem set

Gaitan-Cepeda, L. A., M. Martinez-Gonzalez, et al. (2005). "Oral candidosis as a clinical marker of immune failure in patients with HIV/AIDS on HAART." *AIDS Patient Care STDS* **19**(2): 70–7.

Haydel, M. J., C. A. Preston, et al. (2000). "Indications for computed tomography in patients with minor head injury." *N Engl J Med* **343**(2): 100–5.

Roddey, O. F., Jr., H. W. Clegg, et al. (1995). "Comparison of an optical immunoassay technique with two culture methods for the detection of group A streptococci in a pediatric office." *J Pediatr* **126**(6): 931–3.

Zangwill, K. M., D. H. Hamilton, et al. (1993). "Cat scratch disease in Connecticut. Epidemiology, risk factors, and evaluation of a new diagnostic test." *N Engl J Med* **329**(1): 8–13.

# Multilevel and continuous tests

## Introduction

To this point, we have discussed the accuracy of dichotomous tests – those that are either positive or negative for the disease in question. Now, we want to consider the accuracy of tests with more than two possible results. As discussed in Chapter 2, the results of such tests can be ordinal (if they have an intrinsic ordering, like a Gleason score for pathologic grade of prostate cancer) or nominal (if they do not, such as a blood type). Ordinal variables can be discrete (having a limited number of possible results, like the Gleason score) or continuous, with an essentially infinite range of possibilities (like a serum cholesterol level or white blood cell count). In this chapter, we discuss how making a multilevel or continuous test dichotomous, by choosing a fixed cut-off to divide "positive" from "negative," reduces the value of the test. We also introduce the Receiver Operating Characteristic (ROC) curve used to summarize a multilevel test's ability to discriminate between patients with and without the disease in question. In evaluating a patient, we must use the patient's test result to update his or her pre-test probability of disease. In Chapter 3, we learned the $2 \times 2$ table method for probability updating, but it only applies to dichotomous tests. The LR method will be more useful now that we have moved to tests with more than two results.

## Making a continuous test dichotomous

In Chapter 1, we described the case of a 5-month-old boy with a fever of 39.7°C and no source by history or physical exam. The disease you are concerned about is bacteremia, and the test you are considering is the white blood cell (WBC) count. One possible approach is to make the WBC count into a dichotomous test by choosing a cut-off, such as 15,000/μL, above which the test is considered "positive." Using data from Lee and Harper (1998), we can calculate sensitivity, specificity, LR(+), and LR(−) as shown in Table 4.1.[1]

---

[1] The study by Lee and Harper (1998) provides a nice example to illustrate the concepts in this chapter, but it was done before the era of widespread use of the heptavalent pneumococcal vaccine, so the prior probability

**Table 4.1.** Dichotomizing the WBC as a test for bacteremia in febrile infants (data from Lee and Harper 1998)

| WBC count ($\times 1,000/\mu$L) | Bacteremia | No bacteremia |
|---|---|---|
| $\geq 15\,(+)$ | 109 | 2,028 |
| $< 15\,(-)$ | 18 | 6,601 |
| **Total** | **127** | **8,629** |

$$\text{Sensitivity} = 109/127 = 0.86$$
$$\text{Specificity} = 6601/8629 = 0.76$$
$$\text{LR}(+) = 0.86/(1 - 0.76) = 3.65$$
$$\text{LR}(-) = (1 - 0.86)/0.76 = 0.19$$

We can see that a WBC count $\geq 15,000/\mu$L almost quadruples a febrile infant's pre-test odds of bacteremia. However, this means that we are not distinguishing between a WBC count of $16,000/\mu$L and a WBC count of $28,000/\mu$L, because both are greater than $15,000/\mu$L. The WBC count of $28,000/\mu$L must increase the odds of disease more than the WBC count of $16,000/\mu$L. We would like to be able to account for the higher probability of bacteremia in the infant with the WBC count of $28,000/\mu$L.

For simplicity, let us create an ordinal variable from the WBC count by categorizing the results in a set of intervals: $<5,000/\mu$L; $5,000-9,999/\mu$L; $10,000-14,999/\mu$L; $15,000-19,999/\mu$L; $20,000-24,999/\mu$L; $25,000-29,999/\mu$L, and $\geq 30,000/\mu$L. We have gone from two possible test results to seven possible test results. Instead of a 2 × 2 table, we can create a 7 × 2 table from that same study (Table 4.2).

In the 2 × 2 table for dichotomous tests, the positive result is conventionally put on top, so for consistency, we display the intervals in descending order so that more positive results are higher. Now, the WBC count of $16,000/\mu$L falls into a different category than the WBC count of $28,000/\mu$L.

In Chapter 3's discussion of dichotomous tests, we started by talking about the characteristics of the test: its sensitivity and specificity. Then, we discussed the

**Table 4.2.** 7×2 Table of WBC count results as a test for bacteremia in febrile infants (data from Lee and Harper 1998)

| WBC count ($\times 1,000/\mu$L) | Bacteremia | No bacteremia |
|---|---|---|
| $\geq 30$ | 15 | 67 |
| 25 to $<30$ | 12 | 155 |
| 20 to $<25$ | 34 | 469 |
| 15 to $<20$ | 48 | 1,337 |
| 10 to $<15$ | 15 | 2,767 |
| 5 to $<10$ | 3 | 3,291 |
| 0 to $<5$ | 0 | 543 |
| **Total** | **127** | **8,629** |

of bacteremia they report is too high for vaccinated children. In addition, the WBC count may not perform as well for bacteremia caused by other organisms as it does for pneumococcal bacteremia.

positive and negative LRs, which we use when we have the test result for a particular patient in order to update that patient's odds of disease. For multilevel tests, instead of calculating single values for sensitivity and specificity, we will graphically illustrate the trade-off between them, by plotting Sensitivity versus (1 − Specificity) for each possible test-result cut-off. This graph is called a Receiver Operating Characteristic (ROC) curve. It is a characteristic of the test, not the patient. Then, we will see that, just as a dichotomous test has an LR associated with each of the possible results (positive or negative), a multilevel test has an LR associated with each of the possible results or intervals (such as the WBC count intervals above). When faced with an individual patient and a specific test result, we use the appropriate LR to update that patient's odds of disease.

## ROC curves

When an ordinal or continuous test is made dichotomous, sensitivity and specificity depend on the threshold used to define a positive result. If that threshold is high (e.g., WBC count = 21,000/μL; see Fig. 4.1A), you will have few false positives (positive tests in nonbacteremic infants), but you will fail to identify many cases of disease (bacteremic infants with WBC counts <21,000/μL). If the threshold is low (e.g., WBC count = 12,000/μL; see Fig. 4.1C), you will have more false positives (lower specificity) but fewer false negatives (higher sensitivity). This trade-off between sensitivity and specificity can be shown graphically in an ROC curve (Fig. 4.1).

ROC curves were introduced as part of signal detection theory when radar was being developed during World War II (Swets 1996).[2] Each point on the ROC curve represents a different cut-off for calling the test positive. The "true-positive rate" (Sensitivity) is plotted on the y-axis against the "false-positive rate" (1 − Specificity) on the x-axis. The general idea is that you want to get as many true positives as you can (go *up* the graph) without getting too many false positives (which move you to the right). For convenience, in the discussion below, we will assume that people with disease have *higher* values of the test – that higher test results are abnormal.

If the distribution of test results is similar in people who do and do not have the disease, then no matter what the cut-off is, the number of people with and without the disease who are considered "positive" will be about equal. That is, the true-positive rate will about equal the false-positive rate. In that case, the test discriminates poorly, and the ROC curve will approximate a 45-degree diagonal line (Fig. 4.2).

If the test results are higher in people who have the disease, the curve will go up faster than it moves to the right. The closer the curve gets to the upper left-hand corner of the graph, the better the test (Fig. 4.3).

The area under an ROC curve (AUROC),[3] quantifies the discrimination of the test: 1.0 is perfect; 0.5 is no better than chance. The AUROC has another interpretation as

---

[2] The question was whether a blip on the radar screen represented a true signal (e.g., an airplane) or "noise." If a radar operator tried to raise his proportion of signals identified, he also increased his number of false calls. In other words, lowering the threshold for identifying a signal increased sensitivity but decreased specificity.

[3] This is also sometimes denoted "c" and corresponds to the "c" statistic used to assess the predictive accuracy of a multiple logistic regression model.

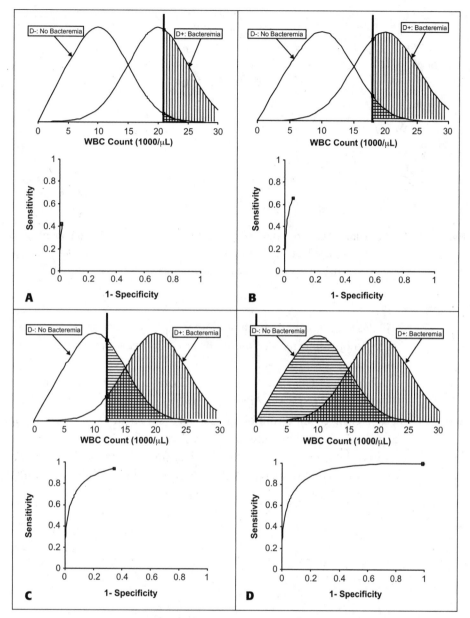

Figure 4.1    Hypothetical probability distributions of WBC count for children with and without bacteremia and how the ROC curve is traced out by serially lowering the threshold for calling the test "positive" from higher (more abnormal) to lower (less abnormal) test results. (**A**) WBC count threshold = 21,000/$\mu$L; False-Positive Rate (1 − Specificity) = 1.4%; True-Positive Rate (Sensitivity) = 42%. (**B**) WBC count threshold = 18,000/$\mu$L; 1 − Specificity = 5%; Sensitivity = 64%. (**C**) WBC count threshold = 12,000/$\mu$L; 1 − Specificity = 35%; Sensitivity = 95%. (**D**) WBC count threshold = 0/$\mu$L (any result is considered "positive"); 1 − Specificity = 100%; Sensitivity = 100%.

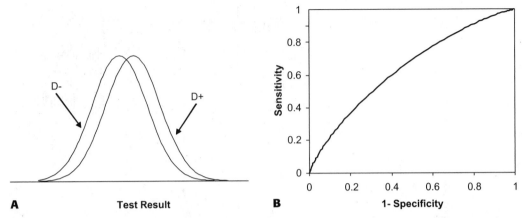

**A**          **Test Result**          **B**          **1- Specificity**

Figure 4.2    Test discriminates poorly between patients with disease (D+) and patients without disease
(D−). (**A**) The distribution of test results in D+ patients is very similar to the distribution in
D− patients. (**B**) This "bad" ROC curve approaches a 45-degree diagonal line.

well: it is the probability that a randomly selected person with the disease will have a
higher (more abnormal) result on the test than a randomly selected person without
the disease.

What if the ROC curve goes under the 45-degree diagonal and AUROC < 0.5?
Then the test is more often high in those who do not have the disease, and you just
need to change your terminology and call lower results "positive" and higher results
"negative." If you wanted to know the shape of the ROC curve without redrawing
it, you could turn it upside down (i.e., you could rotate the paper 180 degrees). You
would not need to recalculate AUROC; it will be just 1 minus the AUROC that you
calculated before.

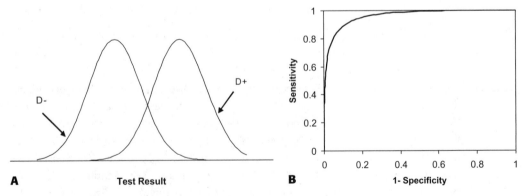

**A**          **Test Result**          **B**          **1- Specificity**

Figure 4.3    Test discriminates well between patients with the disease (D+) and patients without the
disease (D−). (**A**) The distribution of test results in D+ patients differs substantially from
the distribution in D− patients. (**B**) This "good" ROC curve nears the upper left corner of
the grid.

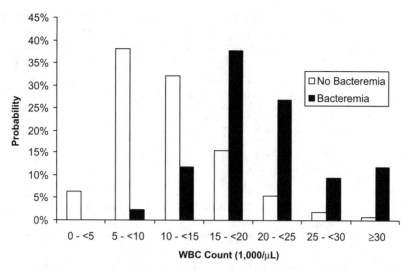

Figure 4.4    Histogram showing distributions of the nonbacteremic and bacteremic populations across the WBC count intervals.

Let us return to our data on febrile infants at risk for bacteremia. The WBC count distributions of the bacteremic and nonbacteremic infants are shown in Figure 4.4.[4]

You can see that, if the WBC count cut-off to divide a "positive" from a "negative" test is 25,000/μL, the specificity of the test is very high. Only a small proportion of the nonbacteremic infants had WBC counts ≥25,000/μL. However, although the proportion of bacteremic infants with WBC counts that high (≥25,000/μL) is greater than the proportion of nonbacteremic infants, it is still small, so the sensitivity would be low.

Table 4.3 provides the same data in tabular form with Sensitivity and 1 − Specificity calculated for you.

Again, the more positive results are higher in the table. The "Bacteremia" and "No Bacteremia" columns correspond to intervals, whereas the "Sensitivity" and "1 − Specificity" columns correspond to cut-offs between "positive" and "negative." Note that Sensitivity is just the cumulative percentage in the "Bacteremia" column and 1 − Specificity is just the cumulative percentage in the "No Bacteremia" column. If we graph Sensitivity against 1 − Specificity, we have the ROC curve in Figure 4.5.

The curve illustrated in Figure 4.5 shows just a few different possible cut-offs, with these few discrete points connected by straight lines. This is the typical appearance for tests with ordinal results or when you create an ROC curve for a test with continuous results by defining a handful of possible cut-offs, as we have here. On the other hand, if a computer plots the ROC curve for a test with continuous (or

[4] As drawn here, this graph tells nothing about the prevalence of bacteremia – that is, the heights of the bars within each group sum to 100%, and we will see that the ratio of the heights of the bars is the LR for a test result interval. Another way to draw histograms like this is to plot numbers of subjects, rather than proportions within each group. Then the height of the bacteremia group's bars would all be a lot lower, and the ratio of the heights of bars would be the posterior odds (in this particular population) rather than the LR.

**Table 4.3.** Sensitivity and specificity of the WBC count as a predictor of bacteremia at different cut-offs for considering the test "positive" (data from Lee and Harper 1998)

| WBC count interval ($\times 1,000/\mu L$) | Percent of bacteremia patients in interval | Percent of no bacteremia patients in interval | Sensitivity (using bottom of interval as cut-off) | 1 − Specificity (using bottom of interval as cut-off) |
|---|---|---|---|---|
| $\geq 30$ | 11.8% | 0.8% | 11.8% | 0.8% |
| 25 to <30 | 9.4% | 1.8% | 21.3% | 2.6% |
| 20 to <25 | 26.8% | 5.4% | 48.0% | 8.0% |
| 15 to <20 | 37.8% | 15.5% | 85.8% | 23.5% |
| 10 to <15 | 11.8% | 32.1% | 97.6% | 55.6% |
| 5 to <10 | 2.4% | 38.1% | 100% | 93.7% |
| 0 to <5 | 0.0% | 6.3% | 100% | 100% |

many discrete) results, it shows what happens when the cut-off is systematically decreased from the highest (or most abnormal) to the lowest (least abnormal) value present in the sample. Figure 4.6 shows two computer-plotted ROC curves for two different WBC counts used to help diagnose bacterial meningitis in infants from 3 to 89 days old (Bonsu and Harper 2003). The WBC count that discriminates well between those with bacterial meningitis and those without bacterial meningitis is the WBC count in the cerebrospinal fluid. The WBC count that discriminates poorly is the WBC count in the peripheral blood. We will return to this figure at the end of this section.

**The walking man approach to understanding ROC curves**

Here is a good way to think about how the computer drew the ROC curves in Figure 4.6. Imagine you have twenty patients, ten of whom have the disease of interest

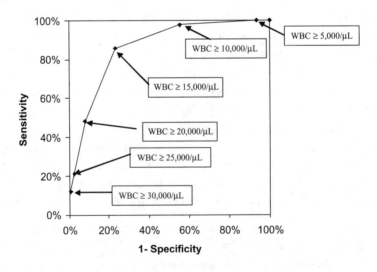

Area Under Curve (AUC) = 0.86

Figure 4.5    ROC curve corresponding to the distributions in Figure 4.4.

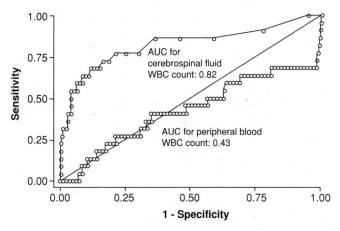

Figure 4.6    Example of computer-drawn ROC curves, in which the cut-off for considering the test "abnormal" is systematically decreased from the highest to the lowest values observed in infants with and without bacterial meningitis. Note that two different WBC counts are considered: the WBC count in the cerebrospinal fluid, which discriminates fairly well between those with and without bacterial meningitis; and the WBC count in the peripheral blood, which discriminates poorly. (From Bonsu and Harper 2003, with permission.) AUC = Area Under Curve.

and ten of whom do not. Perform the test on all of them, and then arrange the test results in order from most abnormal to least abnormal, using "N" to indicate someone with no disease, and "D" to indicate someone who has the disease. (Put ties in parentheses.) Then, for a perfect test, the list would look like this (with spaces added only to enhance readability):

D D D D D    D D D D D    N N N N N    N N N N N

Now picture a little man starting at the lower left corner of the ROC curve. That is the corner that represents 0% sensitivity and 100% specificity – when you say no one has the disease. Put another way, if a high result on the test is abnormal, it is when you say the result has to be higher than the highest value of your sample to be called abnormal. Therefore, everyone is classified as normal, and the sensitivity is 0% but specificity is 100%. Because there are ten patients in each group, make a 10 × 10 grid. Now start at the beginning of the list above. This little man will take a walk on this grid, tracing out an ROC curve. You are going to read the list above out loud to him. Every time you say "D," he will take one step up, corresponding to one more patient with the disease being identified and a 10% increase in sensitivity. Every time you say "N," he will take one step to the right, corresponding to a nondiseased person being identified (false positive) and a 10% decrease in specificity. For every new value of the test, he walks up or over for the number of D or N patients who have that value, then drops a new stone. Each stone represents a point on the ROC curve. You can see, for the perfect test above, he will walk straight up to the upper left-hand corner of the graph, then turn right and walk straight across to the upper right corner, dropping stones all along the way (Fig. 4.7, Perfect Test).

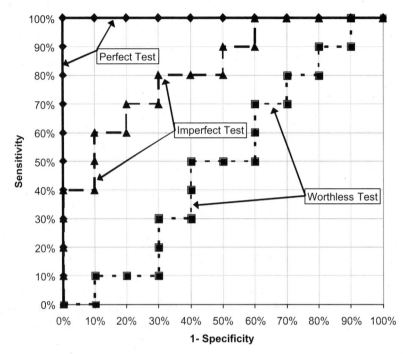

Figure 4.7 Perfect, imperfect, and worthless tests corresponding to the ordered lists of test results given in the text.

Similarly, for a worthless test, the ordering would look something like this:

N D N N D D N D D N N D D N D N D N D N

You can see with this test that he will go up one step about each time he goes over one step, so his path will more or less follow the diagonal line that indicates a worthless test (Fig. 4.7, Worthless Test).

If the test actually provides some information, but is not perfect, the ordered list might look like this, with more Ds at one end and more Ns at the other (Fig. 4.7, Imperfect Test):

D D D D N D D N D N D N N D N D N N N N

You do not need equal numbers of patients per group. If the number of patients is not equal, just divide the vertical scale into d steps, where d is the number with disease, and divide the horizontal scale into n steps, where n is the number without disease. Then just go through your list, going up one step for each D and over one step for each N. (Note: if people with disease have a lower value for the test result, just arrange the values in ascending order, again from most abnormal to least abnormal.)

What about ties, that is, when there are both N and D patients with the same test result? The answer is that, when there is a tie, the ROC curve is diagonal. Recall that the little man only drops a stone after he has walked out all the D and N patients for a particular test value. So if there are three Ns and four Ds that all had the same result, he would take three steps over and four steps up (in any order) before dropping his next stone.

Of course what is happening here is that we are creating the ROC curve by taking each result obtained on the test in order, and saying, "a result more abnormal or equal to this is positive for disease." As we move that number from higher (more abnormal) to lower (less abnormal), we first start picking up more and more diseased individuals (increasing sensitivity), and the little man walks mostly vertically. As we lower this threshold further, we start picking up more nondiseased individuals. For results that are equally likely in diseased and nondiseased people, the little man walks at about a 45-degree angle. Eventually, we get to results that are more common among people who do not have the disease than among people who do (normal values of the test), and he walks more horizontally.

---

**Box 4.1: ROC curves and the Wilcoxon Rank Sum test (also called the Mann–Whitney U-test;) (Hanley and McNeil 1982)**

If you think about the process of the little man tracing out an ROC curve, you can see that the actual values of the test are not important for the shape of the ROC curve or the area under it – only the *ranking* of the values. The ranking determines the order of the Ns and Ds, and hence the pattern of the little man's walk. Thus, it is perhaps not surprising that the statistical significance test for the AUROC comes out exactly the same as that for the Wilcoxon Rank Sum test, a nonparametric alternative to the t-test, used to investigate whether numbers in one group tend to be higher than those in another.

The AUROC and the rank sums can be related as follows. List all of the n patients without disease and d patients with disease in order from most to least abnormal and assign ranks, where 1 is for the most abnormal value and $(n + d)$ is for the least abnormal value. (The way to do ties is assign the average rank to all members of a tie. Thus, if two people are tied for third and fourth, assign both the rank of 3.5; if five people are tied for 7, 8, 9, 10 and 11, assign all of them the rank of 9.) Then take the sum of the ranks of the diseased group; call that S. If the test is perfect, all of the lowest ranks will belong to the diseased group, and S will equal $d(d + 1)/2$ (this is the minumum value of S, $S_{min}$). If all of the people with disease test less abnormal, then S will equal $S_{max} = S_{min} + dn$. The area under the ROC curve, AUROC, is related to these values as follows:

$$AUROC = \frac{S_{max} - S}{S_{max} - S_{min}} = \frac{S_{max} - S}{dn}$$

(Note: if this gives a value <0.5, the ranking was in the wrong order, and you can just change your definition of what direction constitutes abnormal, turn the ROC curve upside down, and subtract the area you got from 1.)

**Abbreviations:**

| | |
|---|---|
| AUROC | area under ROC curve |
| d | number of patients with disease |
| n | number of patients without disease |
| S | sum of ranks in diseased group |
| $S_{min}$ | minimum possible value of S = $d(d + 1)/2$ |
| $S_{max}$ | maximum possible value of S = $S_{min} + dn$ |

### Getting the most out of ROC curves

Take a closer look at the ROC curves in Figure 4.6 and see how much information they contain in addition to the areas under them. First, notice that the points are spread apart on the vertical axis but right next to one another on the horizontal axis. This makes sense if you recall the walking man approach to drawing ROC curves. The grid the little man walks on is divided into d vertical steps and n horizontal steps, where d and n are the numbers with and without disease, respectively. Because meningitis is rare, we expect d to be much smaller than n, so each time he hears "D," he takes a pretty big step up, compared with small steps to the right for each "N." In fact, it is pretty easy to count the number of vertical steps in Figure 4.6 and see that only twenty-two infants in the study had bacterial meningitis.

Now look at the upper right portion of the ROC curve for the peripheral blood WBC count. What is going on there? In that part of the curve, the little man is walking almost straight up. This means that almost all of the patients with very *low* peripheral WBC counts had bacterial meningitis. Although the peripheral WBC count is not a generally good test for meningitis, when it is very low, it does strongly suggest meningitis, that is, the odds of meningitis are substantially increased.

Since the AUROC for the peripheral WBC was <0.5, we might want to turn the ROC curve upside down. Go ahead and do that now with Figure 4.6. What you can see is that, if a low WBC count is defined as abnormal, we can get about 30% sensitivity and close to 100% specificity by using as a cut-off the value at which the ROC curve turns sharply to the right. That sensitivity of about 30% makes sense because you can actually count the little steps and see that seven (32%) of the twenty-two infants with bacterial meningitis had very low peripheral WBC counts.

### LRs for multilevel tests

Recall from Chapter 3 that the general definition of the LR for a test result was the probability of the result in patients with disease divided by the probability of the result in patients without disease. Abbreviating result as r, we can write this:

$$LR(r) = P(r \mid D+)/P(r \mid D-)$$

Because a nondichotomous test has more than two possible results, it has more than two possible LRs. There is no such thing as an LR(+) or an LR(−) for a nondichotomous test, because there is no "+" result and no "−" result.

There is a simple relationship between the interval LR for a multilevel test, as presented in Table 4.4, and the ROC curve: the LR is the slope of the ROC curve over that interval. Take the interval 15 to <20 as an example (Fig. 4.8). The proportion of D+ (bacteremic) patients with WBC counts in this interval is 37.8%, and the proportion of nonbacteremic patients with WBC counts in this interval is 15.5%.

The LR for that interval is $P(r \mid D+)/P(r \mid D-) = 37.8\%/15.5\% = 2.4$. The slope of the ROC curve for that interval is the "rise" of 37.8% over the "run" of 15.5%, also 2.4 (Fig. 4.9).

**Table 4.4.** Likelihood ratios for WBC and bacteremia (from Lee and Harper 1998)

| WBC Count ($\times 1,000/\mu L$) | Bacteremia | No bacteremia | LR |
|---|---|---|---|
| $\geq 30$ | 11.8% | 0.8% | 15.2 |
| 25–30 | 9.4% | 1.8% | 5.3 |
| 20–25 | 26.8% | 5.4% | 4.9 |
| 15–20 | 37.8% | 15.5% | 2.4 |
| 10–15 | 11.8% | 32.1% | 0.37 |
| 5–10 | 2.4% | 38.1% | 0.06 |
| 0–5 | 0.0% | 6.3% | 0.00 |

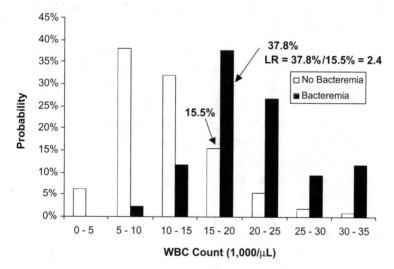

Figure 4.8    Calculation of the LR for the WBC count interval 15 to <20.

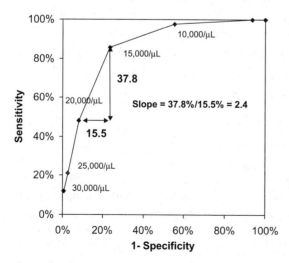

Figure 4.9    The LR for the WBC count interval 15 to <20 is the slope of the ROC curve for that interval.

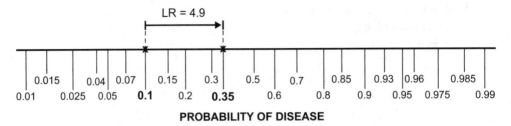

Figure 4.10  Pre-test probability of 10%, LR for a WBC of 23,000/μL of 4.9, yields post-test probability of about 35%.

LRs for the results of multilevel tests like this are combined with prior odds to get posterior odds, the same way as for dichotomous tests. (In fact, we already snuck in an example of this in Chapter 3, Example 3.2, when we used the LR of 100 for a mammogram read as "suspicious for malignancy.")

**Example 4.1** Assume the pre-test probability of bacteremia in a febrile infant is 0.1 (as might be the case in an ill-appearing young infant with a high fever). What would be the posterior probability if the WBC count was 23,000/μL?

1. Convert prior probability to prior odds. Odds = P/(1 − P); because prior probability was 0.10, prior odds = 0.10/(1 − 0.10) = 0.10/0.90 = 0.11.
2. Find the LR corresponding to the result of the test. From Table 4.4, the LR for 20 to <25 × 1,000/μL is 4.9.
3. Obtain the posterior odds by multiplying the prior odds times the LR: Posterior odds = 0.11 × 4.9 = 0.544.
4. Convert posterior odds back to posterior probability. P = Odds/(1 + Odds). So this is 0.544/(1 + 0.544) = 0.353, or about 35%.

You can use the LR slide rule, too. Figure 4.10 shows the same calculation depicted using the LR slide rule's log (odds) scale.

As another example, consider a ventilation/perfusion (V/Q) scan in a 65-year-old man with metastatic cancer, pleuritic chest pain, and shortness of breath. Our internist colleagues (who just love V/Q scans for illustrating LRs) say the prior probability of a pulmonary embolus (PE) in such a patient is about 0.33. The PIOPED (1990) study found the following LRs for V/Q scans:

"High Probability" V/Q Scan.....LR = 13

"Int. Probability" V/Q Scan........LR = 1

"Low Probability" V/Q Scan....LR = 0.4

Normal V/Q Scan.......LR = 0.1

Figure 4.11 shows an "X" at the point on the scale representing the prior probability of 0.33. We can visualize test results as arrows with a direction and length. The direction is to the left if the LR is <1 and to the right if it is >1. The length depends on how far the LR is from 1. It is on a logarithmic scale, so an LR of 100 has the same length as an LR of 0.01 (see Appendix 4.1). In Figure 4.11, the arrows above the scale show how the posterior probability of PE would change with different results on the V/Q scan.

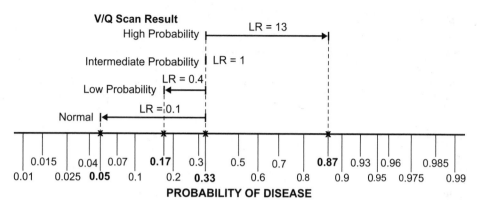

Figure 4.11 LRs for V/Q scan results. The length and direction of the arrows are proportional to the log of the LR. "High Probability": 13; "Intermediate Probability" :1; "Low Probability" : 0.4; "Normal": 0.1.

So if our 65-year-old man with a prior probability of PE of 0.33 had a V/Q scan, you can see that his posterior probability could go as low as about 0.05 or as high as 0.87, depending on the results of the scan (Fig. 4.11).

Note that, in the WBC count and V/Q scan examples above, there are as many LRs as there are results on the test, and there is no LR(+) or LR(−). If you have the result of a multilevel test, and you find yourself looking for the LR(+) or the LR(−) associated with that test result, you need to revise your thinking.

## Optimal cut-off between positive and negative for a multilevel test

The foregoing discussion argued that dichotomizing a multilevel or continuous test by choosing a fixed cut-off to separate positive from negative entails a loss of information. However, for expediency, we still sometimes choose a cut-off for a continuous diagnostic test to separate abnormal from normal. Examples of cut-offs that separate "positive" from "negative" test results include the body temperature (typically 38.5°C) that identifies intravenous drug users to admit for an endocarditis work-up and the plasma glucose level (typically 140 mg/dL) that defines glucose intolerance in pregnancy.

The purpose of dividing a clinical population into higher risk and lower risk groups is to provide differential care: hospitalization for intravenous drug users with fevers; and diet or insulin therapy for pregnant women with glucose intolerance. However, as we learned in Chapter 3, costs are associated with both types of misclassification. These can be expressed by using C and B from Chapter 3: C = the cost of the false positive (a test result that falls on the "high-risk" side of the cut-off value, even though the patient will not benefit from treatment); B = the cost of the false negative (a test result that falls on the "low-risk" side of the cut-off, even though the patient would benefit from treatment). The optimal cut-off exactly balances expected misclassification costs.

One last time, we return to the data on WBC counts in febrile infants at risk for bacteremia. We want to know the WBC cut-off above which we will treat with empiric antibiotics (Kohn and Newman 2001). The first question to ask is about

**Table 4.5.** Posterior odds of bacteremia for 7 WBC categories when the pre-test odds are 15:1,000

| WBC count ($\times 1,000/\mu L$) | LR | Posterior odds: 1,000 |
|---|---|---|
| $\geq 30$ | 15.2 | 228 |
| 25 to <30 | 5.3 | 79 |
| 20 to <25 | 4.9 | 74 |
| 15 to <20 | 2.4 | 37 |
| 10 to <15 | 0.37 | 6 |
| 5 to <10 | 0.06 | 1 |
| 0 to <5 | 0.00 | 0 |

the consequences of error. How many infants are we willing to treat unnecessarily (incurring cost C) to avoid missing one infant with bacteremia (incurring cost B)? Let us suppose that we are willing to treat twenty-five infants with viral fevers to avoid missing one with bacteremia. That means that we have decided that B is twenty-five times as harmful as C; in other words, the ratio of C:B is 1:25, which is our treatment threshold. We want to treat when the odds of disease are 1:25 or greater (e.g., 1:20 or 1:10). (It will help to recognize that 1:25 is the same as 40:1,000.) Our next question is about the pre-test odds of disease. In the data presented above, the odds of bacteremia in the study population were 127:8,629 or about 15:1,000. We know the LR for each of the possible WBC results, so starting with odds of 15:1,000, we can multiply by the LR to calculate the post-test odds for each result, as shown in Table 4.5.

Recall that our threshold for treatment was 40:1,000. We can see that this threshold is exceeded somewhere around a WBC count of 20,000/$\mu L$, so this is the "optimal" cut-off. Using this cut-off assumes, unreasonably, that the pre-test odds of bacteremia and the relative consequences of error are the same for all febrile infants. However, this kind of cut-off calculation might make sense with a screening test for which the pre-test odds of disease actually equal the population prevalence, and the relative consequences of a misclassification error are more or less the same from individual to individual.

Mathematically, the optimal cut-off $r^*$ is the least abnormal r, such that

Pretest Odds $\times$ LR($r^*$) $\geq$ Threshold Odds (C/B)

As the pre-test probability of disease increases, the optimal cut-off decreases (is less abnormal). For example, as the probability of bacteremia increases, the WBC count required to prompt antibiotic therapy is lower. If the pre-test odds of disease are twice as high (30:1,000 instead of 15:1,000), the treatment threshold decreases to 15,000/$\mu L$, as shown in Table 4.6.

## Graphical approach to optimal cut-offs

In Chapter 3, we introduced a graph that showed the expected cost associated with a test/treatment strategy depending on the pre-test probability of disease p[D+].

**Table 4.6.** Post-test odds of bacteremia, given pre-test odds of 30:1,000

| WBC count $(\times 1000/\mu L)^a$ | LR | Posterior odds : 1000 |
|---|---|---|
| $\geq 30$ | 15.2 | 456 |
| 25 to <30 | 5.3 | 158 |
| 20 to <25 | 4.9 | 148 |
| 15 to <20 | 2.4 | 73 |
| 10 to <15 | 0.37 | 11 |
| 5 to <10 | 0.06 | 2 |
| 0 to <5 | 0.00 | 0 |

[a] Note that if we had finer categories of WBC count and sufficient sample size, we could estimate the proper treatment cut-off more precisely.

There were only three strategies: no treat, test, and treat. In Figure 4.12, we reproduce the graph (Fig. 3.5), but this is a "blow-up," showing only the bottom portion of that graph, and we show the test as the WBC count dichotomized at the 15,000/μL cut-off.

One way to look at a multilevel test is to view it as many dichotomous tests, one for each potential cut-off (Figure 4.13). To understand Figure 4.13, recall that the lowest expected cost strategy is the most desirable. Start on the far left end of the probability axis (the x-axis), where probability of disease is 0.0. You can see that, for a range of very low probabilities, the lowest cost strategy is "no treat", that is, do not even test. Then for another interval of low probabilities, the optimal strategy is to test

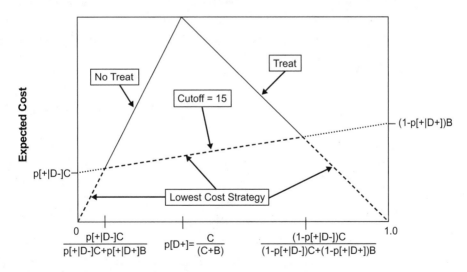

Figure 4.12 Expected cost of the "No Treat," "Test," and "Treat" strategies versus probability of disease. (This is a "blow-up" of Figure 3.5.) The test is the WBC count made dichotomous by choosing a cut-off of $15 \times 10^3/\mu L$.

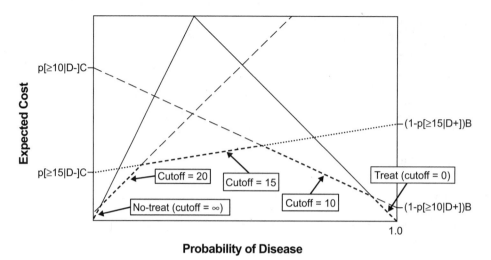

**Probability of Disease**

Figure 4.13 Expected costs of the "test" strategy using various cut-offs to distinguish "positive" from "negative."

using a cut-off of 20; you would treat for a WBC count greater than 20,000/μL. As you move right on the axis and the probability of disease increases, the WBC cut-off decreases to 15 and then 10. Finally, at the far right end of the axis, the probability of disease is so high that you should treat without testing.

We can graph the optimal WBC cut-off as a function of the pre-test probability of disease (Fig. 4.14). As the probability of disease increases, the optimal WBC cut-off decreases from infinity (don't test, don't treat) to 0 (don't test, treat). Make sure you understand conceptually why the WBC count cut-off for treating a febrile infant with antibiotics decreases as the pre-test probability of bacteremia increases. The discrete steps in Figure 4.14 result from dividing the continuous range WBC counts into discrete intervals (30 to 35, 25 to <30, 20 to <25, etc.). For a similar discussion using smooth curves, see Kohn and Newman (2001).

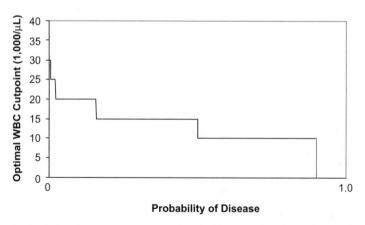

**Probability of Disease**

Figure 4.14 Optimal WBC count treatment threshold as a function of the pre-test probability of disease.

**ROC curves and optimal cut-offs**

You cannot use an ROC curve alone to choose the best cut-off for a multilevel or continuous test. Repeating what we said above, the optimal cut-off, $r^*$, is the least abnormal result, such that

Pretest Odds $\times$ LR($r^*$) $\geq$ Threshold Odds.

Or, substituting $P/(1 - P)$ for pretest odds and C/B for threshold odds,

$[P/(1 - P)] \times LR(r^*) \geq C/B$

Because the LR is the slope of the ROC curve at a particular point, LR(r) may be obtained from the ROC curve. But, the optimal cut-off also depends on the pre-test probability (or odds) of disease and the ratio of misclassification costs, neither of which is depicted in the ROC curve.

Occasionally, someone suggests that the optimal cut-off is the point where the slope of the ROC curve is 1 [i.e., $45°$, LR($r^*$) $= 1$]. This will only be true if the pre-test odds of disease $P/(1 - P)$ are equal to the treatment threshold odds C/B. For example, if failing to treat a D+ individual is twenty-five times worse than treating a D− individual unnecessarily *and* the pre-test odds of disease happen to be 1:25, then the optimal cut-off is where the slope of the ROC curve is 1. This would also be true if misclassification costs were equal (B $=$ C) and the pre-test odds of disease were 50:50. These situations are uncommon, however, so it is seldom true that the optimal cut-off is the point on the ROC curve where the slope is equal to 1.

## Summary of key points

1. For tests with more than two possible results, making a test dichotomous by choosing a fixed cut-off to separate "positive" from "negative" results wastes information. Some positive results will be more abnormal than others, and some negative results will be more normal than others.
2. The distribution of test results among those who do and do not have the disease can be presented graphically using ROC curves.
3. ROC curves allow visualization of the trade-off between sensitivity and specificity as the cut-off for classifying a test as positive changes. They also allow visualization of the LRs for different test results, because the slope of the ROC curve is the LR.
4. The AUROC provides a summary of how well the test discriminates between those who do and do not have the disease.
5. The LR associated with a particular result on a multilevel or continuous test is the probability of that result in people with the disease divided by the probability of that result in people without the disease. Because nondichotomous tests have more than two possible results, they have more than two LRs.
6. When faced with an individual patient with an individual test result, post-test odds of disease equal pre-test odds multiplied by the LR associated with the test result.

7. The optimal cut-off for classifying a test as "positive" depends not only on the shape of the ROC curve, but also on the prior probability of disease and the treatment threshold odds for the disease, C/B.

## Appendix 4.1: Logarithms and the likelihood ratio slide rule

### How does the LR slide rule work?

The LR slide rule relies on the idea that multiplying two numbers (e.g., pre-test odds and LR of a test result) is the same as adding their logarithms. This requires a brief review of logarithms.

### Mathematical digression: logarithms

Recall that the common or base-10 logarithm of a number is defined as the power to which 10 is raised to get that number. $\log(a) = b$, where $a = 10^b : \log(100) = 2$, $\log(10) = 1, \log(1) = 0, \log(0.1) = -1, \log(0.01) = -2$. If you multiply two numbers, x and y, the logarithm of the product is the sum of the logs: $\log(xy) = \log(x) + \log(y)$. For example, $\log(10 \times 100) = \log(10) + \log(100) = 1 + 2 = 3$. Similarly, if you divide two numbers, the logarithm of the quotient is the difference of the logs: $\log(x/y) = \log(x) - \log(y)$. For example, $\log(10/100) = \log(10) - \log(100) = 1 - 2 = -1$.

**Practice Problems:**

1. $\log(2) = 0.3$. What is $\log(5)$?

2. $\log(3) \approx 0.5$. What is $\log(1/3)$?

**Answers:**

1. $5 = 10/2$, so $\log(5) = \log(10/2) = \log(10) - \log(2) = 1 - 0.3 = 0.7$

2. $\log(1/3)) \approx -0.5$

### Natural logarithms

Just as common logarithms are base-10 logarithms, natural logarithms are base-e logarithms, where e is the mathematical constant $2.7183\ldots \ln(a) = b$, where $a = e^b$. The change of base from 10 to e affects the actual numerical value of the logarithm, but nothing else: $\ln(xy) = \ln(x) + \ln(y); \ln(x/y) = \ln(x) - \ln(y)$.

### log(Odds)

You have already become comfortable dealing with odds instead of probabilities. You did this because of the simple relationship between pre-test odds and post-test odds. Now you need to get comfortable with the logarithm of odds, log(Odds), instead of the odds themselves. By taking the logarithms, we can convert the equation for post-test odds from multiplication to addition:

Post-Test Odds = (Pre-Test Odds) × (Likelihood Ratio of Test Result)

Taking logarithms,

log(Post-Test Odds) = log(Pre-Test Odds) + log(Likelihood Ratio of Test Result)

In the chapter, we work Example 4.1 in which a febrile infant with a 10% pre-test probability of bacteremia has a WBC count of 23,000/μL. The LR associated with that result is 4.9. We saw that the post-test probability is 35%. Let us calculate this post-test probability using logarithms and show you how this helps to visualize the process of probability updating.

1. Convert prior probability to prior odds. Odds = P/(1 − P). Because prior probability is 0.10, prior odds = 0.10/(1 − 0.10) = 0.10/0.90 = 0.111.
2. Convert prior odds to log(Odds): log(0.111) = −0.95.

| log (Odds) | 2 | -1.5 | -1 -0.95 | -0.5 | 0 | 0.5 | 1 |
|---|---|---|---|---|---|---|---|
| Odds | 1:100 | 1:33 | 1:9 | 1:3 | 1:1 | 3:1 | 10:1 |
| Probability | 0.01 | 0.03 | 0.10 | 0.25 | 0.5 | 0.75 | 0.91 |

3. Find the log(LR) corresponding to the result of the test. The LR for a WBC of 23,000/μL is 4.9, and log(4.9) = 0.69.
4. Obtain the posterior log(Odds) by adding the log(LR) to the prior log(Odds): Posterior log(Odds) = −0.95 + 0.69 = −0.26.
5. Convert posterior log(Odds) back to posterior Odds: $10^{-0.26} = 0.54$
6. Convert Odds to probability: 0.54/(1 + 0.54) = 0.35, or about 35%.

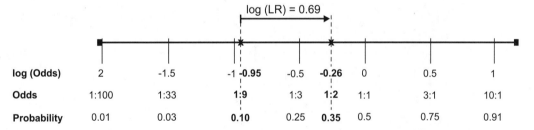

log (LR) = 0.69

| log (Odds) | 2 | -1.5 | -1 -0.95 | -0.5 | -0.26 | 0 | 0.5 | 1 |
|---|---|---|---|---|---|---|---|---|
| Odds | 1:100 | 1:33 | 1:9 | 1:3 | 1:2 | 1:1 | 3:1 | 10:1 |
| Probability | 0.01 | 0.03 | 0.10 | 0.25 | 0.35 | 0.5 | 0.75 | 0.91 |

The key advantage of the log(Odds) scale is our ability to display probability updating as a problem of addition. We just lay the back end of the log(LR) arrow at the pre-test probability, and the arrow tip points out the post-test probability.

The LR slide rule does the conversion between log(Odds) and probability for you by spacing the probabilities according to the logs of their corresponding odds.

# References

Bonsu, B. K., and M. B. Harper (2003). "Utility of the peripheral blood white blood cell count for identifying sick young infants who need lumbar puncture." *Ann Emerg Med* **41**(2): 206–14.

Hanley, J. A., and B. J. McNeil (1982). "The meaning and use of the area under a receiver operating characteristic (ROC) curve." *Radiology* **143**(1): 29–36.

Kohn, M. A., and M. P. Newman (2001). "What white blood cell count should prompt antibiotic treatment in a febrile child? Tutorial on the importance of disease likelihood to the interpretation of diagnostic tests." *Med Decis Making* **21**(6): 479–89.

Lee, G. M., and M. B. Harper (1998). "Risk of bacteremia for febrile young children in the post-Haemophilus influenzae type b era." *Arch Pediatr Adolesc Med* **152**(7): 624–8.

PIOPED (1990). "Value of the ventilation/perfusion scan in acute pulmonary embolism. Results of the prospective investigation of pulmonary embolism diagnosis (PIOPED)." *JAMA*. **263**(20): 2753–9.

Swets, J. A. (1996). *Signal Detection Theory and ROC Analysis in Psychology and Diagnostics: Collected Papers.* Mahwah, NJ, L. Erlbaum Associates.

## Chapter 4 Problems: multilevel and continuous tests

1. You are developing a new home pregnancy test, which gives a digital read-out of pregnancy peptide (in arbitrary units). Results on ten women with early pregnancy and ten nonpregnant controls are shown below:

| Pregnant | Not pregnant |
|----------|--------------|
| 4 | 1 |
| 7 | 1 |
| 15 | 2 |
| 18 | 3 |
| 20 | 5 |
| 23 | 7 |
| 23 | 13 |
| 26 | 16 |
| 30 | 17 |
| 32 | 21 |

a) Draw an ROC curve for this test. (Hint: List results in descending order and use the walking man method.)

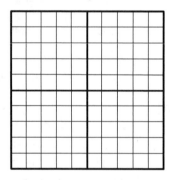

b) Estimate the area under the ROC curve. (Hint: count boxes.)

c) Rank the list in part (a). Remember the highest number gets rank #1. You can write the ranks next to the values in the list.

d) Calculate the rank sum, S, as well as $S_{min}$ and $S_{max}$.

e) Use the formula given in Box 4.1 to determine the AUROC from these ranks. You should get the same answer you got for part (b) above. Isn't that satisfying?

f) Make LRs for test results <10, 10–20, and >20. (Hint: With a tiny sample size like this, you need to pay attention to > vs. ≥)

g) One of your sexually active patients has missed a period. Based on your experience, you estimate there is a 50:50 chance she is pregnant. Her result on the test above is 7 (i.e., <10). How would you revise her odds of pregnancy? What is the probability that she is pregnant?

h) Do you think this test will be clinically useful? Explain.

2. Brennan et al. (2003) reported on the "Prognostic Value of Myeloperoxidase in Patients with Chest Pain." ROC curves from Figure 2C of that paper are reprinted below. The disease being predicted is major coronary events at 30 days.

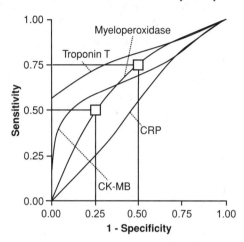

C Major Adverse Coronary Events at 30 Days
Entire Cohort [N=604]

From Brennan et al. *N. Engl. J. Med*, 2003; **349**:1595–1604. Used by permission. Copyright 2003 Massachussetts Medical Society. All rights reserved.

a) From looking at its ROC curve, what can you say about the usefulness of the CRP (C-Reactive Protein) for predicting major adverse coronary events at 30 days?

b) The Methods section of the paper states: "Myocardial infarction [one type of major adverse coronary event] was defined by Troponin T levels of at least 0.1 ng/ml." Explain the connection between this case definition for myocardial infarction and shape of the Troponin T ROC curve.

c) The shape of the ROC curve for myeloperoxidase in the figure suggests that little would be lost by classifying myeloperoxidase levels as high (=abnormal), medium (=indeterminate), and low (=normal). To make the math easy, we've drawn some lines on that ROC curve and included little squares to indicate the cut-offs between high and medium and between medium and low.

   i. What are LRs for low, medium, and high myeloperoxidase results?

   ii. Let's suppose you would treat the patient differently depending on whether you thought the probability of a major adverse coronary event at 30 days was 20% or more. For what range of prior probabilities of a major adverse coronary event at 30 days could the results of the myeloperoxidase test affect your management?

d) The ROC curve for CK-MB (Creatine Kinase – MB fraction) in panel C of the figure has a funny shape. What does the shape tell you about the distribution of CK-MB in subjects with and without major adverse coronary events at 30 days?

3. **Clinical Scenario:** Last night in the Emergency Department you saw a 53-year-old male smoker with a history of chronic obstructive pulmonary disease who presented with acute shortness of breath. The nurse recommended a B-type natriuretic peptide (BNP) test for congestive heart failure, which you obtained. The result was 135 pg/mL. You stole a few minutes to go to PubMed and found the abstract of an article in the *New England Journal of Medicine* (Maisel et al. 2002) that indicates that "the diagnostic accuracy of the B-type natriuretic peptide at a cutoff of 100 pg/ml is 83.4%." Because his value was >100 pg/mL, you concluded that there was a >80% chance that he had heart failure and treated him accordingly. He did not respond as you had hoped, and you were left with some misgivings about the case and your interpretation of the abstract. You resolved to pull the actual article and see what you can learn from it. The main summary figure from the article is below:

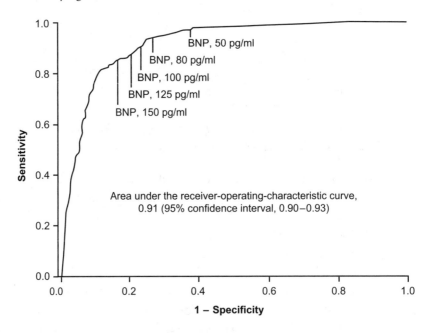

| BNP | | | POSITIVE PREDICTIVE | NEGATIVE PREDICTIVE | |
| | SENSITIVITY | SPECIFICITY | VALUE | VALUE | ACCURACY |
| pg/ml | | | (95 percent confidence interval) | | |
| --- | --- | --- | --- | --- | --- |
| 50 | 97 (96–98) | 62 (59–66) | 71 (68–74) | 96 (94–97) | 79 |
| 80 | 93 (91–95) | 74 (70–77) | 77 (75–80) | 92 (89–94) | 83 |
| 100 | 90 (88–92) | 76 (73–79) | 79 (76–81) | 89 (87–91) | 83 |
| 125 | 87 (85–90) | 79 (76–82) | 80 (78–83) | 87 (84–89) | 83 |
| 150 | 85 (82–88) | 83 (80–85) | 83 (80–85) | 85 (83–88) | 84 |

Receiver-Operating-Characteristic Curve for Various Cutoff Levels of B-Type Natriuretic Peptide (BNP) in Differentiating between Dyspnea Due to Congestive Heart Failure and Dyspnea Due to Other Causes

From Maisel et al, *N Engl J Med*. 2002 Jul 18;**347**(3): 161–7. Used by Permission. Copyright 2002 Massachussetts Medical Society. All rights reserved.

a) In the above table, what is the definition of "test accuracy?"

b) Use the ROC curve for BNP and the table below it to calculate some LRs for the rapid BNP test. (Hint: Use the general formula for LRs, not Sensitivity/ $(1 -$ Specificity.) What LR should you have used for your patient from the night before?

4. Consider a ballot initiative proposed in California several years ago, to allow a jury to convict a defendant if only ten jurors agreed that he or she was guilty, rather than requiring all twelve jurors to agree, as is presently the case. Simplify this problem by ignoring mistrials and considering only two possible verdicts: guilty and not guilty. In this analogy, a truly guilty defendant is like a patient with the disease, an innocent defendant is like a patient without the disease, and a conviction by the jury is like a positive test.

a) If you continue with the diagnostic test analogy, what would you call the proportion of innocent defendants that are acquitted?

b) If your goal were to maximize sensitivity, would you tend to favor the initiative? Why or why not?

c) A key question in evaluating this initiative is: what is the trade-off between "true positives" and "false positives?" That is, how much do you increase your chance of convicting someone who is innocent in order to convict more people who are guilty? This trade-off can be visualized with ROC curves. Draw two hypothetical ROC curves for this problem, labeling the axes and the points "12" and "10" on the curve for the number of jurors needed to convict. Make the first ROC curve one that would lead you to support the initiative, and the other ROC curve one that would lead you to oppose it. (Label the curves "Support" and "Oppose.") Explain your answer.

d) One reason why rational people might disagree on whether to support such an initiative is that their estimates of the shape of the ROC curve differ. Suppose two people agree completely on the ROC curve. What are two other reasons why they might still disagree on whether to support the initiative?

5. The table below comes from a study of febrile infants <3 months old (Pantell, 2004).

| WBC Count (/μL) | Bacterial Meningitis or Bacteremia | | | | LR |
| | Yes | | No | | |
| | Number | % | Number | % | |
| --- | --- | --- | --- | --- | --- |
| 0–4999 | 5 | 7.94 | 96 | 4.41 | |
| 5000–11999 | 21 | 33.33 | 1240 | 56.91 | |
| 12000–19999 | 22 | 34.92 | 691 | 31.71 | |
| >19999 | 15 | 23.81 | 152 | 6.98 | |
| Total | 63 | 100.00 | 2179 | 100.00 | |

a) Fill in the LR for each level of WBC to the right of the table.

b) Among the 775 infants younger than 1 month, the prior probability of bacteremia or meningitis was 4%. What would be the posterior probability if the

WBC were 15,000? (Assume age and WBC are independent predictors, i.e., use the LR from part (a).)

c) Draw an ROC curve for the WBC count as a test for bacteremia or meningitis.

d) Why might the area under this ROC curve not be a good measure of the discrimination of the test?

e) In a febrile infant, which WBC count is most reassuring with regard to the possibility of bacteremia?

f) Assume that, if a febrile infant has a post-test probability of bactermia/meningitis >1%, you will admit and begin empiric antibiotics. Obviously, if the pre-test probability is 50%, you would admit regardless of the WBC count. What is the lowest pre-test probability at which you would admit, regardless of the WBC count?

6. Women 11–14 weeks pregnant who get ultrasound scans often have the fetal nuchal (neck) translucency (NT) measured as a test for chromosomal abnormalities, the most common of which is trisomy 21 (Down syndrome). NT is the measurement (in mm) of the subcutaneous edema (fluid) between the skin at the back of the fetal neck and the soft tissue overlying the cervical spine. Chromosomal abnormalities can be established definitively by using chorionic villus sampling, but this is an invasive test that can accidentally terminate the pregnancy. Cicero et al. (2004) reported NTs in 5,556 fetuses. The tests were done prior to definitive determination of trisomy 21 versus normal chromosomes via chorionic villus sampling. The results are show below.

| Nuchal Translucency (mm) | Trisomy 21 | % | Chromosomally Normal | % | LR |
|---|---|---|---|---|---|
| >5.4 | 104 | 31.2 | 100 | 1.9 | 16.3 |
| 4.5–5.4 | 41 | 12.3 | 84 | 1.6 | 7.7 |
| 3.5–4.4 | 67 | 20.1 | 294 | 5.6 | 3.6 |
| 2.5–3.4 | 83 | 24.9 | 1,500 | 28.7 | 0.87 |
| <2.5 | 38 | 11.4 | 3,245 | 62.1 | 0.18 |
| Total | 333 | 100.0 | 5,223 | 100.0 | |

a) If you are willing to do chorionic villus samples on thirty normal fetuses to identify one trisomy 21 fetus, at what posterior probability of trisomy 21 (after ultrasound) would you do the chorionic villus sampling? (Hint: What we are saying is that it is 30 times as bad to not do chorionic villus sampling and miss a trisomy 21 fetus as it is to do a chorionic villus sampling unnecessarily.)

b) Assume that the threshold calculated in part (a) is your threshold for chorionic villus sampling (the "treatment") and that the only chromosomal abnormality at issue is trisomy 21, with a pre-test probability of 1%. Under these assumptions, what is the threshold NT measurement that should prompt chorionic villus sampling?

c) You just specified an NT threshold that should prompt chorionic villus sampling. If NT at or above this threshold is considered "NT positive" for trisomy

21 and NT below this threshold is considered "NT negative," what are the sensitivity and specificity of the NT test for trisomy 21?

## References for problem set

Brennan, M. L., M. S. Penn, et al. (2003). "Prognostic value of myeloperoxidase in patients with chest pain." *N Engl J Med* **349**(17): 1595–604.

Cicero, S., G. Rembouskos, et al. (2004). "Likelihood ratio for trisomy 21 in fetuses with absent nasal bone at the 11–14-week scan." *Ultrasound Obstet Gynecol* **23**(3): 218–23.

Maisel, A. S., P. Krishnaswamy, et al. (2002). "Rapid measurement of B-type natriuretic peptide in the emergency diagnosis of heart failure." *N Engl J Med* **347**(3): 161–7.

Pantell, R. H., T. B. Newman, et al. (2004). "Management and outcomes of care of fever in early infancy." *JAMA* **291**(10): 1203–12.

# Critical appraisal of studies of diagnostic tests

## Introduction

We have learned how to quantify the reliability (Chapter 2) and accuracy (Chapters 3 and 4) of diagnostic tests. In this chapter, we turn to critical appraisal of studies of diagnostic tests, with an emphasis on problems with study design that affect the interpretation or credibility of the results. After a general discussion of an approach to studies of diagnostic tests, we will review some common biases to which studies of test accuracy are uniquely or especially susceptible and conclude with an introduction to systematic reviews of studies of diagnostic tests.

## General approach

A general approach to critical appraisal of studies of diagnostic tests is to break the study down into its component parts and consider strengths and weaknesses of each, as outlined in Table 5.1. Begin with the research question: is it a question to which you really want to know the answer? Is the test (or history or physical examination finding) being studied one that you have used or could use for your patients? Is the entity being diagnosed one that is important?

Next, consider the study design. All study designs (cross-sectional, case–control, cohort, randomized trial, etc.) have strengths and weaknesses. Watch out for studies of diagnostic tests with a case–control design, in which subjects with the disease are sampled separately from those without the disease. We previously mentioned that the separate sampling of those with and without disease can provide information on test characteristics (sensitivity and specificity) but generally cannot provide information about prior or posterior probability. Other problems with sampling those with and without the disease separately are that the process by which they were classified may have been influenced by the results of the test ("incorporation bias," discussed in the next section) and studies with this design tend to select subjects in whom true disease

**Table 5.1.** Step-by-step critical appraisal of studies of diagnostic tests

| Study Component | Examples | Issues for consideration |
| --- | --- | --- |
| **Research question:** The question that the study is designed to answer. | • How accurate is a bedside test for influenza?<br>• What is the inter-rater reliability of Pap smear readings? | • Is the study question relevant? (Do you care what the answer is?)<br>• Is the test one that you can use for your patients?<br>• Are the outcome variables of interest to you or your patients? |
| **Study design:** How subjects were sampled, what variables were measured, and when. | • Cross-sectional study<br>• Cohort study<br>• Case-control study<br>• Randomized trial | • Are subjects sampled separately by disease status or test results?<br>• Was the predictor variable measured before, at the same time, or after the outcome variable? |
| **Subjects:** How the subjects were identified and selected, and the inclusion and exclusion criteria. | • Consecutive patients 6 months to 6 years old admitted with fever and at least 1 of 4 additional symptoms<br>• Women 35–75 years old presenting for routine Pap smear | • Are the subjects (both with and without disease, if sampled separately) representative of those to whom you wish to generalize the results?<br>• If not, in what direction will differences alter the results? |
| **Predictor variable:** For studies of test accuracy, the test result.<br>How the test was done. | • QuickVue test result obtained by trained and certified nurses<br>• Results of Pap smears read by 4 cytology technicians and 5 cytologists at 2 academic medical centers | • How difficult is it to do the test?<br>• If it requires skill or training, will the skill and training of those doing the test in your setting be similar to what was studied? |
| **Outcome variable:** For studies of test accuracy, the presence or absence of disease. For prognostic tests, the occurrence of a bad outcome, like relapse or death. | • Influenza diagnosed by viral culture or 2 consecutive positive Polymerase Chain Reaction (PCR) tests<br>• Kappa statistic<br>• 5-year all-cause mortality | • Is the gold standard really gold?<br>• Is it clinically relevant – i.e., how well does the gold standard correlate with what you really want to know?<br>• Were those measuring it blinded to results of the test being evaluated? |

(*continued*)

**Table 5.1** (*continued*)

| Study Component | Examples | Issues for Consideration |
| --- | --- | --- |
| **Results and analysis:** What the authors found at the end of the study. May include whether results vary in different subgroups of patients or by center or examiner. | • For studies of reproducibility: kappa, Bland-Altman plots, etc.<br>• For accuracy studies: sensitivity, specificity, predictive value, LRs, AUROC curve, all with confidence intervals | • Were all the subjects analyzed, or were some (e.g., those with ambiguous results or some with negative results) excluded?<br>• If sensitivity, specificity, or LRs were reported for ordinal or continuous tests, were standard cut-offs or intervals used?<br>• If predictive value is reported, is the prevalence in the study representative of your patient population?<br>• Were confidence intervals for relevant quantities included? |
| **Conclusions:** The authors' conclusions regarding the research question, based on the results of the study. | • Authors' conclusions often go beyond estimates of test accuracy or reliability and address whether or when the test is worth doing. | • Do you believe the results are true in the population studied (internal validity)?<br>• Do you believe they apply to patients you see (external validity)?<br>• Did the test provide new information, beyond what was available without the test?<br>• Given your estimates of prior probability and the costs of false-positive and false-negative results, do you agree with authors' conclusions on indications for the test? |

status is more clear-cut than it is in clinical practice ("spectrum bias," discussed later in this chapter).

As in any clinical research study, the extent to which findings can be generalized depends on how the subjects were sampled for the study. Are the prevalence and severity of the disease (and of diseases that could be confused with it) similar to those in your clinical population? If not, in what direction would the differences change the results? If the study is of reproducibility, consider the sampling and representativeness of both the patients on whom the test was done and the people doing the test.

The predictor variable for studies of diagnostic tests is most often the test result. In appraising a study, it is important to look at exactly how the test was done. Are there factors, such as freshness or preparation of the sample, skill of those obtaining the sample, those doing or interpreting the test, or the quality of the equipment used, that might affect the results? If so, in what direction would results be affected?

The outcome variable is the outcome that the predictor variable is supposed to predict or affect. It may be the presence or absence of disease (determined by a gold standard), or the occurrence of a bad outcome, such as death or relapse of disease. Ideally, measurements of the outcome variable should be made by people blinded to the result of the predictor variable, although as will be discussed later, this is not always practical. Because the ultimate goal of testing is to improve outcomes by enhancing decision making, the best studies of diagnostic tests (admittedly few and far between) are those that compare outcomes in patients randomized to receive or not receive the test, as has been done for BNP in emergency department patients presenting with shortness of breath (Mueller et al. 2006) and pulmonary artery catheters in patients with acute lung injury (Wheeler et al. 2006).

The results of the study are what the authors found, generally presented using the parameters described in Chapters 2–4, including kappa, sensitivity, specificity, ROC curves, etc. Because there is a trade-off between sensitivity and specificity, watch for studies that only highlight one or the other; any test can be 100% sensitive if there is no lower limit of specificity and vice versa. These parameters should be accompanied by confidence intervals to quantify the precision of the estimates. We will discuss confidence intervals at length in Chapter 11; for now, we will just say that they show the range of values consistent with the study results.

Finally, consider the conclusions of the study and decide whether they are justified by the results, given any limitations in the other components of the study. If a study concludes that a test is useful, pay particular attention to limitations in its methods that would tend to make the test look falsely good. On the other hand, studies that conclude a test is not useful should be scrutinized for biases that will make the test look worse in the study than it might be in practice.

Conclusions about usefulness of tests often require information and judgments that go far beyond the results of the study. For example, a study that estimates only sensitivity and specificity may conclude that a test is or is not worth doing when the answers to that question depend on the prior probability of the disease, the cost of the test, and the consequences of false-negative and false-positive results, all of which may vary in different populations and may depend on which decision the test is supposed to help with. History and physical examination findings, for example,

**Box 5.1: Example of step-by-step appraisal of a diagnostic test study**

The research question for a recent study (Nassar et al. 2006) was: what is the diagnostic accuracy of clinical examination for detection of noncephalic presentation in late pregnancy? "Noncephalic" means the fetal head is not pointed down. Diagnosing this prior to the onset of labor is important to help decide whether to try an "external version" (pushing on the uterus to turn the fetus) to avoid a breech delivery.

The study design was cross-sectional.

The subjects were 1,633 women with a singleton pregnancy at 35–37 weeks gestation attending antenatal clinics at a Women and Babies hospital in Australia. This represented 96% of the 1,707 eligible women who were approached.

The predictor variable was the clinical examination for presentation by one of more than sixty clinicians (residents or registrars 55%, midwives 28%, obstetricians 17%), with results classified as cephalic or noncephalic.

The outcome variable was presentation determined by portable handheld ultrasonography by operators blinded to the results of the clinical examination.

The results included noncephalic presentation in 130 women (prevalence = 8%), sensitivity $91/130 = 70\%$ (95% CI 62% to 78%), and specificity $1429/1503 = 95\%$ (95% CI 94% to 96%).

The conclusion in the abstract was: "Clinical examination is not sensitive enough for detection and timely management of noncephalic presentation." However, in the text, the authors make the point that costs, resource availability, and feasibility need to be considered before introducing routine ultrasonography to assess fetal presentation.

**Critical appraisal:** This is a nice, clearly reported study.[1] The research question is relevant and the study design is appropriate. The subjects are reasonable: we do not know of any reason why the fetal presentation of these women from Australia should be harder to determine than that of women elsewhere. Because the predictor variable was a clinical finding, and most examinations were done by residents and registrars, the level of skill of the examiners is relevant to generalizability; some readers of the article thought they could do better than the clinicians studied. In response to letters to the editor, the authors provided a breakdown of the sensitivity of different examiners, and there was no clear evidence of improvement with increasing level of experience. However, the authors acknowledge that accuracy could be improved by ongoing training and feedback. A relevant point made in a letter titled *Doctors do not Dichotomize* is that the design of the study did not allow the examiners to include a category for "can't tell." This relates to the decision that the physical examination is supposed to guide. Decisions about external version and operative delivery clearly require a more accurate test. But if the decision is whether to check the presentation with a sonogram, perhaps the examination could be made sufficiently sensitive by including a "not sure" category and then counting "not sure" as a positive test.

may not be sufficiently accurate to determine treatment, but may be sufficient to tip the balance toward or away from additional tests. An example of this is provided in Box 5.1.

---

[1] Except for the reported 95% confidence intervals, most of which are wrong.

## Important biases for studies of diagnostic test accuracy

The general approach outlined above should help you appraise most clinical research studies of diagnostic tests. In this section, we turn to potential problems that are either unique or particularly important to studies of diagnostic test accuracy. In such studies, the test for which accuracy will be determined is called the "index test," and, as described in Chapter 3, the patient's true disease status is determined by the so-called gold standard. Four important biases in studies of diagnostic test accuracy are incorporation bias, verification bias, double gold standard bias, and spectrum bias. If a study estimates the accuracy of a dichotomous test by reporting sensitivity and specificity, these four biases affect the estimates of sensitivity and specificity in different directions, as summarized in Table 5.2.

### Incorporation bias

In order for a study of a diagnostic test to be valid, the index test must be compared to an independent gold standard. If the gold standard is in any way subjective, it must be applied by observers blinded to the results of the index test. It is surprisingly common for the index test to be incorporated into the gold standard, leading to falsely high estimates of both sensitivity and specificity. For example, in their review of 109 studies of diagnostic technologies for acute cardiac ischemia, Lau et al. (2001a; 2001b) found that the studies rarely defined "unstable angina" and generally accepted the clinician's diagnosis. This means that the diagnostic accuracy (sensitivity and specificity) of different technologies to diagnose unstable angina were probably overestimated due to incorporation bias, because the clinician's diagnosis of unstable angina is likely to have been at least partly based on the results of the diagnostic technologies being evaluated.

Obviously, if you are assessing a test's ability to detect disease, and you define disease partly by a positive test, the test is likely to look good. This does not mean that studies susceptible to incorporation bias are useless. Sometimes, in spite of the possibility of this bias, a test still does not look very good, in which case the results can be believed. And sometimes the key to interpreting such studies is simply to understand that they are answering a slightly different question: how well does the test predict the diagnosis of a disease? These studies thus may end up addressing questions about doctors' understanding of the disease, rather than about the disease itself.

### Verification bias

In a study of a diagnostic test, application of the gold standard should not depend on the result of the index test being evaluated. "Verification bias" (also known as referral or work-up bias) occurs when people who are positive on the index test are more likely to get the gold standard, and only those who receive the gold standard are included in the study. Consider a study evaluating the usefulness of ankle swelling to predict a fracture on x-ray in patients with ankle injuries. X-rays are less likely to be ordered in patients with no swelling, and the study includes only those with

**Table 5.2.** Biases in Studies of Diagnostic Test Accuracy

| Bias Type | General description | Specific situations | Sensitivity is falsely... | Specificity is falsely... |
|---|---|---|---|---|
| Incorporation bias | Classification of disease status partly depends on the results of the index test. Gold standard incorporates the index test. | | ↑ | ↑ |
| Verification bias | Patients with positive index tests are more likely to get the gold standard, and only patients who get the gold standard are included in the study. | | ↑ | ↓ |
| Double gold standard bias | Patients with a positive index test are more likely to receive one (often invasive) gold standard, whereas patients with a negative index test are more likely to receive a different gold standard (often clinical follow-up). Bias occurs only if there is a subgroup where the two gold standards give different answers. | For disease that can resolve spontaneously.<br><br>For disease that becomes detectable during the follow-up period. | ↑<br><br><br>↓ | ↑<br><br><br>↓ |
| Spectrum bias | Spectrum of disease and nondisease differs from clinical practice. Sensitivity depends on spectrum of disease. Specificity depends on spectrum of nondisease or of diseases that might mimic the disease of interest. | When disease is skewed toward higher severity than in clinical practice – "sickest of the sick."<br><br>When nondisease is skewed toward greater health – "wellest of the well." | ↑<br><br><br>NA | NA<br><br><br>↑ |

NA = Not Affected

x-rays. This design decreases the numbers of subjects with negative tests (no swelling), both with and without disease (fracture), as represented in cells (**c**) and (**d**) in Figure 5.1. Verification bias will tend to increase the sensitivity ($a/[a + c]$) and decrease the specificity ($d/[d + b]$) compared with what would have been obtained if the gold standard (x-rays) had been applied regardless of the index test result (presence of ankle swelling). Box 5.2 provides a numerical illustration of verification bias.

|  | Fracture | No Fracture |
|---|---|---|
| Ankle Swelling | a | b |
| No Ankle Swelling | c↓ | d↓ |

Figure 5.1    How verification bias leads to overestimation of sensitivity and underestimation of specificity by lowering numbers in cells (**c**) and (**d**).

---

**Box 5.2: Numerical example of verification bias**

We examine two hypothetical studies of ankle swelling as a predictor of fractures in patients with ankle injuries. The first study is a consecutive sample of 200 patients. In this study, all patients presenting to the emergency department with ankle injuries get x-rays, regardless of swelling. The sensitivity and specificity of ankle swelling are 80% and 75%, as shown in the following table:

|  | Fracture | No Fracture |
|---|---|---|
| Swelling | 32 | 40 |
| No Swelling | 8 | 120 |
| **Total** | **40** | **160** |

Sensitivity = 32/40 = 80%    Specificity = 120/160 = 75%

The second study is a **selected** sample, in which only half the patients without ankle swelling are x-rayed. Thus, the numbers in the "No Swelling" row will be reduced by half. This raises the apparent sensitivity from 32/40 (80%) to 32/36 (89%) and lowers the apparent specificity from 120/160 (75%) to 60/100 (60%), as shown in the next table:

|  | Fracture | No Fracture |
|---|---|---|
| Swelling | 32 | 40 |
| No Swelling | 4 | 60 |
| **Total** | **36** | **100** |

Sensitivity = 32/36 = 89%    Specificity = 60/100 = 60%

The verification bias that arises by excluding patients without swelling causes a false increase in sensitivity and decrease in specificity.[2]

---

**Double gold standard bias**

A bias related to verification bias occurs when two distinct gold standards exist and the results of the index test affect which is applied. People who are positive on the index test are more likely to get one gold standard (such as a surgical procedure), whereas people who are negative on the index test are more likely to get a different gold standard (such as clinical follow-up). We call this form of bias "double gold standard bias."[3] In some cases, a double gold standard is unavoidable for ethical or practical reasons. For example, a biopsy can be used as the gold standard in people

---

[2]  This is a bit of an oversimplification, because ideally the subjects with no ankle swelling who do not receive x-rays are not a random sample, but rather a group (judged to be) at low risk based on other findings. Hence, the number of false negatives in this example might be closer to 6 or 7, rather than 4, resulting in a smaller effect on sensitivity than shown here.

[3]  Others call it "referral bias" or "verification bias" and do not distinguish this type of bias from what we called verification bias in the previous section.

with a positive result on a screening test and is hard to justify in those with negative results. But this application of different gold standards depending on the result of the test being studied can introduce problems.

Double gold standard bias is a common problem with cancer screening tests. We will see in Chapter 6 (on screening tests) that many cancers are clinically harmless; they can either resolve spontaneously or just sit there and never cause the patient any problem. If we look harder for cancer only in those whose screening test is positive, we will take credit for getting the right answer on these more benign cancers, no matter what answer the screening test gives. If these patients have a positive screening test and get a biopsy, they are counted as true positives; if they have a negative screening test and never get sick, they are counted as true negatives. Both sensitivity and specificity are falsely increased. In Chapter 6, we will show how this not only makes the test appear to be more accurate (our topic here), but also can make the test appear to reduce mortality among people with the disease. In that context, we will refer to this problem of detecting disease that will never cause clinical problems as "pseudodisease."

The other possibility is that disease could be missed by the first (invasive) gold standard, but nonetheless detected on follow-up. This could occur if the disease was either not present or not detectable initially, as might occur with a fast-growing tumor that could become detectable and lead to symptoms in a short time. In that case, the screening test will always appear to give the wrong answer. If the test is initially positive, and the patient is referred for the invasive gold standard, the test will look like a false positive because the disease has not yet occurred or is not yet detectable by the gold standard. If the test is negative, the patient will be followed, the tumor will present with symptoms, and the test will be considered falsely negative.

With double gold standard bias, the degree of distortion of sensitivity and specificity depends on how closely correlated the test result is with the choice of which gold standard to use, and on the how often the two gold standards give different answers (which depends on the natural history of the disease). Box 5.3 gives a worked example of this type of bias for a disease that might resolve spontaneously.

## Spectrum bias

### Definition and explanation

The best studies of diagnostic tests are those that replicate the conditions of clinical practice, that is, those in which the disease status of the subjects is not known at the outset. Any test can be made to look good if it only needs to distinguish between the very sick and the very well. "Spectrum bias" is the name for the bias that occurs if the subjects for a study of a diagnostic test did not have a reasonable spectrum of the condition being tested for and of the "nondisease" that may mimic it.

We warned you in Chapter 1 that the assumption that disease was dichotomous is an oversimplification, and that in real life, diseased and nondiseased populations may be heterogeneous. In fact, we can be a bit more specific: sensitivity (or, for nondichotomous tests, the distribution of test results in the diseased group) will depend on the spectrum of disease, and specificity (or the distribution of results in

**Box 5.3: Numerical example of double gold standard bias**

In a study of ultrasonography to diagnose intussusception (a telescoping of the intestine upon itself) in young children (Eshed et al. 2004), all children with a positive ultrasound scan for intussusception received a contrast enema (Gold Standard #1), whereas the majority of children with a negative ultrasound were observed in the emergency department (Gold Standard #2). The results of the study are shown below:

|  | Intussusception | No Intussusception |
|---|---|---|
| Ultrasound+ | 37 | 7 |
| Ultrasound− | 3 | 104 |
| **Total** | **40** | **111** |
|  | Sensitivity = 37/40 = 93% | Specificity = 104/111 = 94% |

The 104 subjects with a negative ultrasound listed as having "No Intussusception" actually included 86 who were followed clinically and did not receive a contrast enema. If about 10% of these subjects (i.e., 9 children) actually had an intussusception that resolved spontaneously but would still have been identified if they had a contrast enema, and all subjects had received a contrast enema gold standard, those 9 children would be considered false negatives rather than true negatives , with a resulting sensitivity of 37/49 = 76% and specificity of 95/102 = 93%, as shown below:

|  | Intussusception | No Intussusception |
|---|---|---|
| Ultrasound+ | 37 | 7 |
| Ultrasound− | 3 + 9 = 12 | 104 − 9 = 95 |
| **Total** | **49** | **102** |
|  | Sensitivity = 37/49 = 76% | Specificity = 95/102 = 93% |

Thus, compared with the single gold standard of the contrast enema, the double gold standard leads to higher estimates of both sensitivity and specificity because it counts as true negatives some subjects who would be considered false negatives by the contrast enema.

Now consider the thirty-seven subjects with positive ultrasound scans, who had intussusception based on their contrast enema. Suppose about 10% (i.e., 4) of those intussusceptions would have resolved spontaneously if given the chance. Then, if the single gold standard were clinical observation, four children considered true positives by the contrast enema would become false positives, with a small decrease in specificity from 93% to 90%. The loss of these four true positives also decreases sensitivity a little, from 93% to 92%. Thus, compared with the single gold standard of clinical follow-up, the double gold standard again leads to higher estimates of both sensitivity and specificity because it counts as true positives some subjects who would be considered false positives by clinical follow-up.

|  | Intussusception | No Intussusception |
|---|---|---|
| Ultrasound+ | 37 − 4 = 33 | 7 + 4 = 11 |
| Ultrasound− | 3 | 104 |
| **Total** | **36** | **115** |
|  | Sensitivity = 33/36 = 92% | Specificity = 104/115 = 90% |

Thus, for spontaneously resolving cases of intussusception, the ultrasound scan will appear to give the right answer whether it is positive or negative, increasing both its apparent sensitivity and specificity.

the nondiseased group) will depend on the spectrum of nondisease. A study that disproportionately includes patients with more severe disease will often have a falsely high sensitivity, whereas a study in which the patients without the disease are very healthy (or do not have anything resembling the target disease) will give a falsely high specificity. Conversely, sensitivity and specificity will be lower if patients with less severe disease are to be distinguished from patients with other, similar diseases. This comes as a bit of bad news for those who were hoping that they could begin tabulating a list of LRs for different results of various tests, because LRs may vary in different patient populations, depending on the typical severity of disease in that population, as well as the distribution and severity of other conditions that could mimic the disease in the nondiseased group.

As an example of spectrum bias, suppose you are interested in LRs for the erythrocyte sedimentation rate (ESR) for diagnosing appendicitis in patients with abdominal pain. The LR for a particular ESR result is P(result|appendicitis)/P(result|no appendicitis). But P(result|no appendicitis) clearly depends on what the patients who do not have appendicitis actually do have. A study of the ESR in young women with abdominal pain who are at risk of acute salpingitis, a disease associated with high values of the ESR, will give different LRs from a study in children or in men. The distribution of ESRs in the no appendicitis groups will differ, even if the distribution of ESRs in subjects with appendicitis is the same.

### Prevalence of disease, spectrum bias, and nonindependence of test characteristics

In this section, we show how changes in the spectrum of disease and nondisease may vary with disease prevalence. In previous chapters, we assumed that test characteristics (sensitivity, specificity, and LRs) do not vary with the prevalence of disease. When differences in disease prevalence are associated with differences in disease (and nondisease) severity, this assumption may be incorrect.

For example, in the United States, which is an area of relatively low prevalence of iron deficiency, possible tests for iron deficiency anemia, such as pallor on physical examination, a low hematocrit, or low mean corpuscular volume, are likely to have lower sensitivity than in Africa, where the prevalence of iron deficiency anemia is higher. This is because the severity of iron deficiency in Africa is likely to be greater, so that the African patients with iron deficiency will be more iron deficient, and the tests above are more likely to be abnormal in those with the disease (i.e., have higher sensitivity).

The same considerations apply to specificity, except that in this case, the "nondiseased" populations in the two regions are likely to differ. Specificity does not depend on the prevalence of the disease, but it does depend on the prevalence of diseases that can be confused with the disease in question. Specificity of the tests or findings for iron deficiency anemia could be lower in Africa because other diseases (like malaria or hookworm) that might make children anemic (and therefore pale) are more common there, and "tests" like pallor will be abnormal with these other diseases as well.

In the iron deficiency example, sensitivity increases with prevalence, because greater prevalence is associated with greater disease severity. But the opposite could also be true. If the (apparent) prevalence of disease depends on the level of surveillance, then an area with high prevalence might also be an area where the average severity of disease is less, because the additional cases picked up by closer surveillance are likely to be milder than those that presented with symptoms. In that case, sensitivity of some tests could be lower in the high-prevalence area. For example, consider the sensitivity of digital rectal examination for detecting prostate cancer. In a place where prostate-specific antigen screening is widespread, the prevalence of prostate cancer would be higher, and the population of prostate cancer patients would presumably include many more in whom no tumor was palpable, leading to a lower apparent sensitivity of physical examination.

When you read a paper that tries to measure sensitivity and specificity, think about whether the spectrums of disease and nondisease in the study subjects are similar to those in patients you are likely to see. As a general rule, the more severe the disease in the patients who have it, the greater the sensitivity, whereas the healthier the "nondiseased" group, the greater the specificity.

### Spectrum bias as a cause of test nonindependence

We just discussed examples where diseases had different prevalences and different test characteristics in different populations due to what we have called spectrum bias. In this section, we further generalize this point, showing that the populations in which test characteristics differ can be defined not only by time and place, but also by results of history, physical examination, or other tests. In this case, we see that spectrum bias is one reason for another problem, which we will encounter again in Chapter 8: nonindependence of tests.

In a classic article on spectrum bias (Lachs et al. 1992), the authors studied the leukocyte esterase and nitrite[4] on a urine dipstick as predictors of a urinary tract infection (UTI), defined as a urine culture with greater than $10^5$ bacteria/mL. They divided the 366 adults subjects in the study into those with high ($>50\%$) and low ($\leq50\%$) prior probability of UTI, based on the signs and symptoms recorded by clinicians before obtaining the urine dipstick result, which was classified as positive if either the leukocyte esterase or nitrite was positive. They found marked differences in both sensitivity and specificity in 2 groups defined by prior probability (Table 5.3).

How can we account for these results? One possibility is that the patients with higher prior probability of UTI had more severe UTIs. Thus, their UTIs were easier to diagnose, and sensitivity was higher. Similarly, maybe some of those with high

**Table 5.3.** Differences in test characteristics of the urine dipstick in women at high and low prior probability of UTI, based on signs and symptoms (from Lachs et al. 1992)

|                  | Sensitivity | Specificity | LR+ | LR− |
| ---------------- | ----------- | ----------- | --- | --- |
| High Prior Prob. | 92%         | 42%         | 1.6 | 0.19 |
| Low Prior Prob.  | 56%         | 78%         | 2.5 | 0.56 |

---

[4] The leukocyte esterase is a test for white blood cells in the urine; the nitrite test is for bacteria.

prior probability of UTI had urine cultures with just under $10^5$ bacteria/mL. In that case, their lack of UTI would be harder to diagnose, leading to a lower specificity.

A related possibility is that, distinct from disease severity, the index test (dipstick) is measuring something that has already been measured by another test: in this case, the clinical assessment based on signs and symptoms. Perhaps there is a subset of patients with UTI who have inflammation of the lower urinary tract. If this inflammation is what leads to both pain with urination and abnormal urine tests, then, in a way, painful voiding (obtained from the history) is measuring the same aspect of the disease (urinary tract inflammation) as the inflammation identified with dipstick for leukocyte esterase. In that case, we would expect the two tests – clinical assessment of dysuria and a dipstick positive for leukocyte esterase – to be nonindependent, as discussed in Chapter 8. Once you know that a woman has dysuria, you do not learn as much from finding out that she has leukocyte esterase on her urine dipstick, and vice versa. Nonindependence tends to make the sensitivity of the index test appear better, whereas the specificity will generally decrease. The results in Table 5.3 are quite consistent with this explanation.

### Overfitting
" If you torture data sufficiently, it will confess to almost anything."

– Fred Menger

"Overfitting" refers to use of models that are made overly complicated in order to fit the data that have been collected. It is analogous to gerrymandering of congressional districts, which provides perhaps the best way to visualize the problem (Fig. 5.2). Overfitting is mainly a problem when a combination of tests is chosen from many candidate tests to identify a disease or predict a prognosis, so we will discuss it in more detail in Chapter 8, which covers multiple tests and multivariable-decision rules. If you develop a prediction rule by choosing the best combination of tests and

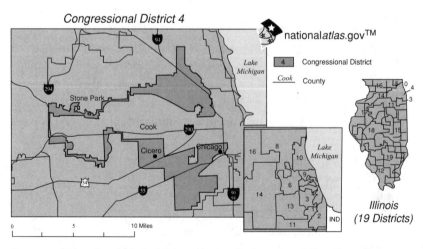

Figure 5.2    Gerrymandering, in which legislators choose their voters, rather than vice versa, provides a visual image of overfitting. This is the 4th Illinois Congressional District. (From: http://nationalatlas.gov/printable/images/pdf/congdist/IL04_110.pdf. Accessed 7/25/08.)

findings from a large number of such variables investigated, you can often develop what might look like a good prediction rule (especially if the sample size is small). But this takes advantage of chance variations in the data that will probably disappear if others try to validate the prediction rule on a new dataset.

A mild form of overfitting bias can occur in studies of a single continuous test when an "optimal" cut-off value is chosen to separate positive from negative results *after* looking at the data. In Chapter 4, we pointed out one problem with making a continuous or multilevel test dichotomous by choosing a fixed cut-off value: this practice discards information by equating slightly abnormal results with extremely abnormal results. Another problem is that the fixed cut-off is chosen to minimize some kind of cost function, often the total number of misclassifications.[5] However, the cost-minimizing cut-off for one group of patients will not be the same as for another group of patients, both because the prevalence of disease will differ between the two datasets and because of chance variations in the distributions of test results.

## Systematic reviews of diagnostic tests

Clinicians wishing to practice evidence-based diagnosis are often faced with a problem: when we look in the literature to find values for sensitivity, specificity, LRs, or other test characteristics, we find studies with varying results. Or, perhaps more commonly, we look in a textbook chapter or a typical review article and find statements like "the XYZ test has sensitivity from 63% to 100% and specificity from 34% to 88%," followed by a string of references. For many tests, the range of reported estimates for sensitivity and specificity is so large that the resulting LRs could be consistent with either an informative or useless test. What do we do?

One approach is to pull all of the articles and critically appraise them, using the general approach you have learned in this book or by using a checklist for diagnostic test study quality (Whiting et al. 2006; Bossuyt et al. 2003; Straus et al. 2005). However, most of us do not have time to do this, and even if we did, it would be hard to synthesize the results. To address this problem, systematic reviews of diagnostic tests are starting to appear, although methods and standards for them are still developing (Deeks 2001; Pai et al. 2004; Mallett et al. 2006). As with other systematic reviews, systematic reviews of diagnostic tests should have four key features: 1) a systematic and reproducible approach to finding and selecting the relevant studies; 2) a summary of the results of each of the studies; 3) an investigation seeking to understand any heterogeneity between the studies; and 4) a summary estimate of results, if appropriate.

One difference between systematic reviews of studies of diagnostic tests and other systematic reviews is that reviews of diagnostic tests commonly attempt to estimate two parameters (sensitivity and specificity), rather than one (e.g., a risk ratio). These two parameters are related: as one goes up, the other often goes down, especially

---

[5] Choosing a cut-off that minimizes total number of misclassifications assumes that misclassifying a normal individual as diseased is just as bad as misclassifying a diseased individual as normal. It is often the case that it is much worse to misclassify a diseased individual as normal than vice versa.

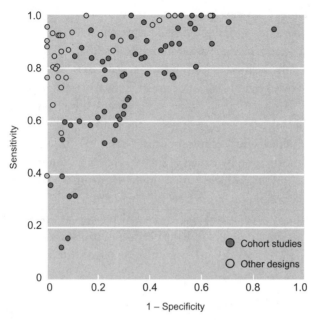

Figure 5.3    Studies of MRI for the diagnosis of multiple sclerosis. Cohort studies (solid circles) produced lower estimates of accuracy than studies using other designs. (From Whiting et al. 2006, used with permission)

if one of the reasons for differing estimates is a difference in the cut-off (or some underlying hidden threshold[6]) used to define a positive result. One approach to this is to plot the sensitivity and specificity obtained from different studies on the same axes used to draw an ROC curve (Sensitivity vs. 1 – Specificity; see Chapter 4). This gives a visual representation of the extent to which differences in reported sensitivity and specificity could be the result of differences in the threshold for a positive test.

It is particularly helpful if characteristics of the studies help explain the location of their points on the ROC plane. For example, Figure 5.3 is taken from a systematic review of magnetic resonance imaging for the diagnosis of multiple sclerosis (Whiting et al. 2006). It shows that studies with a cohort design tend to have lower accuracy estimates: almost all of the points in the upper left corner of the ROC plane (corresponding to the highest estimates of accuracy) came from studies with weaker designs.

There are methods of drawing Summary Receiver Operating Characteristic (SROC) curves through groups of studies, plotted as in Figure 5.3 (Littenberg and Moses 1993; Macaskill 2004). Generally, this is most appropriate if studies with similar designs, in similar populations, and/or with similar gold standard definitions are grouped together, making the results more homogeneous. Possible reasons for heterogeneity in accuracy estimates can also be investigated statistically, using analyses in which each study constitutes an observation, characteristics of the study (like design, blinding, spectrum of disease, etc.) are the predictor variables, and the results of the study are the outcomes. Whether the review uses these sophisticated methods,

---

[6] Even apparently dichotomous tests can have different thresholds. For example, some observers may call a urine dipstick positive for only a minimal color change, while others may require the color change to be more definite.

or simply identifies and summarizes studies, your goal as the reader of a systematic review of a diagnostic test is to obtain estimates of test characteristics based on the most valid studies, in populations and under testing conditions that best duplicate the conditions under which you would be using the test.

## Making use of biased studies

A key step in reading journal articles is not just to identify potential biases, but to determine how the biases could affect the conclusions. A problem with some checklists for critically appraising studies of diagnostic tests is that they can lead to rejection of some studies as "flawed," even though the studies may provide useful information. For example, if a study concludes that a diagnostic test is not useful in a particular situation, and biases in the design of the study would have led to the test looking better than it really is, the study's conclusion is not undermined. On the other hand, if biases in the study design would tend to make the test look bad, the conclusion that the test is not useful may simply be due to these biases.

For example, if a test distinguishes poorly between people with severe disease and healthy medical students, it is likely to do even worse in patients with a more clinically relevant spectrum of disease and nondisease. Similarly, if a study subject to verification bias still reports that sensitivity is poor, that conclusion is probably valid. In these examples, the key is to notice that the potential bias would make the test look falsely good. On the other hand, consider the study of ultrasonography to diagnose intussusception (Eshed et al. 2004). The ultrasonographers were not the world experts; in fact, many of them were junior radiology residents new to the procedure. If the authors had reported poor accuracy, the generalizability of the results to setting with more experienced ultrasonographers would have been questionable. However, since the reported accuracy was good, this lack of ultrasonographer experience is of less concern.

## Summary of key points

1. As with any clinical research study, critical appraisal of a study of a diagnostic test starts with consideration of the research question, study design, study subjects, predictor variable, and outcome variable.
2. In studies of diagnostic test accuracy, the predictor variable is typically the result of the index test (the test being studied) and the outcome variable is the patient's true disease state as determined by the gold standard.
3. Studies evaluating diagnostic tests are susceptible to particular biases.
4. Incorporation bias occurs when classification of the patient as diseased depends partly on the result of the index test. It biases both sensitivity and specificity up.
5. Verification bias occurs when patients who are positive on the index test are more likely to be referred for the gold standard and hence to be included in the study. It biases sensitivity up and specificity down.

6. Double gold standard bias occurs when there are two different gold standards applied selectively based on index test results – for example, an invasive test that is applied when the index test is positive and clinical follow-up that is applied when the index test is negative. If there is a subgroup of patients for whom the invasive test would be positive but the clinical follow-up would be negative (e.g., because of spontaneous resolution of disease), the use of these two gold standards, instead of one or the other, will bias both sensitivity and specificity up. On the other hand, if there are subjects for whom the invasive gold standard is negative, but clinical follow-up is positive (e.g., because of rapidly progressive disease not initially present), both sensitivity and specificity will be biased down.

7. Spectrum bias occurs when the spectrum of disease and nondisease in the study population differs from that in the clinical population in which the test will be used. If the group of patients with the disease has severe disease ("the sickest of the sick"), sensitivity will be biased up. If the group of patients without the disease is very healthy ("the wellest of the well"), specificity will be biased up.

8. When there are multiple studies of the same test, it may be possible to do a systematic review and develop summary estimates of test sensitivity and specificity and to summarize the results using an SROC curve.

9. Even flawed studies of diagnostic tests can be useful as long as the flaws affect sensitivity and specificity in predictable ways.

## References

Bossuyt, P. M., J. B. Reitsma, et al. (2003). "Towards complete and accurate reporting of studies of diagnostic accuracy: the STARD initiative." *Br Med J* **326**(7379): 41–4.

Deeks, J. J. (2001). "Systematic reviews in health care: Systematic reviews of evaluations of diagnostic and screening tests." *Br Med J* **323**(7305): 157–62.

Eshed, I., A. Gorenstein, et al. (2004). "Intussusception in children: can we rely on screening sonography performed by junior residents?" *Pediatr Radiol* **34**(2): 134–7.

Lachs, M. S., I. Nachamkin, et al. (1992). "Spectrum bias in the evaluation of diagnostic tests: lessons from the rapid dipstick test for urinary tract infection." *Ann Intern Med* **117**(2): 135–40.

Lau, J., J. P. Ioannidis, et al. (2001a). "Diagnosing acute cardiac ischemia in the emergency department: a systematic review of the accuracy and clinical effect of current technologies." *Ann Emerg Med* **37**(5): 453–60.

Lau, J., J. P. Ioannidis, et al. (2001b). *Evaluation of Technologies for Identifying Acute Cardiac Ischemia in Emergency Departments.* Rockville, MD, The Agency for Healthcare Research and Quality. Available at http://www.ncbi.nlm.nih.gov/books/bv.fcgi?rid=hstat1.chapter.37233.

Littenberg, B., and L. E. Moses (1993). "Estimating diagnostic accuracy from multiple conflicting reports: a new meta-analytic method." *Med Decis Making* **13**(4): 313–21.

Macaskill, P. (2004). "Empirical Bayes estimates generated in a hierarchical summary ROC analysis agreed closely with those of a full Bayesian analysis." *J Clin Epidemiol* **57**(9): 925–32.

Mallett, S., J. J. Deeks, et al. (2006). "Systematic reviews of diagnostic tests in cancer: review of methods and reporting." *Br Med J* **333**(7565): 413.

Mueller, C., K. Laule-Kilian, et al. (2006). "Cost-effectiveness of B-type natriuretic peptide testing in patients with acute dyspnea." *Arch Intern Med* **166**(10): 1081–7.

Nassar, N., C. L. Roberts, et al. (2006). "Diagnostic accuracy of clinical examination for detection of non-cephalic presentation in late pregnancy: cross sectional analytic study." *Br Med J* **333**(7568): 578–80.

Pai, M., M. McCulloch, et al. (2004). "Systematic reviews of diagnostic test evaluations: What's behind the scenes?" *ACP J Club* **141**(1): A11–3.

Straus, S., W. Richardson, et al. (2005). *Evidence-Based Medicine: How to Practice and Teach EBM.* New York, Elsevier/Churchill Livingstone.

Wheeler, A. P., G. R. Bernard, et al. (2006). "Pulmonary-artery versus central venous catheter to guide treatment of acute lung injury." *N Engl J Med* **354**(21): 2213–24.

Whiting, P., R. Harbord, et al. (2006). "Accuracy of magnetic resonance imaging for the diagnosis of multiple sclerosis: systematic review." *Br Med J* **332**(7546): 875–84.

## Chapter 5 Problems: studies of diagnostic tests

1. Consider the following excerpt from the abstract of an article about diagnosing Von Willebrand's disease (Werner et al. 1992):

**ABSTRACT**

... To determine the best tests to identify patients with von Willebrand disease (vWD), we reviewed the laboratory studies of 24 children with vWD... The diagnosis of vWD required the presence of a personal and family history of bleeding symptoms and a documented abnormality of vWF [von Willebrand Factor] activity or vWF antigen. vWF activity, vWF antigen, factor VIII procoagulant (factor VIII:c) and blood type were [also] determined in 104 symptom-free children.

... The vWF activity, vWF antigen, and factor VIII:c were abnormal in 79%, 58%, and 33% [of vWD patients], respectively. Receiver-operating-characteristic analysis showed the vWF activity to be superior to either the vWF antigen or factor VIII:c in establishing the diagnosis of vWD. The combination of the activity, bleeding time, and partial thromboplastin time successfully identified 92% of the patients as abnormal. Determination of vWF activity should be included routinely in the evaluation of hemostasis in children with symptomatic disease.

   a) What were the index tests in this study?
   b) How was disease status determined – that is, what was the gold standard?
   c) What parameter (sensitivity, specificity, predictive value, etc.) are the percentages (79%, 58%, and 33%) reported in the second paragraph?
   d) What is the problem with the study design and how would it affect the estimates in part c?

2. Below are excerpts from the abstracts from two studies that gave discrepant answers to the question: Is urine microscopy needed in patients whose urine dipstick is negative?

**#1. Morrison, M.C., and G. Lum**. (1986). "Dipstick testing of urine: can it replace urine microscopy?" *Am J Clin Pathol* **85**(5): 590–4.

**Abstract**. One thousand consecutive urine specimens were studied to assess the sensitivity of a commercially available dipstick to predict the presence or absence of microscopic abnormalities... The Chemstrip-9$^{TM}$ had a sensitivity of 82%, specificity of 42%, and a false negative rate of 36%. Clinical review of patients with false negative results showed that approximately one-third to one-half of these patients had either spinal cord injury or genitourinary problems... Our data suggest that in our patient population, we should not eliminate microscopic urine examination based on abnormal dipstick findings.

**#2. Hamoudi, A.C., S.C. Bubis, C. Thompson**. (1986). "Can the cost savings of eliminating urine microscopy in biochemically negative urines be extended to the pediatric population?" Am J Clin Pathol **86**(5): 658–60.

**Abstract**. The authors determined the value of performing urine microscopy on biochemically negative urine specimens in a pediatric population. Four reactions of the Chemstrip-9$^{TM}$ were used as biochemical indicators, namely, protein, occult blood, leukocyte esterase, and nitrite. Out of 1,016 urine specimens thus studied, 310 were true positive. Eleven specimens reacted biochemically in the absence of significant microscopic findings (false positive), 668 specimens were negative by the Chemstrip-9$^{TM}$ and were either negative microscopically or had less than five white blood cells (WBCs) per high power field (HPF) and were considered true negatives. Twenty-seven specimens had negative biochemical indicators, in spite of positive microscopy... The sensitivity of the four parameters for predicting significant microscopy of urinary sediment is 92% and the specificity is 98%. The predictive value of a negative result is 96.1%, and that of a positive result is 96.5%. The authors therefore conclude that urine microscopy is unnecessary in biochemically negative urine specimens from pediatric patients who are asymptomatic for urinary tract disease.

a) Make 2 × 2 tables for the Chemstrip-9 compared with urine microscopy for both studies. Put the "disease" (urine microscopy result: abnormal or normal) on the top and the test (urine dipstick) on the left side. (Note: In the Morrison study, 573 of the 1000 specimens had abnormal urine microscopy. Because of rounding, your numbers will only be approximate.)

b) What is meant by the "false negative rate of 36%" in the Morrison study? (Is this the standard definition?)

c) What are at least three possible explanations for the apparently discrepant results of these two studies? Which do you think are most likely to explain the results? (Hint: Use the structure suggested at the beginning of the chapter.)

3. Women presenting to the emergency department with abdominal pain and a positive pregnancy test may have an ectopic pregnancy (about 10%), an

abnormal intrauterine pregnancy (about 30%), or a normal intrauterine pregnancy (about 60%). An excerpt from the abstract of a study on this topic is reprinted below (Marill et al. 1999):

> The objectives of this study were to determine the optimal cutoff value and utility of a single serum beta human chorionic gonadotropin hormone (HCG) level in assessing the likelihood of ectopic pregnancy. A retrospective chart review was performed at an urban county hospital. The optimal cutoff value was determined by comparing all available patients diagnosed with ectopic pregnancy and *patients diagnosed with threatened abortion in the Emergency Department who subsequently delivered a baby at the same hospital*... [emphasis added]

The "patients diagnosed with threatened abortion ... who subsequently delivered a baby at the same hospital" were patients who presented with abdominal pain but ultimately turned out to have a normal intrauterine pregnancy. These patients tend to have higher HCGs than patients with abnormal intrauterine (non-ectopic) pregnancies. No women with abnormal intrauterine pregnancies were included in the non-ectopic study sample. The authors found the sensitivity of an HCG <40,000 mIU/mL for ectopic pregnancy was 99%, and the specificity was 85%. (That is, 85% of the women who subsequently delivered a baby at the same hospital had an HCG $\geq 40,000$ mIU/mL.)

a) Is spectrum bias a potential problem in this study? Why or why not?

b) Is the sensitivity estimate too high, too low, or about right?

c) Is the specificity estimate too high, too low, or about right?

4. The abstract of the study of ultrasound to diagnose intussusception summarized in Box 5.3 is excerpted below (Eshed et al. 2004).

> BACKGROUND. Ultrasonography (US) is an important tool in the screening and diagnosis of patients with suspected intussusception.
>
> MATERIALS AND METHODS. Between January 1999 and February 2003, 151 patients with suspected intussusception underwent screening US. The mean age of the patients was 13.8 months...
>
> RESULTS. Sixty-five patients had both US and air enema. Forty-four patients had a positive US result; 37 (84%) were true positive and 7 (16%) were false positive. Twenty-one patients had a negative US result; 18 (86%) were true negative and 3 (14%) were false negative. Eighty-six patients [with negative ultrasound scans] underwent screening US only and were then kept under observation in the emergency room. They were all diagnosed as having a non-surgical condition [i.e., as true negatives]. The total accuracy rate was 93%, sensitivity was 84%, specificity was 97%, positive predictive value was 93% and negative predictive value was 94%...

(For the questions below, assume that the statement, "They were all diagnosed as having a non-surgical condition," means that none of the 86 patients who only had a negative screening ultrasound and clinical follow-up (but no air enema) were felt to have an intussusception. Also assume that, if air enema was performed at all, it was performed immediately after the ultrasound. Parts (**a–c**) review material covered in Chapter 3.)

a) Create a 2 × 2 table that summarizes the results of the study. (You can check your answer in Box 5.1.)

b) Check the authors' calculations of sensitivity, specificity, and accuracy of ultrasound for diagnosis of intussusception in this study.

c) Can positive and/or negative predictive value be estimated from a study with this sampling scheme? If so, what are they? If not, why not?

d) The authors did not perform air enemas on all of the children; in some, they just watched them. Name the bias this could cause (using the terminology from this text).

e) Assume that intussusception never resolves spontaneously – that is, that nobody who would have had a positive enema (if one were done) would ever have negative clinical follow-up. Also assume no new cases of intussusception develop after the air enema. What would be the effect of the bias you named above on estimates of sensitivity and specificity of ultrasound from this study?

f) Now repeat part (**e**) assuming that intussusception does sometimes spontaneously resolve – that is, that some of those with negative clinical follow-up would have had a positive enema, if one were done. (Maintain the assumption that no new cases develop.)

g) Now repeat part (**e**), only this time assume that intussusception can develop during a short follow-up period after the enema has been done.

5. In Chapter 4, Problem 3, we mentioned the B-natriuretic peptide (BNP) test for congestive heart failure (CHF) and the study (Maisel et al. 2002) that reported that, using a cutoff of 100 pg/mL, the test had a sensitivity of 90%, a specificity of 76%, and an LR(+) of about 3.8. In Chapter 4, we learned that using a single cut-off to dichotomize a continuous test like BNP is unwise; the range of BNP values should be divided into several intervals, each with an associated LR.

a) Another issue (Schwam 2004) with the study is that some of the dyspnea patients without acute CHF didn't have any realistic clinical chance of having CHF. They had an obvious diagnosis of asthma, upper respiratory infection, or pneumonia. Also, the authors seem to have excluded from the analysis 72 patients with a history of left ventricular dysfunction but no acute CHF. These excluded patients had higher BNP levels than other non-CHF (D–) patients (average 346 pg/mL vs. 110 pg/mL). How would these problems affect the reported sensitivity, specificity, and LR(+)?

b) The gold standard in this study was the consensus diagnosis of two cardiologists who reviewed the patient's chart, including medical history, ECG, chest x-ray, and follow-up studies. The two cardiologists were blinded to BNP and to the emergency department diagnosis. Ignoring BNP for the moment, it turned out that increased heart size on chest x-ray had high sensitivity and specificity for CHF. Do you think these estimates of sensitivity and specificity are biased? If so, name the bias and how it affects the estimates.

6. Kharbanda et al (2005) reported sensitivity and specificity of several history and physical findings to diagnose appendicitis among children presenting to an urban emergency room. Children were included if they underwent surgical consultation for possible appendicitis. The "gold standard" was pathology for patients who had an appendectomy and phone follow-up for those who did not have surgery. The finding "pain with percussion, hopping or cough" had sensitivity of (only) 78%. Indicate whether the following statements are true or false and explain your answer.

a) The sensitivity may be falsely low because children who could hop around without pain would be less likely to receive surgical consultation, and hence would be under-represented in the study (verification bias).

b) The sensitivity may be falsely low because of double gold standard bias: the gold standard was different for those who did and did not receive surgery, and a child who could hop without pain would be unlikely to receive surgery, giving what was probably a mild case of appendicitis time to resolve on its own.

## References for problem set

Eshed, I., A. Gorenstein, et al. (2004). "Intussusception in children: can we rely on screening sonography performed by junior residents?" *Pediatr Radiol* **34**(2): 134–7.

Maisel, A. S., P. Krishnaswamy, et al. (2002). "Rapid measurement of B-type natriuretic peptide in the emergency diagnosis of heart failure." *N Engl J Med* **347**(3): 161–7.

Marill, K. A., T. E. Ingmire, et al. (1999). "Utility of a single beta HCG measurement to evaluate for absence of ectopic pregnancy." *J Emerg Med* **17**(3): 419–26.

Schwam, E. (2004). "B-type natriuretic peptide for diagnosis of heart failure in emergency department patients: a critical appraisal." *Acad Emerg Med* **11**(6): 686–91.

Werner, E. J., T. C. Abshire, et al. (1992). "Relative value of diagnostic studies for von Willebrand disease." *J Pediatr* **121**(1): 34–8.

# Screening tests

## Introduction

You may wonder why we have a separate chapter on screening tests. After all, now that you have learned about sensitivity, specificity, likelihood ratios, Receiver Operating Characteristic curves and so forth, it seems like you should be well equipped to evaluate screening tests. However, whereas diagnostic tests are done on sick people to determine the cause of their symptoms, screening tests are generally done on healthy people with a low prior probability of disease. The problem of false positives and possible harms of unnecessary treatment looms larger. The questions of whether the patient benefits from being diagnosed and whether this benefit justifies the possible harms and costs of the test are more salient for screening. Finally, because decisions about screening are often made at the population level, political and other factors may be more influential. Thus, in this chapter, we focus explicitly on the question of whether doing the test improves health, not just whether it gives the right answer, and we pay particular attention to biases and nonmedical factors that can lead to excessive screening.[1]

## Definition and types of screening

Our favorite definition of screening is that suggested by Eddy (1991): *"the application of a test to detect a potential disease or condition in people with no known signs or symptoms of that disease or condition."* The "test" being applied may be a laboratory test or x-ray, or it may be nothing more than a standard series of questions, as long as the goal is to detect a disease or condition of which the patient has no known symptoms.

---

[1] We do not wish to come across as complete screening nihilists. In fact, both of us have loved ones whose lives we believe may have been saved by screening. However, this is an area where we are concerned that enthusiasm has sometimes exceeded science, where there is a potential for harm, and where we see a growth industry that could consume ever greater resources with diminishing return. Hence our emphasis here tends to be on taking a critical approach to studies of screening, and on not overestimating the value of screening.

**Table 6.1.** Types of screening

| | Unrecognized symptomatic disease | Presymptomatic disease | Risk factor |
|---|---|---|---|
| Examples | • Refractive errors in children<br>• Depression<br>• Iron deficiency | • Syphilis<br>• Neonatal hypothyroidism<br>• Many types of cancer<br>• Glaucoma<br>• Abdominal Aortic Aneurysm | • High blood pressure<br>• High blood cholesterol |
| Number Labeled | Few | Few | Many |
| Number Treated | Few | Few | Many |
| Duration of Treatment | Varies, may be short | Varies, may be short or long | Usually long |
| Number Needed to Treat | Few | Few | Many |
| Ease of Showing Benefit | Often easy | Often difficult | Usually very difficult |
| Potential for Harm | False positives | • False positives<br>• Pseudodisease<br>• Labeling | • Risks from treatment, including delayed adverse effects<br>• Labeling |

This definition has two advantages over the definitions you will see elsewhere, which specify that screening involves "testing for asymptomatic disease." First, "*no known symptoms*" is not quite the same as asymptomatic, because some people may have symptoms they do not recognize as such. Second, the Eddy definition includes testing not just for diseases, but for "*conditions.*" The goal of many screening tests is not to detect disease, but to detect risk factors – that is, to detect the condition of being at increased risk for one or more diseases.

Based on this definition, we can divide screening into three types:
• Screening for *unrecognized symptomatic disease,*
• Screening for *presymptomatic disease,* and
• Screening for *risk factors.*

The goals of these types of screening differ, thus the study designs, numbers of subjects, and amount of time needed to study them differ as well (Table 6.1). There is, however, some overlap between these categories. For example, glaucoma may be asymptomatic or cause unrecognized visual field loss, and osteoporosis might be considered a disease or just a risk factor for fractures.

Screening for unrecognized symptomatic disease is generally the most easily evaluated type of screening, because both the accuracy of the test and the benefits of early detection can be assessed in relatively short-term studies, often with modest sample sizes. Vision screening in children is a good example: children who have trouble with the eye chart are referred for further evaluation. If they are confirmed to have refractive errors, glasses are prescribed. No randomized trials are needed to tell that glasses will help the child see better, because the effect is immediate. Other examples of this type of screening are screening for depression or iron deficiency anemia. When patients are already symptomatic, demonstrating a benefit from identifying and treating them does not require a long trial with many subjects.

Screening for presymptomatic disease is harder to assess. As is the case with unrecognized symptomatic disease, because the disease is already present at the time of screening, the accuracy of the screening test can be measured in the present, without a long follow-up period. But because the disease is initially asymptomatic, demonstrating benefits of treatment generally will require a follow-up study (often a randomized trial), to show that early diagnosis and treatment of disease reduces the frequency or severity of symptoms later. Examples include screening for cystic fibrosis, abdominal aortic aneurysms (AAAs), and breast cancer. On the other hand, if the natural history and pathophysiology of the disease are clear and the effects of treatment are dramatic (e.g., as with screening for syphilis or neonatal hypothyroidism), randomized trials of treatment may not be needed.

It is most difficult to decide whether to screen for risk factors for disease, because both the ability of the test to predict disease and the ability of treatment to prevent it generally must be assessed by using longitudinal studies, often with very large sample sizes. The first step is quantifying how well the measurement of the risk factor (e.g., a blood cholesterol measurement) predicts the risk of disease (heart attacks or strokes); the second step involves determining whether and by how much treatment lowers that risk. Because deaths or other serious events occur in only a small proportion of subjects (even for relatively common diseases like heart disease), this second step may require following many thousands of subjects for many years. An intermediate step, determining how well treatment lowers the level of the risk factor, is generally insufficient, because (as we will discuss in the next section) lowering the level of a risk factor may not lead to the expected lowering of the risk of disease (Guyatt et al. 2008). A dramatic example of this was the Cardiac Arrhythmia Suppression Trial, in which patients were screened for premature ventricular contractions (PVCs), a risk factor for sudden death after a heart attack. The PVCs were diminished by treatment with antiarrhythmic drugs, but unfortunately, this did not translate into fewer sudden deaths. In fact, the death rate was nearly 3 times higher in those treated, leading to an estimated 50,000 excess deaths in the U.S. (Moore 1995).

There is another important difference between screening for risk factors and screening for diseases. Most of what we learned about quantifying the accuracy of diagnostic tests in the previous chapters does not work well for risk factors. Sensitivity, specificity, and prior and posterior probability all refer to "prevalent disease": disease that the person either already has or does not have. The time dimension for study designs for measuring these parameters is generally cross-sectional (measurements made at about the same time) as opposed to longitudinal (measurement of predictor followed by measurement of outcome).[2] On the other hand, for risk factor screening, we are generally trying to predict incidence (not

---

[2] As discussed in Chapter 5 under "Double Gold Standard Bias," sometimes studies of the *accuracy* of cancer screening tests include a longitudinal component (for those who test negative). Studies of the *efficacy* of these tests have to be longitudinal.

prevalence) of disease. Thus, it is awkward to speak about sensitivity and specificity when quantifying the accuracy of risk factor screening tests, because the gold standard cannot be immediately applied. We will discuss this issue at greater length in the next chapter, which is about prognostic tests.

## Importance of a critical approach to screening tests

### Possible harms from screening

Although screening tests and resulting treatments, when properly selected and done, may have substantial benefits, there are also significant possible harms from screening. The potential to do harm is particularly great for risk factor-screening tests, because the number treated and duration of treatment may be much greater than for other screening tests. Some of the possible harms of screening apply to all persons screened, some only to those with specific test results, and others extend beyond those screened. These possible harms from screening, although perhaps generally underappreciated, are not conceptually difficult, so we will just list them with examples in Table 6.2, rather than discuss them at length.

### Reasons for excessive screening

The possible costs and risks of screening are more than sufficient to justify a cautious approach. But there is another reason as well: awareness of the strong forces likely to lead to excessive screening. The main force may be the desire to do good – to do something that will help people live longer and healthier lives. But other forces tending to increase screening are worth considering as well (Table 6.3). Unlike the potential market for tests and treatments for symptomatic diseases, which is limited by the prevalence of the symptoms, the potential market for screening tests and resulting treatments has no such limits. The number of people at risk for each disease times the number of years for which they are at risk creates a vast potential market for screening tests, including the machines and personnel required to do them. The "patients" identified by screening become a similarly vast market for the drugs or other interventions intended to reduce their risk. In the case of disease screening, the market for treatments is limited by the number of people found to have the disease. The market for treatments for risk factors, in contrast, has no such limits, as there may be a measurable (or imagined) health benefit to treatment even at levels of the risk factor that are very prevalent in the population. Thus, we should not be surprised that companies selling products related to screening tests or to treating the diseases they are intended to diagnose or hospitals that have invested in these technologies should be very interested in moving the public toward more screening.

Pressure for increased screening does not arise solely from for-profit companies. For academic researchers like us, the greater the number of people who have, get, or worry about our disease of interest, the greater the importance of the research and the researcher, and the greater the opportunities for funding, collaborators, publications, and travel. Similarly, nonprofit organizations (like the American Liver

**Table 6.2.** Possible harms from screening

| Group at risk or affected and type of harm | Examples |
| --- | --- |
| **A. Everyone tested** | |
| • Time, cost of test | • CT scan for early lung cancer |
| | • Genetic testing for predisposition to breast and ovarian cancer |
| • Pain, discomfort, anxiety, or embarrassment from the screening test or anticipation thereof | • Venipuncture |
| | • Digital rectal examination |
| | • Sigmoidoscopy |
| | • Mammography |
| • Late adverse effects | • Cancer from radiation for mammography (Law and Faulkner 2001) |
| **B. People with a negative test result** | |
| • Inappropriate reassurance leading to delay in diagnosis of target disease (false negative) or to unhealthy decisions with regard to other risk factors (false or true negative) | • Delay in evaluation of hearing loss in baby with falsely normal newborn hearing screen |
| | • Patients with normal cholesterol levels deciding they do not need to exercise or stop smoking |
| **C. People with a positive test result** | |
| • Time, cost, pain, discomfort, anxiety, and complications of follow-up testing – generally much worse than costs and risks of initial tests | • Breast or prostate biopsies |
| | • Perforation from colonoscopy following fecal occult blood testing |
| • Costs and risks of treatment for those testing positive; may exceed benefits, even in "true positives" | • Increased fractures when osteoporosis is treated with sodium fluoride (Riggs et al. 1990) |
| | • Increased mortality from use of clofibrate for high blood cholesterol (WHO 1980) |
| | • Increased mortality in patients with asymptomatic PVCs after myocardial infarction when treated with antiarrhythmic drugs (Epstein et al. 1993) |
| • Unnecessary treatment of "pseudodisease" | • Prostatectomies, mastectomies, or lung resections for biopsy-proven cancer that would not have caused problems anyway |
| • Loss of privacy or insurability | • Testing for hepatitis C, HIV, or syphilis |
| • Labeling or other psychological distress; failure to be reassured after normal follow-up testing | • Increased absenteeism in steelworkers found to have hypertension (Haynes et al. 1978) |
| | • Self-restriction of activities following low bone density measurements in elderly women (Rubin and Cummings 1992) |
| | • Altered parent–infant relationship following false-positive newborn hypothyroidism screening (Fyro and Bodegard 1987) |
| | • Continued anxiety following false-positive mammograms (Barton et al. 2004) |

**Table 6.2** (*continued*)

| Group at risk or affected and type of harm | Examples |
|---|---|
| **D. People not tested** | |
| • Injuries to testing personnel | • Radiation, needle sticks, etc. |
| • Harms to contacts, partners, family members | • False-positive or false-negative tests for sexually transmitted diseases |
| | • Finding of infant blood group inconsistent with supposed paternity |
| • Time cost of patients and physicians informing themselves about tests the patient chooses not to have done | • Expensive screening tests being marketed directly to consumers (Lee and Brennan 2002) |
| • Removal of resources from where they would do more good (Eddy 1997) | • Mammography for the wealthy in poor countries (Braveman and Tarimo 1994) |

Foundation or the American Cancer Society) tend to favor screening tests for their disease or organ system. Aside from any medical benefits from screening, it has the potential to identify large groups of people likely to be interested in the work of the organization and to make donations. As discussed below, some of those most in favor of screening may believe that their lives were saved by screening tests.

Although managed care organizations might be expected to favor limiting screening (because, in most cases, it increases their costs), even they have reasons to encourage screening. Performance of screening tests, because it is popular with the public, easily measured, and little affected by complex, variable presentations of patients with symptoms, tends to be disproportionately weighted on quality "report cards" like the Health Plan Employer Data and Information Set (HEDIS 2009). In addition, health plans may find it advantageous to emphasize preventive care, if doing so attracts healthier patients.

Finally, the general public tends to be supportive of screening programs. Part of this is wishful thinking. We would like to believe that bad things happen for a reason, and that there are things we can do to prevent them (Marantz 1990). We also tend to be much more swayed by stories of individual patients (either those whose disease was detected early or those in whom it was found "too late") than by boring statistics about risks, costs, and benefits (Newman 2003). Because, at least in the U.S., there is no clear connection between money spent on screening tests and money not being available to spend on other things, the public tends not to be swayed by arguments about cost efficacy (Daniels 1986; Mariner 1995; Eddy 1997). In fact, in the general public's view of screening, even wrong answers are not necessarily a bad thing.

Schwartz et al. (2004) did a national telephone survey of attitudes about cancer screening in the U.S. They found that 38% of respondents had experienced at least one false-positive screening test. Although more than 40% of these subjects referred to that experience as "very scary" or the "scariest time of my life," 98% were glad they had the screening test! As our gynecologist colleague George Sawaya (who

**Table 6.3.** Powerful non-medical forces that could lead to increased enthusiasm for screening

| Stakeholder | Reasons to favor screening[a] | Example |
|---|---|---|
| Companies selling tests or testing equipment | Sell more tests or testing machines | • Osteoporosis testing machines<br>• Office cholesterol machines<br>• Private companies marketing genetic tests or body scans |
| Companies selling products to treat the condition | Sell more product | • Schering–Plough has funded public awareness campaigns to encourage PSA and hepatitis C screening [they make Eulexin (flutamide) used to treat prostate cancer and Intron (inteferon) used to treat hepatitis C] |
| Clinicians or hospitals who diagnose or treat the condition | More patients, procedures, income, importance | • Gynecologists tend to recommend more Pap smears and urologists more PSA testing than generalists<br>• Thoracic surgeons or radiologists may favor CT screening for lung cancer |
| Politicians | • Appear sympathetic to those who have or are at risk of the condition<br>• Be responsive to special interests or contributors | • U.S. Senate vote 98–0 overturning National Cancer Institute panel's recommendations that mammography decisions for 40- to 49-year-old women be individualized (Ernster 1997) |
| Nonprofit disease research and advocacy groups | • Increased importance of disease and hence of organization's work<br>• More people with the disease or risk factor who become interested are active constituents and potential donors<br>• Increase attractiveness for donations from industry | • American Liver Foundation Hepatitis C Screening promotion (paid for by Schering–Plough)<br>• American Cancer Society recommendations for cancer screening often more aggressive than those of the U.S. Preventive Health Services Task Force |
| Academics who study the condition | • Increased importance, recognition, and funding for research for the condition<br>• Accessible funding from industry | • Hypercholesterolemia, osteoporosis, and virtually everything else |
| Patients/the public | • Wishful thinking – wanting to believe bad things happen for a reason and that there are things we can do to prevent them<br>• Individualistic perspective – lack of concern about costs if someone else is paying them | • Belief in and demand for PSA testing and mammography disproportionate to evidence of benefit<br>• View that those (even elderly) not wishing to be screened are "irresponsible" (Schwartz et al. 2004) |

[a]  Aside from the desire to help people, which is assumed to be a reason for all.

studies Pap smears) puts it, "the patients are so grateful when we come to the rescue and put out the fire that they forget that we were the ones who set it in the first place."

We know of no similar survey that addresses how patients feel about false-negative results, but some may still be happy they had the test. Patients whose cancer is diagnosed at a late stage who did not get screened are likely to wonder if they could have been saved if they had been screened. Those who were screened and were (presumably falsely) negative will at least have the comfort of knowing it was not their fault and of not being blamed by their doctors, family, and friends (Marantz 1990). Another disturbing result of the survey by Schwartz et al. was that, even though (as of 2002) the U.S. Preventive Health Services Task Force felt that evidence was insufficient to recommend prostate cancer screening, more than 60% of respondents said that a 55-year-old man who did not have a routine PSA test was "irresponsible," and more than a third said this for an 80-year old man! Thus, regardless of the efficacy of screening tests, they have become an obligation if one does not wish to be blamed for getting some illnesses.

### Reasons for underscreening

We have emphasized many reasons to worry about excessive screening, but insufficient screening can occur as well. All of the potential problems that screening can cause (Table 6.2) are reasons why it might not be done even when a net benefit could be projected: it costs money, takes time, patients may fear discomfort or loss of privacy, etc. If screening leads to improved health but net increases in costs, managed care organizations could deliberately make it difficult to do the tests. Some hospitals may lack the confidence, competence, and capacity to deal with positive results. In order to make screening work, the systems for dealing with positive results and providing services to identified patients need to be in place.

## Critical appraisal of studies of screening tests

### The big picture

The general idea of a lot of screening (and diagnostic tests) is that, if you do the test, it will help you diagnose the disease, and if you diagnose the disease, you will improve outcome. If we want to know whether to do a test, we would really like to know whether people who get the test have a better outcome than people who do not (Fig. 6.1). Unfortunately, most studies do not address that question directly. Instead, studies either 1) correlate testing or test results with diagnosis or stage (e.g., studies that estimate diagnostic yield, sensitivity, specificity, Receiver Operating Characteristic curves, likelihood ratios, etc.) or 2) correlate diagnosis or stage with ultimate outcome. The latter studies are those susceptible to lead- or length-time biases, which we will discuss below.

For simplicity, assume that we are screening for presymptomatic disease, and in a subset of patients, the disease is fatal a predictable time period after symptoms develop (Fig. 6.2). The disease is detectable by screening some time after its biological

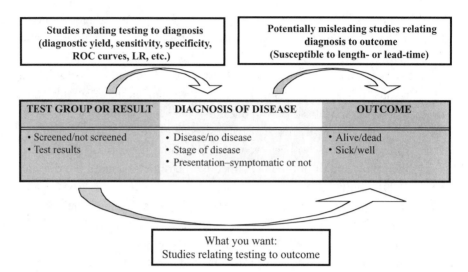

Figure 6.1    Predictor and outcome variables in studies of screening. The best studies bridge the gap and compare outcomes in those screened and not screened.

onset but before symptoms develop (Herman et al. 2002). The rationale for screening is that intervention during this detectable preclinical phase ("latent phase") forestalls or prevents symptom onset and prolongs life.

The best way to assess screening is to randomize people into two groups: one that receives the screening test and one that doesn't. As we will discuss in Chapter 9, randomization ensures against systematic differences between the two groups with respect to disease risk, health habits, and other factors that can affect the outcome of interest (e.g., life expectancy). Both the screened and unscreened groups will include

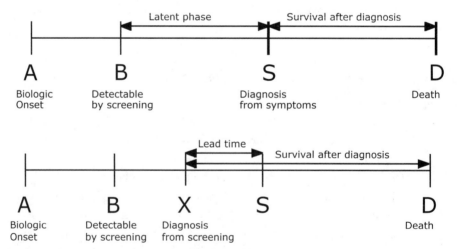

Figure 6.2    *Upper Panel:* Natural history of disease in people affected by lead-time bias. Disease progresses from biological onset (A) until it is detectable by screening (B), through the latent phase, until diagnosis from symptoms (S), through the clinical phase, until death (D). *Lower Panel:* Lead-time bias: early detection does not prolong overall survival, but does prolong the time from diagnosis to death. The period between diagnosis from screening (X) and when diagnosis would have occurred from symptoms (S) is the lead time.

many individuals who do not have the disease in question. If screening affects the life expectancy of these nondiseased individuals at all, it is likely to have a negative effect.[3] Both groups will also include individuals with the disease. In the unscreened group, the disease will be diagnosed at symptom onset, but in the screened group, at least some cases of the disease may be diagnosed by screening. If screening genuinely allows interventions that forestall or prevent symptoms and prolong life, and if this effect exceeds the negative effect of screening on nondiseased individuals, the overall death rate should be lower and life expectancy should be longer in the screened group. So, the ideal study would be a randomized trial of screening versus no screening that compares the overall mortality between the two randomization groups. Although such a study may not be practical, keeping this ideal study design in mind can help you understand biases common in observational studies, to be discussed below.

### Observational studies of screening tests

Observational studies of screening deviate in various ways from the ideal randomized trial of screening versus no screening. Some compare the outcome (such as death from prostate cancer) among persons who have been screened with those who have not been screened, but the assignment to the screened and unscreened groups is not random, and there are systematic differences between them. Others limit the comparison to those with the disease. The screened patients with the disease (even if it was missed on screening and diagnosed by symptoms) may be compared with the unscreened patients with the disease (all of whom were diagnosed by symptoms). Finally, those diagnosed by screening may be compared with those diagnosed by symptoms (whether or not they were ever screened). Observational studies are subject to several important biases that can make screening tests appear to be more beneficial than they are.

### Volunteer bias

When assignment to the screening group is not random, comparisons between people who are and are not screened may be invalid because people who volunteer for screening are generally different from people who do not. The screened group may be at higher risk of poor outcome, if, for example, they volunteered for screening because of a symptom they did not disclose (people with symptoms are generally excluded from studies of screening tests). More typically, they may be at lower risk of poor outcome, because of healthier habits or better access to health care. For example, Otto et al. (2004) compared the number of deaths over a 5-year period of men who agreed to be in a randomized trial of prostate cancer screening with the number expected for that population and found that it was 13% lower. To address volunteer bias, investigators measure and attempt to control for factors that might be associated with both receiving the screening test and outcome (e.g., family history, education level, number of health maintenance visits, etc.), but the only way to

---

[3] This is almost always the case, but a possible exception is the Multicenter Aneurysm Screening Study described in Problem 6–6.

eliminate the possibility of volunteer bias is to randomize the study subjects either to receive or not to receive the test.

### Lead-time bias

Lead time is the apparent increase in survival obtained when a disease is detected before it would have become symptomatic and been detected clinically (Fig. 6.2). Lead-time bias affects the subset of the population destined to die of the disease whether or not they are screened. The trouble is, even if screening and/or treatment are completely ineffective, if you start counting years of survival from the date of diagnosis, moving the date of diagnosis earlier will make survival seem longer (Fig. 6.2). Lead-time bias is thus a problem when postdiagnosis survival is compared between persons whose disease was detected by screening and those whose disease was detected by development of symptoms. Lead-time bias cannot occur in a randomized trial of screening or a cohort study that compares the entire screened group with the entire unscreened group; survival time is counted from either randomization (in the trial) or inception (in the cohort), rather than from date of diagnosis.

### Length-time bias

This bias gets its name from the fact that heterogeneity in the natural history of a disease can lead to subjects spending a variable **length** of **time** in the presymptomatic phase. A clearer name for it could be "different natural history bias." Length-time bias may occur whether the study considers one-time screening or screening at regular intervals, but only when it compares survival time from diagnosis between those diagnosed by screening versus those diagnosed by symptoms.

When thinking about length-time bias, assume that the entire population is being screened for disease; there is no unscreened group. If the disease being screened for is heterogeneous (e.g., some tumors are indolent, whereas others rapidly metastasize and kill), the cases that are more slowly progressive (and have a longer latent phase) will be preferentially diagnosed by screening. In comparison to individuals whose disease is diagnosed by symptoms, those with disease diagnosed by screening have more indolent disease, and hence show improved survival. This is illustrated in Figure 6.3 in which three of the subjects have much more rapidly progressive diseases, as represented by the compressed progression time from disease onset (A) to detectability by screening (B) to development of symptoms (S) to death (D).

Because screening tests done at any particular point in time can only get the head start on detection if they catch the disease in its latent phase (between times B and S in Fig. 6.3), patients whose diseases spend a short time in that state are less likely to be identified by screening and more likely to present with symptoms. These patients will have a poorer prognosis due to the rapidly progressive nature of their disease. Thus, the basic problem is that, although detection by the screening test will be associated with a better prognosis, the causal inference is incorrect: both early detection and the improved prognosis are due to the better expected natural history of the disease (Fig. 6.4).

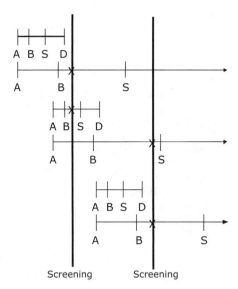

Figure 6.3 Length-time bias. If some cases of disease are rapidly progressive (indicated by short intervals between A, B, S, and D), they are less likely to be caught between B and S when a screening test is done, and hence more likely to present with symptoms. (A, biological onset; B, detectable by screening; X, detected by screening; S, symptom onset; D, death). In the figure, 3/6 = 50% of the cases are rapidly progressive and have a bad prognosis. However, this is true of only 1/4 = 25% of the cases detected by screening.

Length-time bias is only operative when disease is heterogeneous *and* survival from diagnosis is compared between persons whose disease was detected by screening and those whose disease was detected in other ways. Length-time bias will generally be accompanied by at least some lead-time bias. (In Fig. 6.3, the time between the vertical screening lines and points S is the contribution of lead-time bias.) However, the reverse is not always true: lead-time bias will occur even if the natural history of the disease is entirely homogeneous and there is no length-time bias.

Finally, as long as a study (randomized trial or cohort study) compares the entire screened group with the entire unscreened group (between-groups comparison), lead-time and length-time bias are not issues.

### Stage migration bias

Newer, more sensitive diagnostic tests can lead to the diagnosis of disease at an earlier or milder stage, and also to patients being classified as being in a higher stage of disease than would have been known previously (Fig. 6.5). For example, a more sensitive bone scan might lead to some patients being classified as having stage IV

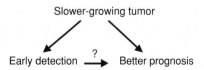

Figure 6.4 A noncausal relationship between early detection and a better prognosis is the cause of length-time bias.

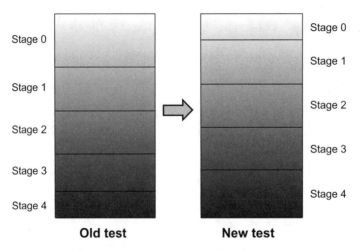

Figure 6.5    Stage migration bias. Newer, more sensitive tests lead to less severe disease and a better prognosis at each stage.

prostate cancer, when previously they would have been thought to be in a less advanced stage. These patients likely have a longer life expectancy than those with the more significant bone metastases detectable by a less sensitive scan. The end result is that stage-specific survival (e.g., survival of patients with stage IV disease before and after the new test) will appear to improve with the more sensitive test, even if no one lives longer. The survival of those at lower stages is improved by having the patients with a worse-than-average stage-specific prognosis leave their stage and be classified in a higher stage. Survival at higher stages is increased because of the entry of subjects from lower stages with better-than-average, stage-specific prognosis for their new stage. However, if a change in the distribution to more advanced stages is the cause of the improvement in stage-specific survival, overall survival will be the same (Feinstein et al. 1985). If a study reports stage-specific improvement in survival with a new screening test, comparing overall survival between screened and unscreened groups is a good way to check for stage migration bias.

Stage migration bias can also occur in the absence of changes in diagnostic testing, simply because of changes in the diagnostic criteria for different stages over time. This was demonstrated for breast cancer, when changes in classification of lymph node involvement between the 5th and 6th editions of the American Joint Committee on Cancer staging system dramatically altered stage-specific survival (Olivotto et al. 2003; Woodward et al. 2003).

### Pseudodisease

In Chapter 5 on biases in studies of test accuracy, we described double gold standard bias, in which some patients could be designated as D+ on surgical pathology but as D− on clinical follow-up if they have either transient or dormant disease. For patients like this, if a positive index test leads to biopsy but a negative index test leads to clinical follow-up, the index text will always appear to give the right answer. Here, we are not worried about overestimating the accuracy of an index text, but rather, overestimating the effectiveness of a screening program. In this context, the problem is the possibility of detecting "pseudodisease" – that is, disease that never would have affected the patient had it not been diagnosed. (This is also called overdiagnosis.) It is difficult to identify pseudodisease in an individual patient, because it requires completely ignoring the diagnosis. (If you treat pseudodisease, the treatment will always appear to be curative, and you won't realize the patient had pseudodisease rather than real disease!) In some ways, pseudodisease is an extreme type of stage migration bias. Patients who were not previously diagnosed as having the disease are now counted as having it. Although the incidence of the disease goes up, the prognosis of those who have it improves.

We would like to believe that pathologists can look at a biopsy and reliably distinguish benign from malignant tissue. However, there is abundant evidence that this is not always the case – some tumors that microscopically are diagnosed as breast, prostate, and even lung cancers do not behave as cancerous (Welch 2004).

Lack of understanding of pseudodisease, including the lack of people who know they have had it, is a real problem, because most of us understand the world through stories (Newman 2003). Patients whose pseudodisease has been "cured" become strong proponents of screening and treatment and can tell a powerful and easily understood story about their experience. On the other hand, there aren't people who can tell a compelling story of pseudodisease – men who can say, "I had a completely unnecessary prostatectomy," or women who say, "I had a completely unnecessary mastectomy," even though we know statistically that many such people exist.

The existence of pseudo–lung cancer was strongly suggested by the results of the Mayo Lung Study, a randomized trial of chest x-rays and sputum cytology to screen for lung cancer among 9,211 male cigarette smokers (Marcus et al. 2000). Because it was a randomized trial and screening should lead to early detection of lung cancer but not affect its cumulative incidence (over a sufficiently long follow-up period), the number of new lung cancers in the 2 groups should have been the same, with (if screening worked) more tumors at lower stages in the screened group and more tumors at higher stages in the control group. In fact, however, after a median follow-up of 20.5 years, there was still a highly significant 29% *increase* in the cumulative incidence of lung cancer in the screened group. There was an excess of tumors at an early, resectable stage, but no decrement in late-stage tumors. The screened group therefore had more lung "cancer" resections, but no overall decrease in lung cancer deaths. In fact, there was a trend ($P = 0.09$) toward an increase in deaths attributed to lung cancer in the screened group (Marcus et al. 2000).

Pseudodisease has been divided into two types (Black and Welch 1997). Type I pseudodisease is related to length-time bias. Just as some individuals can have particularly aggressive forms of the disease, others can have particularly indolent forms, which are detectable on screening but would never cause the patient any symptoms. Type II pseudodisease occurs even if the natural history of the disease is homogeneous. Some people with preclinical disease will die from another cause before the disease becomes symptomatic. This is why screening an octogenarian for cancer rarely makes sense.

## Randomized trials of screening tests

We have said that the best way to determine whether a test is of benefit is to perform a randomized trial in which subjects are randomized to be tested or not. These have been done only for a few major screening tests, like mammography and stool occult blood testing. A drawback to randomized trials is that they may need to be very large and of long duration. Aside from the fact that the target diseases may be quite uncommon, the sample size has to be increased even further to make up for the bias toward the null (finding no effect) that occurs as a result of crossover between groups: some subjects randomized to screening will decline it, and some randomized to usual care will get screened anyway. One controversy that comes up particularly for randomized trials of screening tests is the choice of outcome variables.

### Total mortality versus cause-specific mortality

There are good arguments for saying that, in order to know that a screening test is beneficial, we need to see a decrease in total mortality in a group randomized to screening as opposed to just a decrease in cause-specific mortality.[4] Whereas mortality is easy to ascertain objectively, cause-specific mortality is subject to judgment and might be influenced by the screening test. It also may be difficult or impossible to know whether some deaths occurred as late effects of the treatment or of the screening test itself. This is a particular problem with large, population-based studies where death certificates are used. Although blinding those assigning cause of death to treatment group assignment will reduce that problem, it will not eliminate it, because screening produces information and events that become part of the patient's medical history.

Black et al. (2002) describe two major biases that result from using cause-specific rather than overall mortality as the outcome. "Sticky diagnosis bias" refers to the likelihood that, once a disease (particularly cancer) is diagnosed, deaths are more likely to be attributed to it. For example, sometimes patients die of unclear causes. If they previously had a cancer diagnosed by screening, their death would be more likely to be attributed to that cancer. The diagnosis of cancer "sticks" to the patient. This is a bias that will make a comparison of cause-specific mortality look *worse* for screening. Those in the screened group will tend to have higher cause-specific mortality attributed to the cancer they were screened for, even if they die of other conditions.

On the other hand, another possibility is what Black et al. call "slippery linkage bias." This occurs when the linkage between deaths due to screening, follow-up, or treatment "slips," so that deaths that may have occurred as a result of screening are not counted in the cause-specific mortality for the disease. This can occur from late complications from the screening test itself or from complications of treatment. For example, if a patient in a randomized trial of fecal occult blood testing to screen for colon cancer eventually dies after a series of complications that began with a

---

[4] This discussion is focused on screenings whose goal is to prolong life.

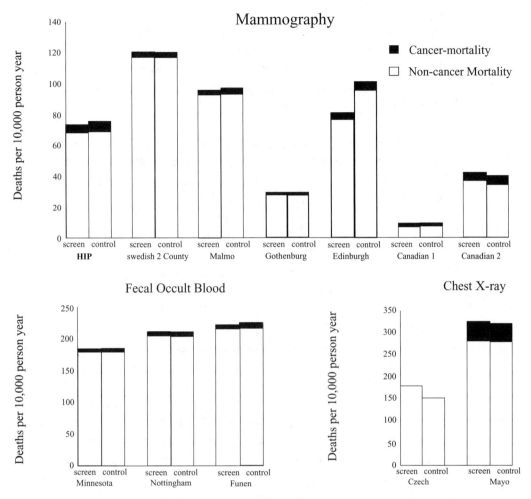

Figure 6.6    Cancer and noncancer mortality in randomized trials of cancer screening. From Black et al. (2002).

colonic perforation during colonoscopy for a false-positive fecal occult blood test, the death would not be counted as a colon cancer death, although it was caused by screening for colon cancer. Similarly, there is good evidence from randomized trials that radiation therapy for breast cancer is associated with a late increase in coronary heart disease death rates (Early Breast Cancer Trialists' Collaborative Group 2000). These deaths may occur with greater frequency in screened women, who are more likely to receive radiation, but will be difficult or impossible to link to screening.

There really is only one problem with using total mortality as an endpoint in screening trials, but it is a big one: deaths from causes unrelated to screening or the target condition will generally swamp deaths affected by screening, making it virtually impossible to identify beneficial (or harmful) effects. This is illustrated graphically in Figure 6.6. When only a few percent of deaths are likely to be due to the target condition, it is difficult to detect any effect on total mortality.

### Biases that make screening tests look worse

We have focused on biases that tend to make tests look better than they really are.[5] This is because, at least historically, people doing studies of tests have often been advocates of the tests, so these were the biases to be most concerned about. But as more people (like us) who are skeptical about tests write articles about them, we should consider biases that can make tests look *worse* in a study than they might be in practice:

1. **Inadequate power:** It is easy to fail to find any benefit of a test if your sample size is too small or duration of follow-up too short. Another way to reduce your power is to look at total mortality, rather than cause-specific mortality.

2. **People performing the test are unskilled:** If the test takes some skill, by studying it in a setting where it is not done well, you can find that it doesn't work.

3. **People who test positive are not properly followed up or treated:** For example, if one wanted to show that fecal occult blood testing was worthless, one could study it in a setting where many patients were not followed up or where those who were followed up were not well treated.

### Back to the big picture

So what should we do to avoid recommending screening tests that might do harm, while not taking a completely nihilistic stance? First, every effort must be made to perform studies that answer the main question of whether screening leads to better outcomes among patients. Because the ideal study design (randomized trial with total mortality as the outcome) is rarely feasible, keep several criteria in mind when considering the alternatives. First, studies should attempt to capture morbidity and mortality due to the screening test itself. Second, we should recognize that the need to examine total mortality varies with the screening test and the intervention. For fecal occult blood screening, for example, where the test involves no exposure to radiation and the treatment is primarily surgical, we have fewer concerns about late adverse effects than with mammography. Treatment resulting from mammography may involve radiation and/or systemic treatment with hormone analogs or chemotherapeutic agents that may have significant effects on causes of death other than breast cancer that may not be apparent for years. Finally, large, relatively simple, randomized trials and, when possible, much lower cost observational alternatives, like natural experiments, are desirable to address specific concerns about increases in mortality from causes other than the disease being screened for. Randomized trials and their alternatives will be discussed in Chapters 9 and 10.

## Summary of key points

1. The purpose of screening tests is to identify unrecognized symptomatic disease, presymptomatic disease, or risk factors for disease.

---

[5] Except Sticky Diagnosis Bias, which makes the screening test look worse in terms of cause specific mortality.

2. A critical approach to screening tests is important because screening tests can cause harm and because there are many forces and biases that tend to favor screening.
3. The most definitive way to assess screening tests is with randomized trials that have total mortality as the outcome, but these are seldom feasible, necessitating care when interpreting observational studies and trials focused on cause-specific mortality.

## References

Barton, M., D. Morley, et al. (2004). "Decreasing women's anxieties after abnormal mammograms: a controlled trial." *J Natl Cancer Inst* **96**: 529–38.

Black, W. C., D. A. Haggstrom, et al. (2002). "All-cause mortality in randomized trials of cancer screening." *J Natl Cancer Inst* **94**(3): 167–73.

Black, W. C., and H. G. Welch (1997). "Screening for disease." *AJR Am J Roentgenol* **168**(1): 3–11.

Braveman, P., and E. Tarimo (1994). *Screening in Primary Health Care: Setting Priorities with Limited Resources*. Geneva, World Health Organization.

Daniels, N. (1986). "Why saying no to patients in the United States is so hard. Cost containment, justice, and provider autonomy." *N Engl J Med* **314**(21): 1380–3.

Early Breast Cancer Trialists' Collaborative Group (2000). "Favourable and unfavourable effects on long-term survival of radiotherapy for early breast cancer: an overview of the randomised trials." *Lancet* **355**(9217): 1757–70.

Eddy, D. (1991). *Common Screening Tests*. Philadelphia, PA, American College of Physicians.

Eddy, D. M. (1997). "Breast cancer screening in women younger than 50 years of age: what's next?" *Ann Intern Med* **127**(11): 1035–6.

Epstein, A. E., A. P. Hallstrom, et al. (1993). "Mortality following ventricular arrhythmia suppression by encainide, flecainide, and moricizine after myocardial infarction. The original design concept of the Cardiac Arrhythmia Suppression Trial (CAST)." *JAMA* **270**(20): 2451–5.

Ernster, V. L. (1997). "Mammography screening for women aged 40 through 49–a guidelines saga and a clarion call for informed decision making." *Am J Public Health* **87**(7): 1103–6.

Feinstein, A. R., D. M. Sosin, et al. (1985). "The Will Rogers phenomenon. Stage migration and new diagnostic techniques as a source of misleading statistics for survival in cancer." *N Engl J Med* **312**(25): 1604–8.

Fyro, K., and G. Bodegard (1987). "Four-year follow-up of psychological reactions to false positive screening tests for congenital hypothyroidism." *Acta Paediatr Scand* **76**(1): 107–14.

Guyatt, G., D. Rennie, et al. (2008). *Users' Guides to the Medical Literature: A Manual for Evidence-Based Clinical Practice, 2nd Edition*. New York, NY, McGraw Hill Medical, pp. 113–143.

Haynes, R. B., D. L. Sackett, et al. (1978). "Increased absenteeism from work after detection and labeling of hypertensive patients." *N Engl J Med* **299**(14): 741–4.

HEDIS (2009). "The Health Plan Employer Data and Information Set (HEDIS®)." Available from: http://www.ncqa.org/tabid/784/Default.aspx. Accessed 10/3/08.

Herman, C. R., H. K. Gill, et al. (2002). "Screening for preclinical disease: test and disease characteristics." *AJR Am J Roentgenol* **179**(4): 825–31.

Law, J., and K. Faulkner (2001). "Cancers detected and induced, and associated risk and benefit, in a breast screening programme." *Br J Radiol* **74**(888): 1121–7.

Lee, T., and T. Brennan (2002). "Direct-to-consumer marketing of high-technology screening tests." *N Engl J Med* **346**(7): 529–531.

Marantz, P. R. (1990). "Blaming the victim: the negative consequence of preventive medicine." *Am J Public Health* **80**(10): 1186–7.

Marcus, P. M., E. J. Bergstralh, et al. (2000). "Lung cancer mortality in the Mayo Lung Project: impact of extended follow-up." *J Natl Cancer Inst* **92**(16): 1308–16.

Mariner, W. K. (1995). "Rationing health care and the need for credible scarcity: why Americans can't say no." *Am J Public Health* **85**(10): 1439–45.

Moore, T. J. (1995). *Deadly Medicine: Why Tens of Thousands of Heart Patients Died in America's Worst Drug Disaster.* New York, Simon & Schuster.

Newman, T. B. (2003). "The power of stories over statistics." *Br Med J* **327**(7429): 1424–7.

Olivotto, I. A., P. T. Truong, et al. (2003). "Staging reclassification affects breast cancer survival." *J Clin Oncol* **21**(23): 4467–8.

Otto, S. J., F. H. Schroder, et al. (2004). "Low all-cause mortality in the volunteer-based Rotterdam section of the European randomised study of screening for prostate cancer: self-selection bias?" *J Med Screen* **11**(2): 89–92.

Riggs, B. L., S. F. Hodgson, et al. (1990). "Effect of fluoride treatment on the fracture rate in postmenopausal women with osteoporosis." *N Engl J Med* **322**(12): 802–9.

Rubin, S. M., and S. R. Cummings (1992). "Results of bone densitometry affect women's decisions about taking measures to prevent fractures." *Ann Intern Med* **116**(12 Pt 1): 990–5.

Schwartz, L. M., S. Woloshin, et al. (2004). "Enthusiasm for cancer screening in the United States." *JAMA* **291**(1): 71–8.

Welch, H. G. (2004). *Should I Be Tested for Cancer? Maybe Not, and Here's Why.* Berkeley, CA, University of California Press.

WHO (1980). "W.H.O. cooperative trial on primary prevention of ischaemic heart disease using clofibrate to lower serum cholesterol: mortality follow-up. Report of the Committee of Principal Investigators." *Lancet* **2**(8191): 379–85.

Woodward, W. A., E. A. Strom, et al. (2003). "Changes in the 2003 American Joint Committee on Cancer staging for breast cancer dramatically affect stage-specific survival." *J Clin Oncol* **21**(17): 3244–8.

## Chapter 6 Problems: screening tests

1. For each of the following study descriptions, name and briefly explain the bias most likely to account for the results.

   a) A study on early treatment of lupus-related kidney disease (nephritis) compared patients who had a kidney biopsy early in their clinical course with patients biopsied late in their course. The study measured time to renal failure from the time of the biopsy and found that those biopsied earlier had a longer time to renal failure.

   b) One way to screen for *colon* cancer is to have patients collect a small amount of stool on a Hemoccult® card that can be chemically tested for the presence of blood. A study of fecal occult blood screening finds a dose-response between the number of Hemoccult® cards returned and decreased risk of *lung* cancer death.

c) A new policy requires all asthmatics to have a $pCO_2$ measured in the emergency department, with automatic admission to the ICU rather than the ward if the $pCO_2$ exceeds 45 mm Hg. (A $pCO_2 > 45$ mm Hg is an indication of increased severity.) Death rates from asthma in both the ICU and on the ward decline.

2. A 2006 paper in the *New England Journal of Medicine* (Henschke et al. 2006) reported 88% estimated 10-year lung cancer-specific survival among 412 patients with pathologically proven stage I lung cancer detected by CT screening. They contrasted this with about 5% survival among lung cancer patients in general. Which of the following statements about this finding are true? [True/False for (a–d); include explanation for (e).]

a) Because survival was counted beginning at the time of diagnosis, some improvement in survival would be expected due to *lead-time bias*, even if there was no advantage to early detection.

b) "Sticky diagnosis bias" could be an explanation for these findings in favor of screening.

c) Because tumors identified on screening tests tend to be slower-growing and have a more benign prognosis than tumors that present with symptoms, *length-time bias* could contribute to these favorable results.

d) *Overdiagnosis* of lung cancer (pseudodisease) in these participants is unlikely because all diagnoses were confirmed pathologically.

e) These results show that CT screening reduces lung cancer mortality by 80% or more. Explain your answer.

3. The Multicenter Aneurysm Screening Study (Ashton et al. 2002) was a randomized trial of the effectiveness of ultrasound screening for Abdominal Aortic Aneurysm (AAA) in reducing aneurysm-related mortality. Men aged 65–74 were randomized either to be invited to receive a screening abdominal ultrasound scan or not. Aneurysm-related and overall mortality in the two randomization groups are reported below:

**Multicenter Aneurysm Screening Study**

|  | N | AAA-Related Deaths | % | Total Deaths | % |
|---|---|---|---|---|---|
| Invited | 33,839 | 65 | 0.19% | 3,750 | 11.08% |
| Not Invited | 33,961 | 113 | 0.33% | 3,855 | 11.35% |
| Total | 67,800 | 178 |  | 7,605 |  |

a) Does screening appear to be effective in reducing aneurysm-related deaths?

b) You can see that, in those invited for screening, there were 48 fewer AAA deaths $(113 - 65)$ and 105 fewer total deaths $(3855 - 3750)$. Thus, there were $105 - 48 = 57$ fewer *non*-AAA deaths in those invited for screening. Which of the following do you think are the most likely explanations for this: Volunteer or Selection Bias; Lead-Time Bias; Length-Time Bias; Stage Migration Bias;

Misclassification of Outcome; Misclassification of Exposure; Cointerventions; or Chance?

c) The authors also did a *within groups* analysis in the invited group only, comparing those who did and did not get the ultrasound scan. Results are summarized below, same format as before:

**Multicenter Aneurysm Screening Study – Invited Group Only**

|             | N      | AAA Death | %     | Total Death | %      |
|-------------|--------|-----------|-------|-------------|--------|
| Scanned     | 27,147 | 43        | 0.16% | 2,590       | 9.54%  |
| Not Scanned | 6,692  | 22        | 0.33% | 1,160       | 17.33% |
| **Total**   | **33,839** | **65** |       | **3,750**   |        |

The total mortality rate in the invited patients who were scanned (9.54%) was 45% lower than that of the invited patients who were not scanned (17.33%) Again, which of the following explanations are most likely responsible for this difference: Volunteer or Selection Bias; Lead-Time Bias; Length-Time Bias; Stage Migration Bias; Misclassification of Outcome; Misclassification of Exposure; Cointerventions; or Chance?

d) This was a randomized trial, so the safest way to analyze the data is by group assignment – an "Intention to Treat" analysis. Nonetheless, it is sometimes of interest to compare groups according to how they were actually treated – an "As Treated" analysis. Do you believe the "As Treated" comparison of AAA deaths (not total deaths) between the scanned and not scanned patients within the Invited group is biased? Why or why not?

4. Torres et al. (1994) studied a population of 86 children who had been diagnosed and treated for posterior fossa medulloblastoma (a brain cancer). After initial treatment, these 86 children were screened for recurrence with a brain scan every 6 months, or scanned sooner if they developed symptoms or signs suggestive of recurrence. There were 23 children with recurrences: 4 were detected on interval screening and 19 presented with symptoms or signs of recurrence between surveillance scans. All 23 recurrences resulted in death. In the group of 4 recurrences that were detected by a regular screening scan (not prompted by signs or symptoms), the median survival was 20 months. In the group of 19 recurrences that presented with symptoms or signs, the median survival was only 4 months (P = 0.03). In the Letters to the Editor about this article, there was some debate about whether lead-time and/or length-time bias could explain this survival difference.

a) Could lead-time bias explain the entire survival difference? If not, how much of the survival difference could be explained by lead-time bias?

b) Could length-time bias explain the survival difference?

5. Mastroiacovo et al. (1992) studied the all-cause mortality of children with Down syndrome (DS) in Italy. As expected, they found that the strongest predictor of death was congenital heart disease (CHD). They noted that DS patients with CHD in northern Italy had greater survival than those with CHD in southern Italy. Also, DS patients without CHD in northern Italy had greater survival than

those without CHD in southern Italy. The authors suspect that medical care for the children in the South might not be as good. In the discussion, they state:

The insufficient resources for pediatric care available in the South could explain the low proportion of CHD diagnosed among DS infants there (10.6% as compared with 21.7% in the North).

Is it possible that the overall survival for DS patients (combining patients with and without CHD) in southern Italy could be just as high as in northern Italy? Explain.

## References

Ashton, H. A., M. J. Buxton, et al. (2002). "The Multicentre Aneurysm Screening Study (MASS) into the effect of abdominal aortic aneurysm screening on mortality in men: a randomised controlled trial." *Lancet* **360**(9345): 1531–9.

Henschke, C. I., D. F. Yankelevitz, et al. (2006). "Survival of patients with stage I lung cancer detected on CT screening." *N Engl J Med* **355**(17): 1763–71.

Mastroiacovo, P., R. Bertollini, et al. (1992). "Survival of children with Down syndrome in Italy." *Am J Med Genet* **42**(2): 208–12.

Torres, C. F., S. Rebsamen, et al. (1994). "Surveillance scanning of children with medulloblastoma" *N Engl J Med* **330**(13): 892–5.

# Prognostic tests and studies

## Introduction

In previous chapters, we discussed issues affecting evaluation of diagnostic tests: how the reason to make a diagnosis may determine which tests should be done, how test reliability and accuracy are assessed, how to combine the results of tests with prior information to estimate the probability that a patient has a disease, and how to assess studies of diagnostic tests. In this chapter, we consider those same kinds of questions, with respect to prognostic tests.

## Prognostic versus diagnostic tests

Prognosis is "a forecasting of the probable course and termination of an illness" (Webster's Unabridged Dictionary 2001). The main difference between prognostic tests and diagnostic tests is that, with prognostic tests, a time dimension is involved. With diagnostic tests, we are concerned with determining who does and does not have a disease. In this chapter, we begin with people who have a disease and try to predict their prognosis – that is, what will happen to them in the future. Thus, studies of prognostic tests generally have to be longitudinal in nature. That is, they need to follow a group of patients over time and allow measurement of incidence rather than just prevalence.

As was the case with studies of diagnostic tests, in which we compared test results among patients with and without the disease (a dichotomous variable), the outcome variable of a prognostic test study is generally also dichotomous – survival versus death, disease-free survival versus disease recurrence, and so on; each subject either does or does not develop that outcome. However, due to the time component, the result of a prognostic test is often not dichotomous. That is, studies of prognostic tests, even when the outcome variables are dichotomous, do not generally report results like "will die" and "will survive." Instead, they generally report quantitative results – for example, when a given marker is present, 1-year mortality is 30%, compared with 60% when it is absent. Thus, whereas a diagnostic test gives either the right or the wrong answer for an individual patient, the accuracy of prognostic tests, whose results are translated into probabilities of an outcome, can generally only be assessed in groups of patients followed over time. If a test suggests that a patient has a 30% chance of dying in the next year, it is not clear when the patient would need to die in order for the test to give the "right" answer.

An exception to this rule is that, if the time period of interest is very well defined (and usually short), accuracy can be assessed on individual patients. For example, if the time period of interest is the days following resuscitation from a cardiac arrest, one might measure predictors of survival to hospital discharge. A predictive index could be dichotomized or clinical prediction rule developed, which would, in fact, be either right or wrong. When the time course for a prognosis is short, prognostic tests are like diagnostic tests.

It is also possible to assess the accuracy of a prognostic test in individual patients when the outcome variable of interest is continuous. For example, you might predict that a woman with osteoporosis will lose 0.5 cm of height per year, or that a pregnant woman with diabetes will have a 4-kg baby. For patients with incurable disease, an estimated survival time (typically in months) is also a continuous outcome. In the case of a continuous outcome, the accuracy in individual patients can be assessed by the difference between what was predicted and what was observed, and the mean and distribution of these differences can be studied in groups of patients. A graph with the difference between observed and predicted outcomes on the y-axis versus observed outcome on the x-axis produces a calibration plot very similar to the Bland–Altman plots used for method comparison studies (discussed in Chapter 2).

## Prognostic tests versus risk factors

In Chapter 6, we distinguished between screening for unrecognized symptomatic disease, presymptomatic disease, and risk factors. Evaluating the effectiveness of screening for risk factors generally requires larger and longer studies, comparing outcomes in the screened and unscreened groups. The study must allow time for the screening test to accurately identify those at higher risk, for those subjects to receive an effective intervention to decrease that risk, and for some of them to develop the outcome.

Because prognostic tests are predicting associations between test results and outcomes over time, they are more similar to risk factor-screening tests than to diagnostic tests. However, in contrast with risk factors, prognostic associations are of interest even if they are not causal. As we will discuss in the next chapter, the best way to estimate the probability of disease is often by combining information from several different tests. Similarly, the best way to estimate prognosis is often by combining information from several variables. Multivariate techniques, such as logistic regression, are often useful for studies of prognostic tests, just as they are for observational studies of risk factors. However, with prognostic tests, this is often to determine to what extent a new, more difficult or more expensive test adds information to what was already available, rather than to distinguish between causal associations and those due to confounding, which is the priority for studies of risk factors.

Studies of risk factors for disease generally yield relative measures of association: risk ratios, odds ratios, and hazard ratios. These measures express how many times more likely a patient with the risk factor is to develop the outcome than a patient without the risk factor.[1] They do not tell us the patient's absolute risk of the outcome, such as how likely this particular patient is to develop the outcome over the next 5 years. But patients with diseases want to know their absolute risks. They do not just want to know if their chance of dying in the next 5 years is half (or twice) as high as someone else's; they want to know what their chance of dying actually *is* – that is, their prognosis.

## Quantifying the accuracy of prognostic tests

### Calibration versus discrimination

Prognostic test accuracy has two dimensions: *calibration* and *discrimination*. Calibration refers to how well the probability estimated from the test result matches the actual probability, whereas discrimination refers to how well the test differentiates between patients more and less likely to have the outcome.

Because each individual patient will either have the outcome or not, calibration is measured by comparing the predicted probability estimated from results of prognostic tests on a group of patients to the actual probability – that is, to the proportion of a group of patients that develops the outcome in a specified time period. For example, if we assemble a cohort of HIV+ patients with CD4 counts <500, the predicted 5-year mortality might be 45%. If the observed mortality in that group of patients after 5 years were 40% to 50%, calibration would be good: the observed probability of mortality in the group would match the expected probability.

Calibration is typically measured by dividing the population into groups (often deciles of risk) and comparing predicted and observed frequencies of the outcome. This is most appropriately done by visual inspection, either of the numbers themselves or of a graph of observed versus expected probabilities, as illustrated in Box 7.1. Statistical tests of calibration are also available, but they have the disadvantage that they provide P-values for the discrepancy between observed and predicted probabilities but no summary estimate of "effect size" – that is, how far apart these probabilities actually are. Thus, if the sample size is very large, P-values can be statistically significant even when the calibration is good, and conversely, if the sample size is too small, poor calibration will not be statistically significant. (We discuss this problem with P-values and the distinction between P-values and effect size in Chapter 11.)

Just good calibration is not sufficient, however. If you were to include an entire population in the test of calibration and simply use the population value for probability of death from the disease as your estimate for each person, your calibration would be perfect – each person in the population would have the same, correct

---

[1] We will review the difference between risk ratios and odds ratios, and when it is important, in Chapter 9.

**Box 7.1: Calibration and discrimination for prognosis of low back pain**

Dutch investigators studied predictors of prognosis in patients presenting to general practitioners with low back pain (Jellema et al. 2007). They developed a clinical prediction rule that provided an estimated probability of an "unfavorable course," defined as back pain perceived by the patient as at most "slightly improved," at subsequent follow-up visits. The prediction rule was based on answers to a baseline questionnaire covering things like radiation of the pain, previous history of back pain, and general health. (Clinical prediction rules are discussed in Chapter 8.) They also asked the general practitioners to estimate the probability of restricted functioning at 3 months to the nearest 10% (i.e., on an 11-point scale: 0%, 10%, 20%, 30% ... 100%). The calibration of the two methods is illustrated in Figures 7.1a and 7.1b. Calibration was good for both – most of the points are close to the line that represents perfect calibration. However, you can see that discrimination of the clinical prediction rule (Fig. 7.1a) was better than the practitioners' estimates, because it yielded a wider range of predicted probabilities. Remember, discrimination is the ability to move probabilities away from the mean probability toward 0 and 1. This improved discrimination was reflected in a higher area under the ROC curve (AUROC): 0.75 (95% CI 0.69 to 0.81) for the clinical prediction rule, compared with 0.59 (95% CI 0.52 to 0.66) for the general practitioner's estimate.

probability of dying. However, discrimination would be poor. You would be unable to tell which people were most likely to die and which were least likely to die.

Discrimination refers to how well the test can separate the subjects' probability of the outcome from the average probability of the group to values closer to zero (no chance of developing the outcome) and 1 (certain to develop the outcome). In the example of HIV+ people with CD4 counts <500, discrimination could be improved

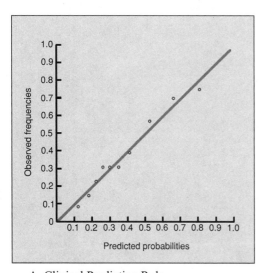

A. Clinical Prediction Rule

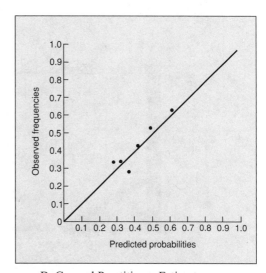

B. General Practitioner Estimate

Figure 7.1    Predicted probability plotted against observed frequency of continued low back pain among patients seen by Dutch general practitioners. Both sets of predicted probabilities are well calibrated, but the clinical prediction rule discriminates better, as shown by a wider range of predicted probabilities (predicted probabilities closer to 0 and 1 for more subjects). From Jellema et al. (2007).

by further dividing the CD4 count into smaller categories, so that subjects with CD4 counts <50, who have the worst prognosis, would not be lumped together with those with counts from 400 to 499, whose prognosis is better.

A commonly used approach to quantifying the discrimination of a prognostic test is to pick a particular time period (e.g., 5 years) and then treat the outcome as a simple dichotomous variable (e.g., alive or dead at 5 years). We can then express the discrimination of a prognostic test with our old friend from Chapter 4, the AUROC, where instead of comparing test results in disease and nondiseased, the results are compared in those who did and did not develop the outcome (e.g., 5-year survival), and the varying definition of a positive test is what traces out the ROC curve (Box 7.2). A test with perfect discrimination would produce

---

**Box 7.2**

Mackillop and Quirt (1997) performed a cohort study of oncologists' ability to predict "cure" (5-year disease-free survival) in 96 cancer patients. At the beginning of the study, the doctors assigned a probability of cure to each patient. After 5 years of follow-up, 26 patients had survived without recurrence. Figure 7.2 (*top*) shows their distribution of doctor-assigned probability of cure. Figure 7.2 (*bottom*) shows this same distribution for the 70 patients who had a recurrence or died.

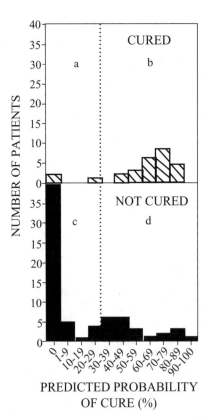

Figure 7.2   Frequency distribution of doctor-assigned, 5-year, disease-free survival ("cure") in 26 patients who did survive without recurrence (*top*) and 70 patients who suffered a recurrence or died (*bottom*). From Mackillop and Quirt (1997), Figure 3. Used with permission.

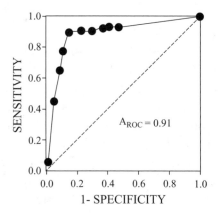

**Figure 7.3**    ROC curve summarizing doctors' ability to discriminate between patients who go on to survive for 5 years without recurrence and patients who die or have recurrences within 5 years. From Mackillop and Quirt (1997), Figure 4. Used by permission.

an ROC curve like a perfect diagnostic test: straight up and then straight across, with an AUROC of 1.0. We emphasize that the AUROC only measures how well the prognostic test discriminates between survivors and nonsurvivors; it says nothing about calibration. Recall from Chapter 4 that the ROC curve depends only on the ranking of individual measurements (in this case, risk estimates) and not their absolute values. Given any pair of patients – one who survived 5 years and one who did not survive – the AUROC is the probability that the survivor would be ranked more highly with regard to survival probability than the non-survivor.

For example, Figure 7.3 shows the ROC curve that results from sequentially raising the threshold for "will survive 5 years without recurrence" from 0% to 100% in the study described in Box 7.2. The AUROC is 0.91, meaning that, of all the $(26 \times 70 = 1820)$ possible cured–uncured pairs, the cured patient was ranked by the oncologist as more likely to be cured than the uncured patient 91% of the time.

Although use of the AUROC to quantify discrimination is common and easy to understand, dichotomizing survival at one point leads to loss of information. For example, dichotomizing survival at 5 years equates a death at 1 week with a death at 4.9 years, and a death at 5.1 years with $>10$-year survival. One approach to this problem is to make a whole family of ROC curves, for outcomes occurring at different time periods (e.g., 1-, 2-, 3-, 4-, 5-year survival, etc.).

Providing an estimate of discrimination is also difficult when not all outcomes are known. This can happen when subjects are lost to follow-up or die of other causes, as often happens in long-term studies of cause-specific mortality in older subjects. One approach to the latter problem is to focus on total mortality, but if many of the deaths are due to causes other than the disease of interest, the results will in part reflect the association (or lack thereof) between the prognostic factors and these other causes of death.

## Risk ratios, rate ratios, and hazard ratios

Prognostic test studies often report results using risk ratios, rate ratios, or hazard ratios. These measures all express the likelihood of developing the outcome in people who have a risk factor compared with those who do not. As with the use of ROC curves, the use of risk ratios requires dichotomizing the outcome, which leads to loss of information about when the outcome occurred and about people who were lost to follow-up. Rate ratios and hazard ratios can take into account variable follow-up periods and times to the outcome, so these measures are preferable when follow-up time is variable and there are issues such as competing mortality. Rate ratios and hazard ratios will be biased if loss to follow-up is associated with both the prognostic factor and the outcome of interest. Also, as we noted above, risk, rate, or hazard ratios alone are less clinically useful, because most clinical decisions should be based on absolute rather than relative risks.

## Assessing the value of prognostic information

Much prognostic information is available at little cost or risk; variables such as age, current symptom burden, extent of disease, and functional status are often highly predictive of prognosis. On the other hand, when we are considering risky or expensive prognostic tests, we should consider how to assess the value of such tests in order to make better decisions about their use.

Unfortunately, quantifying (or even estimating) the value of prognostic information is difficult, because the proper effect of prognostic information on decisions may be unclear. For example, if you inform a patient that her estimated 5-year survival from breast cancer is 80%, but a new test might change that to either 70% or 90%, how will that affect her subsequent decisions? The patient with only a 70% survival probability might opt for treatment with a more aggressive regimen, but this more aggressive treatment may not have been shown to be effective. If, in fact, the treatment is ineffective or even does harm, then the test that led to your giving that treatment was (at best) of no value. Similarly, if the test result led to treatment being withheld in the patient with 90% predicted survival, and that patient would have benefited from the treatment, again, the test was not valuable, and, in fact, caused the patient harm. Remember, the main value of a test is in allowing us to make better decisions. This implies enough knowledge of risks, costs, and benefits of treatment to create a treatment threshold. But if the treatment threshold is not known with any precision at all (e.g., it is thought that treating is worthwhile if the risk of death over the next 5 years is somewhere between 10% and 80%), then performing prognostic tests that allow better estimation of prognosis within this range does not help with the treatment decision.

The gap between prognostic information and the information needed to make decisions is illustrated by a study of breast cancer patients' estimates of their prognosis with and without adjuvant chemotherapy (Ravdin et al. 1998). The patients' estimates of recurrence risk and the benefits of treatment were much too high, translating to an absolute risk reduction of about 30%, when the correct number was closer to 7.5%. However, the median absolute reduction of risk at which the women would choose adjuvant chemotherapy was only 0.5% to 1%, so in most cases, it does not appear that inaccurate estimates of prognosis affected their decisions. Similarly, a randomized trial that included provision of accurate prognostic information to patients and clinicians found no improvement in patient care or outcomes (SUPPORT 1995).

We should still make every effort to help patients obtain an accurate prognosis. Patients may value prognostic information beyond its ability to help with clinical decision making, and in some patients, accurate information could favorably affect decisions. But if the prognostic test is difficult or expensive, we should consider whether its result will be helpful and for what purpose.

You can think about No Treat–Test and Test–Treat thresholds for a prognostic test in the same way as for a diagnostic test if you dichotomize the outcome (e.g., 5-year mortality).

1. First, think about what treatment or management decision(s) the test is supposed to help resolve.
2. Then, consider the concept of the "treatment threshold." This is the post-test probability of developing the outcome that determines whether or not to initiate treatment. For example, at what (posterior/post-test) probability of a bad outcome (e.g., death, recurrence, etc.) would you recommend more aggressive treatment?
3. Now use available clinical data to estimate a prior (pre-test) probability – in this case, not that the patient *has* a disease, but instead that the patient will *develop* the particular outcome you wish to avoid within a specified time period. This is based on your history, physical examination, and all other information except the prognostic test you are considering.
4. Now consider the probability that the additional prognostic information will change your decision, and estimate the value of that change. For example, if having a positive test for the latest pricey genetic marker would increase the estimated risk of recurrence from 30% to 60%, would that change your mind about what treatment you recommend? If so, what is the chance that the marker will be positive, and how confident are you that the change in treatment would improve the patient's life expectancy?

All of this is difficult to do – much more difficult than deciding whether to perform a throat culture to help decide whether to treat with penicillin. But this is what you would need to do to be able to assign a value to a prognostic test. This difficulty is what makes us generally skeptical about expensive prognostic tests.

## Critical appraisal of studies of prognosis and prognostic tests

As was the case with diagnostic tests, we summarize several issues that arise commonly in evaluating studies of prognosis. Most of these issues arise for other types of studies as well, so we will only highlight them briefly here.

## Sample selection and generalizability

It is important to understand how the subjects in a study of prognosis were identified. Patients whose disease is identified by screening will generally do better than those who present to community physicians with symptoms, who will do better than those referred to tertiary centers. Prognostic studies that obtain their subjects from these different sources will yield different results. This occurs both as a result of the selection process leading to referral and as a result of differences in the time point in the course of the disease at which they are enrolled. Therefore, a key question to ask in appraising a study of a prognostic test is how the subjects came to be included in the study at the time they did, and whether the patients to whom you wish to generalize the results would have any reason to be under-represented in the study.

## Effects of treatment

If the illness being studied is treatable, then its prognosis will be affected not only by the selection process for subjects in the study, but also by how they were treated. If you want to generalize to your patients, not only must the patients in the study be similar to yours at the onset of the study, they need to be treated similarly throughout the course of the study. Watch out for studies in which differences in treatment due to perceived differences in prognosis muddy the ability to determine what factors actually are most predictive of prognosis. A study of prognostic factors in elderly ICU patients would likely find associations with mortality either for factors that really do predict mortality or for factors that treating physicians strongly believe will predict mortality, because having many of the latter factors may lead to withdrawal of life support.

## Loss to follow-up

Patients lost to follow-up add uncertainty to estimates of prognosis. This is a particular problem if there is reason to believe their prognosis might be different from the prognosis of those whose outcome is known. One way to get some limits on the degree to which subjects lost to follow-up could affect the study results is to recalculate the proportion with the outcome (e.g., survival), first assuming that all those missing had the outcome, and then assuming none did. For example, consider a follow-up study of 200 patients, of whom 120 survived, 60 died, and 20 could not be accounted for at 5 years. If the subjects lost to follow-up are simply not counted, survival would be $120/180 = 67\%$. If all 20 patients lost to follow-up are assumed to have died, the observed survival would be $120/200 = 60\%$, and if none had died, it would be $140/200 = 70\%$. Thus, the largest effect of loss-to-follow-up in this example would be to increase apparent survival from 60% to 67%, or decrease it from 70% to 67%. If this very conservative approach still yields useful prognostic information, you are on firm ground. A less conservative approach would be to assign the missing subjects the lowest and highest plausible event rates (rather than the rates of 0% and 100% used above).

This same approach applies when estimating possible effects of loss-to-follow-up on an estimate of the relative risk associated with presence of a particular prognostic factor. The largest possible effect that loss to follow-up could have can be estimated by assuming that all those lost to follow-up had a bad outcome in one group and a good outcome in the other group, or vice versa.

## Blinding

We will discuss blinding in greater detail in Chapter 9. For now, we note that blinding is most important for subjective outcomes and when the prognostic factors of interest may affect treatment. For example, consider a study of predictors of the need for hospitalization in children presenting to the emergency department with acute asthma. If the goal is to study the prognostic value of the initial oxygen saturation, those making the decision to admit should be kept blinded to that value, so that it could not itself affect the decision to admit.

## Overfitting

We mentioned this problem in Chapter 5, and drew an analogy with the Illinois 4th Congressional District (fig. 5.2). If you look at enough variables, you are bound to find some combination that is associated with adverse outcome in one particular sample. Similarly, if the investigators select the cut-off that defines abnormal results based on what works best in the sample, the value of the test will be overestimated. To be convincing, the prognostic factors identified in one study need to be restudied in another dataset, separate from the one from which they were derived, using the same cut-offs to define abnormal results (Hilsenbeck et al. 1992). The need for a *validation* dataset will be discussed again in Chapter 8.

## Multiple and composite outcomes

A problem similar to overfitting occurs when multiple outcome variables are measured in a study, and the ones that are predicted by the test are selectively highlighted or reported. This multiple comparison problem also arises in randomized trials, and will be discussed in Chapters 9 and 11. Similarly, sometimes several outcomes are grouped together into a composite outcome – again, a common strategy in clinical trials. As in a randomized trial, it is important to know whether the investigators specified the composite outcome in advance, and whether there is evidence that the composite outcome variable might be dominated by a more common or more subjective but less important outcome, such as nonfatal myocardial infarction or the development of unstable angina rather than death. If more subjective outcomes are predicted best, you should double check to make sure that they were ascertained by blinded observers. (Such blinding can be difficult, as previously discussed in Chapter 6, when we reviewed "sticky diagnosis" bias.)

## Sample size

Especially if bad outcomes are rare, there may be too few cases to be able to learn much about factors that affect prognosis. From the patient's point of view, this does not necessarily make the study problematic, because patients are most interested in *absolute* risk. If a large study has very few bad outcomes, the confidence intervals around relative risks may be very wide, suggesting that the study did not provide much information. But the confidence intervals around absolute risks may be narrow enough to be clinically meaningful. We discuss this issue at length in Chapter 11.

### Quantifying new information

It is easy to identify findings and markers that statistically significantly predict prognosis. However, the key questions are how much new information a test provides, beyond what was already known, and how valuable that information is. Watch out for two ways the apparent predictive ability of a test can be inflated. First, if measurements of other variables that predict prognosis are coarse or imprecise, the apparent contribution of the new test will be larger, because information from the other variables will be incompletely taken into account in multivariate models. Second, the apparent predictive ability of a test can be inflated by comparing risk at extremes of the test, such as reporting the hazard ratio for a comparison between the highest and lowest quintiles of the measurement. Box 7.3 illustrates both of these problems.

### Publication bias

Publication bias occurs when studies that have favorable results are published preferentially over those that do not. Although publication bias is a problem for all types of studies, it may be a particular problem for studies of prognostic markers. This is fairly understandable – it is hard to get very excited about submitting or reading a paper about factors that are worthless for predicting prognosis. On the other hand, if you look at enough possible prognostic factors in enough different ways, it is easy to find some that are good predictors of prognosis. These positive factors may be mentioned in the abstract of a paper, and other researchers will be able to easily find any previous studies in which they were predictive by doing a PubMed search. In contrast, all of the possible prognostic factors that were *not* associated with outcome in a study will be harder to find. They may or may not be listed in a table or mentioned in the "Methods" section of the current paper, but more significantly, evidence of their lack of association with outcome is unlikely to be found with a PubMed search. Publication bias is a significant problem for meta-analyses of studies of prognostic tests (Kyzas et al. 2005).

Keep in mind that clinically useful information about prognosis does not just come from studies that focus primarily on prognosis. Much valuable information can be obtained from the outcomes in either control or treated groups in randomized trials (depending on whether the patient of interest will be treated or not). Randomized trials (as discussed in Chapter 9) have the advantages that ascertainment of outcome is more complete and more objective than is typical of less rigorous designs.

## Genetic tests

Because there seems to be so much interest and excitement (and hype!) about new genetic tests, we should clarify how they differ from other tests discussed in this book. A large part of the excitement about genetic tests relates to the possibility of greater understanding of underlying molecular mechanisms of disease. The hope is

**Box 7.3: Example of a prognostic test study**

Paik et al. (2004) reported on the ability of a multigene assay to predict recurrence of tamoxifen-treated, node-negative breast cancer. They used the assay to create a "recurrence index," which they then classified as low-, intermediate-, or high-risk. The 10-year Kaplan–Meier estimates of distant recurrence rates were 6.8%, 14.3%, and 30.5% in the three groups, respectively. When entered into a Cox proportional hazard model, the recurrence index was a strong, independent predictor of prognosis, with a hazard ratio of 3.21 per 50-point change in the index (P < 0.001).

A strength of this study is that all of the decisions about how to create the index from the results of individual gene tests, including the cut-offs, were made in advance. This should reduce overfitting. However, the reported hazard ratio of 3.2 is impossible to interpret without knowledge of the meaning of a 50-point change in the index. (The hazard ratio for a 25-point change would be $\sqrt{3.2}$, or about 1.8.) In this study, a 50-point difference in the index was a large difference: 51% of the subjects had scores less than 18 and only 12% had scores over 50. On the other hand, the authors simply dichotomized age (at 50 years) and tumor size (at 2 cm).[2] By failing to capture all information in these covariates, they may have inflated the apparent predictive power of their new index. A Letter to the Editor by Goodson (2005) brings up a similar point with respect to the pathological grading of the tumors. Again, if the pathologists grading the tumors are not very good at that task, the recurrence index will look better in comparison. Supplementary appendices to the paper indicate that the agreement on tumor differentiation (in three categories) was only fair (kappa = 0.34–0.37), supporting Goodson's concern. Finally, the authors do not indicate the degree to which adding their test to what was already available improved discrimination, how this would improve decisions, or how these better decisions might improve outcomes. These are relevant considerations because, at the time of the study, the test (patented and/or owned by many authors of the study; Paik et al. 2004) was being sold for $3,500 (Tanvetyanon 2005).

that, by identifying alleles of specific genes that cause or predispose to disease, we may be able to learn what these genes do and understand how variations in their expression can lead to ill health. Although so far the track record of successes in this area is underwhelming, there is no doubt that some genetic tests have value for this purpose. Because the goal in that situation is improved understanding of disease rather than assisting with clinical decisions, assessment of these tests and the studies that describe them requires specific content knowledge about the underlying biology and is not covered in this book.

In contrast, other genetic tests may have the potential to improve health by allowing better estimates of the probability of various diseases either being present already or developing in the future or of the prognosis of existing disease. The evaluation and interpretation of these genetic tests is the same as for any other test – it involves asking the same questions about the information different test results provide: how likely a particular patient is to have a result that is informative, how the test will improve clinical decisions, and the estimated impact of these improved decisions on clinically relevant outcomes.

---

[2] The investigators could have treated tumor size the way they treated their recurrence index, as a continuous variable, and reported the hazard ratio per 10-cm increase in tumor size!

In interpreting studies of genetic tests, and gauging which of the two purposes above may be most relevant, it is helpful to ignore low P-values and look for clinically meaningful measures of effect size. For example, consider a recent report of risk alleles for multiple sclerosis (MS) identified by a genome-wide study (Hafler et al. 2007). No disease-causing mutations for MS have been identified; it is thought that multiple common polymorphisms work in concert to increase susceptibility to the disease. The investigators reported associations between MS and multiple single-nucleotide polymorphisms. Most P values for the single-nucleotide polymorphisms they found were in the $10^{-4}$ to $10^{-8}$ range, although the authors reported a P-value of $8.94 \times 10^{-81}$ for the HLA-DRA locus.[3] However, the corresponding odds ratios for most of the risk alleles were only 1.08 to 1.25, and the odds ratio for the HLA-DRA locus was only 1.99. It is hard to make a case that odds ratios of this magnitude could be helpful clinically, and the authors do not do so. Rather, the hope is that these results may contribute to better understanding of the pathogenesis of MS.

## Summary of key points

1. Prognostic tests differ from diagnostic or screening tests because their goal is to predict events that may happen in the future, rather than to identify conditions already present.
2. Studies of the value and accuracy of prognostic tests generally require longitudinal follow-up of groups of patients.
3. How the groups are selected and the completeness of follow-up are important aspects of the critical appraisal of such studies.
4. The potential value of prognostic tests is related to both their *calibration* to the actual prognosis of the patient and their *discrimination* between those more and less likely to develop the outcome.
5. Prognostic information can be summarized with baseline (absolute) risk, risk ratios, rate ratios, hazard ratios, and/or ROC curves for outcomes at various points in time.
6. The value of invasive or expensive tests used to assess prognosis depends on what decisions the additional prognostic information will help with, the importance of these decisions, and the likelihood that they will be changed by a more accurate estimate of prognosis.
7. Genetic tests whose purpose is to inform clinical decision making are critically appraised and used in the same way as other prognostic tests.

## References

Goodson, W. H., 3rd (2005). "Molecular prediction of recurrence of breast cancer." *N Engl J Med* **352**(15): 1605–7; author reply 1605–7.

Hafler, D. A., A. Compston, et al. (2007). "Risk alleles for multiple sclerosis identified by a genomewide study." *N Engl J Med* **357**(9): 851–62.

[3] We find it amusing that the significance was reported with 3 digits when the exponent was − 81!

Hilsenbeck, S. G., G. M. Clark, et al. (1992). "Why do so many prognostic factors fail to pan out?" *Breast Cancer Res Treat* **22**(3): 197–206.

Jellema, P., D. A. Van Der Windt, et al. (2007). "Prediction of an unfavourable course of low back pain in general practice: comparison of four instruments." *Br J Gen Pract* **57**(534): 15–22.

Kyzas, P. A., K. T. Loizou, et al. (2005). "Selective reporting biases in cancer prognostic factor studies." *J Natl Cancer Inst* **97**(14): 1043–55.

Mackillop, W. J., and C. F. Quirt (1997). "Measuring the accuracy of prognostic judgments in oncology." *J Clin Epidemiol* **50**(1): 21–9.

Paik, S., S. Shak, et al. (2004). "A multigene assay to predict recurrence of tamoxifen-treated, node-negative breast cancer." *N Engl J Med* **351**(27): 2817–26.

Ravdin, P. M., I. A. Siminoff, et al. (1998). "Survey of breast cancer patients concerning their knowledge and expectations of adjuvant therapy." *J Clin Oncol* **16**(2): 515–21.

SUPPORT (1995). "A controlled trial to improve care for seriously ill hospitalized patients. The study to understand prognoses and preferences for outcomes and risks of treatments (SUPPORT). The SUPPORT Principal Investigators." *JAMA* **274**(20): 1591–8.

Tanvetyanon, T. (2005). "Molecular prediction of recurrence of breast cancer." *N Engl J Med* **352**(15): 1605–7; author reply 1605–7.

Webster's unabridged dictionary (2001). New York, Random House Reference.

## Chapter 7 Problems: prognostic tests

1. Box 7.2 presents the findings from a study of oncologists' ability to discriminate between those cancer patients who are likely to survive, disease-free, for 5 years and those who are likely to die or have a recurrence (Mackillop and Quirt 1997). The authors assessed calibration as well as discrimination by comparing the predicted probability of cure to the actual disease-free survival rate in 5 subgroups of the 96 patients.

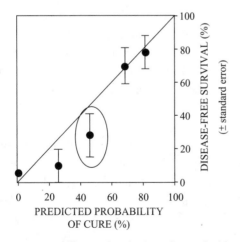

From Mackillop and Quirt (1997). Used with permission.

a) The circled point represents doctor-predicted versus actual cure (± standard error) for 12 patients to whom the doctors assigned a 40% to 59% chance of cure. Were the doctors overly optimistic or pessimistic?

b) What about the subgroup of patients (N = 48) to whom the doctors assigned a near 0% chance of cure? Were the doctors right?

2. Cytomegalovirus (CMV), like the chickenpox virus, varicella, is a virus to which most women have already been exposed before pregnancy. However, as with varicella, a pregnant woman with a first-time infection can pass the virus to the fetus. This congenital infection can lead to complications, including hearing loss. One way to test for congenital infection is to look for the virus in the baby's urine (viuria). Fowler et al. (1992) studied the risk of hearing loss in infants and children with congenital CMV.[4]

Here is an excerpt from the paper's Methods section.

Of the children in the study, 172 were identified through the obstetrical services at hospitals where we screened newborns for viuria to detect congenital CMV infection. Twenty-five additional congenitally infected newborns were referred to us by other hospitals or because the mother had evidence of infection on serologic screening or had illness during pregnancy or because elevated cord-blood levels of IgM or rheumatoid factor or symptoms of congenital infection in the newborn led to virologic testing.

a) Comment on the inclusion criteria for the 172 + 25 = 197 subjects in the study. What effect might the sample selection process have had on the results?

b) Overall, hearing loss occurred in 24 of 197 (12%) infants in this study. If you are seeing an infant with congenital CMV picked up on routine screening, what would you calculate as the lowest and highest risks of sensorineural hearing loss consistent with this study? (Ignore random error, i.e., do not do confidence intervals. We are just looking for the effect of the sampling scheme.)

c) Repeat part (b), but this time assume the infant was referred because of symptoms of congenital CMV.

3. In Box 7.1, we summarized a Dutch study of prognosis of low back pain (Jellema et al. 2007). In that study, a clinical prediction rule derived by the authors on the 314 subjects in the study had better discrimination than the general practitioner's (GP's) estimate of prognosis. Nonetheless, the authors concluded that "risk estimation by GPs . . . at present, seems to be the best available option."

a) Why do you suppose this conclusion was so cautious? Do you agree?

b) A close look at Figure 7.1b shows that there are only 6 points on the graph of predicted versus observed probabilities of a bad outcome. Normally, predicted probabilities are divided into deciles for these plots. If you assume that is the case, can you explain why there are only 6 points on this graph? (Hint: Recall the GPs rated their estimated probability rounding to the nearest 10%.)

4. Greenland et al. (2004) recently compared the Framingham Risk Score (FRS), obtained from history and physical examination and lipid levels, with a Coronary

---

[4] Thanks to Ruth Gilbert and Stuart Logan of the Evidence-based Child Health Centre in London for this example.

Artery Calcium Score (CACS) obtained from CT scanning in 1,461 asymptomatic adults at least 45 years old.

The FRS is an estimate of the 10-year risk of nonfatal myocardial infarction or death. The authors found that the CACS was predictive of this combined outcome among those with a FRS of more than 10%, but not in those with an FRS less than 10%, and they recommended against doing CACS when the FRS was less than 10%.

In a Letter to the Editor, Pletcher et al. (2004) wrote:

"In fact, such an interaction would be difficult to detect, and this study adds little evidence, given the low number of persons in the study with an FRS < 10% (n = 98) and the low number of events in this subgroup (n = 1)."

a) Do you think this lack of power affects the conclusion that CACS is not indicated in this low-risk group?

b) Pletcher et al. also point out that the FRS was less predictive of events in the Greenland et al. study, compared with previous studies, and postulated that this could occur if treatment decisions based on the FRS blunted its predictive ability. What could the authors do to address this possibility?

5. People with cancer that spreads to bone can have fractures and severe bone pain. Brown et al. (2003) investigated a measure of bone resorption, urinary N-telopeptide excretion (Ntx), as a predictor of these complications. Bisphosphonates are drugs used to strengthen bones and reduce fractures in people with osteoporosis.

From the abstract:

A total of 121 patients had monthly measurements of Ntx during treatment with bisphosphonates. All skeletal-related events, plus hospital admissions for bone pain and death during the period of observation, were recorded... **Patients with baseline Ntx values $\geq 100$ nmol/mmol creatinine (representing clearly accelerated bone resorption) were 19.48 times (95% CI 7.55, 50.22) more likely to experience a skeletal-related event/death during the first 3 months than those with Ntx < 100 ($P < 0.001$).** In a multivariate logistic regression model, Ntx was highly predictive for events/death. N-telopeptide appears useful in the prediction of patients most likely to experience skeletal complications and thus benefit from bisphosphonate treatment.

a) The "events" that the Ntx predicted included death. How might this have affected the results?

b) Here are the study results at 3 months:

|  | **Skeletal Complication (0–3 months)** | | |
| --- | --- | --- | --- |
| **NTX** | **Yes** | **No** | **Total** |
| $\geq$**100** | 41 | 15 | **56** |
| <**100** | 8 | 57 | **65** |
| **Total** | 49 | 72 | **121** |

Do you agree with the authors' statement? ("Patients with baseline Ntx values $\geq 100$ nmol/mmol creatinine... were 19.48 times... more likely to experience a skeletal-related event/death during the first 3 months than those with Ntx <100 . . . ")

c) The last sentence of the abstract states: "N-telopeptide appears useful in the prediction of patients most likely to experience skeletal complications and thus benefit from bisphosphonate treatment."

Do you agree that the study provides information on who might most benefit from bisphosphonates? Why or why not?

6. *TP53* is the gene for tumor-suppressor protein p53. In a multicenter, 7-year prospective cohort study, disruptive *TP53* mutations in tumor DNA (i.e., mutations leading to loss of function of p53) were associated with reduced survival after surgical resection in patients with squamous-cell cancer of the head and neck (Poeta et al. 2007).

a) Of the 420 subjects, 232 had died by the end of the follow-up period. Of these, 121 died from head and neck cancer, 62 from other causes, and 49 from unknown causes. The authors used overall survival as the outcome for all analyses. How would the use of overall (vs. cause-specific) survival affect the results?

b) How else could the authors have handled the subjects who died of other and unknown causes?

c) One question that arises for genetic tests is how much *new* information they provide. For example, if disruptive *TP53* mutations worsened prognosis by leading to more advanced stage at presentation, much of the prognostic information from *TP53* might be captured from stage at presentation. In fact, in this study, the nodal stage at presentation was highly predictive of survival. Bivariate (just one variable plus the outcome) and multivariate hazard ratios for nodal stage (N1–N3 vs. N0 or NX) and *TP53* (disruptive mutation vs. no mutation) are shown in the table below.

|                           | HR (95% CI)       |                   |
| ------------------------- | ----------------- | ----------------- |
| **Prognostic Factor**     | **Bivariate**     | **Multivariate**  |
| **Nodal Stage N1–N3**     | 2.0 (1.4–2.4)     | 2.4 (1.8–3.3)     |
| **Disruptive TP53 mutation** | 1.7 (1.3–2.4)  | 1.7 (1.3–2.4)     |

What can you conclude about whether the *TP53* gene provides *new* information about prognosis in head and neck cancer patients?

d) Assuming the hazard ratios reported in this study are valid and generalizable, what else would you need to know in order to decide whether to order this test on your patients?

## References for problem set

Brown, J. E., C. S. Thomson, et al. (2003). "Bone resorption predicts [0.3k] for skeletal complications in metastatic bone disease." *Br J Cancer* **89**(11): 2031–7.

Fowler, K. B., S. Stagno, et al. (1992). "The outcome of congenital cytomegalovirus infection in relation to maternal antibody status." *N Engl J Med* **326**(10): 663–7.

Greenland, P., L. LaBree, et al. (2004). "Coronary artery calcium score combined with Framingham score for risk prediction in asymptomatic individuals." *JAMA* **291**(2): 210–5.

Jellema, P., D. A. Van Der Windt, et al. (2007). "Prediction of an unfavourable course of low back pain in general practice: comparison of four instruments." *Br J Gen Pract* **57**(534): 15–22.

Mackillop, W. J., and C. F. Quirt (1997). "Measuring the accuracy of prognostic judgments in oncology." *J Clin Epidemiol* **50**(1): 21–9.

Pletcher, M. J., J. A. Tice, et al. (2004). "Use of coronary calcification scores to predict coronary heart disease." *JAMA* **291**(15): 1831-2; author reply 1832–3.

Poeta, M. L., J. Manola, et al. (2007). "TP53 mutations and survival in squamous-cell carcinoma of the head and neck." *N Engl J Med* **357**(25): 2552–61.

# Multiple tests and multivariable decision rules

## Introduction

In Chapter 3, when we introduced dichotomous tests, the LR of a positive result [LR(+)], and the LR of a negative result [LR(−)], we also made a point of distinguishing between prevalence and prior probability. Recall that prior probability is the more general term. The prior probability is equal to the prevalence of the disease in the population only when we do not know anything else about the patient. This is often the case for screening tests applied to large populations without obtaining information on individuals that allows differentiation between them. Although we tend to focus on laboratory or imaging tests, any new information about the patient can be used to update the prior probability of disease from what is known about the prevalence of disease in the population. As soon as we obtain individual-level information by taking a history and doing a physical examination, we develop a different estimate for the prior probability than the prevalence of the disease.

In this chapter, we discuss combining multiple types of information – elements of history, findings on physical examination, laboratory results, or radiographic images. We cover (at least theoretically) how we might get from prevalence to prior probability based on the history and physical examination, and then to posterior probability based on additional information from diagnostic tests. We begin by reviewing the concept of test independence, and then we discuss how to deal with departures from independence, which are probably the rule rather than the exception.

## Test independence

**Definition:** Two tests are "independent" if the LR for any combination of results on the two tests is equal to the product of the LR for the result on the first test times the LR for the result on the second test.

**Explanation:** What independence means is that, *among people who have the disease,* knowing the result of Test 1 tells you nothing about the probability of a certain result on Test 2, and that the same is true *among people who do not have the disease*. When we say the two tests are independent, we mean they are independent *once disease status is taken into account*. That is why we keep putting that part in italics. This is called "stratifying" on disease status. If we did not do this, then patients with an abnormal result on Test 1 would be more likely to be abnormal on Test 2 simply because they would be more likely to have the disease. Mathematically, the way to express this is to say the tests are "conditionally independent," by which we mean they are independent once the condition of having the disease or not is accounted for.

Using probability notation, independence means that, for every possible result $r_B$ of Test B, the probability of a patient with disease having that result, $P(r_B|D+)$, is the same regardless of the result that the patient has on Test A. If Tests A and B are dichotomous and the patient actually has the disease, independence requires that a false negative on Test B is no more likely because the patient had a false negative on Test A. It is easy to think of counterexamples – nonindependent tests – where a false negative on Test A makes a false negative on Test B more likely. For example, a patient with acute cardiac ischemia who does not have ST elevation on the electrocardiogram (ECG) is also less likely to have a positive troponin.[1]

Similarly, in a patient without disease, independence means the probability of the result, $P(r_B|D-)$, is the same regardless of the result on Test A. For dichotomous tests on a patient without the disease, independence requires that a false positive on Test B is no more likely because the patient had a false positive on Test A. Again, counterexamples are numerous. An abdominal pain patient *without* appendicitis who nevertheless has a fever is also more likely to have an elevated WBC count.

If neither $P(r_B|D+)$ nor $P(r_B|D-)$ depends on the result of Test A, then the LR for result $r_B$ on Test B, $P(r_B|D+)/P(r_B|D-)$, does not depend on the result of Test A. When this is the case, the tests are independent. We can start with any prior odds of disease and multiply by the LR for the result of Test A to get posterior odds of disease. Then, we use these odds as the prior odds for Test B, multiply by the LR for the result of Test B, and get the posterior odds after both Test A and Test B.

Perhaps it is easiest to understand independence by giving some examples of nonindependent tests. Suppose you are doing a study to identify predictors of pneumonia in nursing home residents with fever and cough. You determine that cyanosis has an LR of 5 and that an oxygen saturation of 85% to 90% has an LR of 6. If the patient is cyanotic *and* has an oxygen saturation of 87%, does that mean we can multiply the prior odds by $5 \times 6 = 30$ to get the posterior odds? No. Once we know that the patient is cyanotic, we do not learn that much more about the probability of pneumonia from the oxygen saturation, and vice versa.

There are at least three related reasons why tests can be nonindependent. The first is that they are measuring similar things. The cyanosis and low oxygen saturation example illustrates this. Some patients with pneumonia will be hypoxemic and some will not, and both the patient's color and the oxygen saturation are giving

---

[1] Troponin is a serum marker for heart muscle damage. It is actually a continuous test, but for current purposes it can be viewed as dichotomous.

information on that one aspect of pneumonia: hypoxemia. Jaundice, dark urine, light stools, and direct hyperbilirubinemia provide a similar example of tests that are measuring the same basic pathophysiologic manifestation of hepatitis, and therefore will not be independent.

A second reason is that the disease is heterogeneous. Pneumonia is heterogeneous in that some cases are associated with hypoxemia and some are not. Similarly, some cases of hepatitis are icteric and some are not. But disease heterogeneity can lead to test nonindependence even when the tests do not measure the same pathophysiologic aspect of the disease. For example, another cause of heterogeneity is disease severity. The most severe acute coronary syndromes are ST elevation myocardial infarctions, and these are also the acute coronary syndromes most likely to result in elevated troponins. Varying disease severity is an obvious cause of nonindependence for diseases with an arbitrary definition. For example, if we define coronary heart disease based on at least 70% stenosis of a coronary vessel, patients with 71% stenosis are more likely to have false-negative results on most tests than those with 98% stenosis, regardless of what pathophysiologic alteration is actually being measured.

Third, the nondisease may be heterogeneous. Lack of coronary disease is going to be much more difficult to diagnose in a patient with 69% stenosis than it is in patients with 10% stenosis. Alternatively, the nondisease group could be heterogeneous because it includes patients with other diseases that make the tests falsely positive. For example, if we were looking at LRs for bacterial meningitis in patients with headache and fever, the comparison group might include both patients with no meningitis at all and patients with viral meningitis. If that were the case, we would expect findings that pointed to meningitis in general [e.g., headache, stiff neck, photophobia, cerebrospinal fluid (CSF) pleocytosis] also to be nonindependent, because all of these would be more likely to be falsely positive in the subset of non–bacterial meningitis patients who had viral meningitis. Above, we gave the example of fever and WBC count as tests for appendicitis in patients with abdominal pain. A patient without appendicitis who does have fever is also more likely to have a high WBC count, because the same nonappendicitis condition causing his fever is also likely to cause an increased WBC count.

### Visualizing nonindependence using the LR slide rule

When tests are independent, their LRs can be multiplied, which is the same as adding on the LR slide rule's log(odds) scale (see Chapter 3). In other words, the arrows for their results can be laid end-to-end. If the tests are not independent – for example, if they measure the same pathophysiologic aspect of a disease – you cannot get the LR arrow for the combined results by laying the LR arrows for the individual results end-to-end.

For example, consider aspartate transaminase (AST) and lactate dehydrogenase (LD) enzyme levels[2] in the diagnosis of hepatocellular injury (liver inflammation). Conditions that cause a false-positive result on one (e.g., hemolysis, muscle injury)

---

[2] AST = Aspartate Transaminase, LD = Lactate Dehydrogenase. Both are important metabolic enzymes that are commonly elevated in hepatitis, but they can also be elevated when non-liver cells, such as blood cells

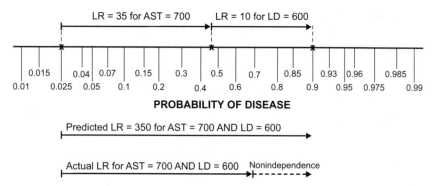

Figure 8.1     LR slide rule arrows demonstrate the concept of nonindependence. In diagnosing hepatocellular injury, the AST and LD are not independent because they can both be elevated in other conditions like hemolysis and muscle damage; therefore, the LR arrow for the combination of both AST = 700 and LD = 600 cannot be obtained by laying the LR arrows for each of these results end-to-end.

also make a false-positive result on the other more likely. Therefore, although the LR for AST = 700 might be 35, and for LDH = 600 might be 10, the LR for both AST = 700 *and* LD = 600 is likely to be a lot less than (10 × 35 =) 350, because the tests are not independent. This is illustrated in Figure 8.1.

## Combining the results of two dichotomous tests: an example

We start with an example of combining results from two prenatal sonographic tests for trisomy 21 (Down syndrome): nuchal translucency (NT) and examination for the nasal bone. Trisomy 21 can be established definitively by using chorionic villus sampling, but this is an invasive test that can accidentally terminate the pregnancy. Both NT and nasal bone examination are noninvasive tests done by ultrasound at approximately 13 weeks gestation. Examination of the nasal bone is a truly dichotomous test; absence of the nasal bone (NBA) is suggestive of trisomy 21 and therefore constitutes "positive" nasal bone exam for trisomy 21. NT is the measurement (in mm) of the subcutaneous edema between the skin at the back of the fetal neck and the soft tissue overlying the cervical spine. We pointed out in Chapter 4 that choosing a cut-off to make a continuous or multilevel test into a dichotomous test discards information. However, for purposes of exposition, we will use the cut-off of 3.5 mm to make NT a dichotomous test; we will consider an NT ≥3.5 mm "positive" for trisomy 21.

Cicero et al. (2004) reported NTs and nasal bone examinations on 5556 fetuses. The tests were done prior to definitive determination of trisomy 21 versus normal karyotype via chorionic villus sampling. The results are shown in Table 8.1.

Assume that the fetuses screened have a trisomy 21 prevalence of 6%. If a fetus has a NT ≥3.5 mm, the post-test probability of trisomy 21 is 31%. Ignoring the NT, if the fetus has NBA, the post-test probability is 64%. See if you can reproduce

and muscle cells are damaged. The units of both are International Units per Liter (IU/L). We left the units out in this text to improve readability.

**Table 8.1.** NT and NBA in fetuses with and without trisomy 21 as determined by chorionic villus sampling[a]

|  |  | Trisomy 21 | | |
|  |  | Yes | No | LR |
| --- | --- | --- | --- | --- |
| NT ≥ 3.5 mm | Yes | 212 | 478 | 7.0 |
|  | No | 121 | 4745 | 0.4 |
| **Total** |  | **333** | **5223** |  |

|  |  | Trisomy 21 | | |
|  |  | Yes | No | LR |
| --- | --- | --- | --- | --- |
| NBA | Yes | 229 | 129 | 27.8 |
|  | No | 104 | 5094 | 0.3 |
| **Total** |  | **333** | **5223** |  |

[a] From Cicero et al. (2004).

these calculations. They are displayed in Figure 8.2 on the LR Slide Rule's log(Odds) scale.

The calculations in Figure 8.2 apply if we consider either the NT ≥3.5 mm *or* NBA. What if we consider both? First, let us assume the two tests are independent. If the two tests are independent, we can multiply their LRs, so the LR for a combined positive result, NT ≥3.5 mm *and* NBA, would be 7.0 × 27.8 = 194. Using this LR and a pre-test probability of 6% results in a post-test probability of 92.5%. Figure 8.3 displays this calculation.

Now, rather than assuming independence, let us look at the actual data from the sample. If we consider both NT and the examination for the nasal bone together, there are four possible results. Table 8.2 shows the data and LRs associated with those four results.

Look at the top row of the table, where both tests are positive for trisomy 21. If both tests are positive, the LR is 68.8, not 7.0 × 28.8 = 194. Therefore, if the pre-test probability of trisomy 21 is 6% and both tests are positive, the post-test probability is 81%, not 92.5% (see Fig. 8.4).

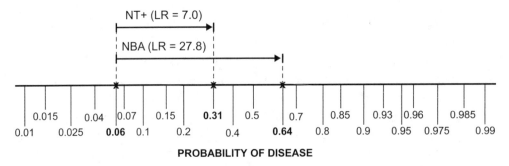

Figure 8.2    Starting with a 6% pre-test probability of trisomy 21, an NT ≥3.5 mm (NT+) increases the probability to 31%; ignoring the NT result, NBA increases the probability to 64%.

**Table 8.2.** The combination of NT and nasal bone examination results in fetuses with trisomy 21 and chromosomally normal fetuses

| NT ≥ 3.5 mm | NBA | Trisomy 21 | | | | |
|---|---|---|---|---|---|---|
| | | Yes | % | No | % | LR |
| Yes | Yes | 158 | 47.4% | 36 | 0.7% | 68.8 |
| Yes | No | 54 | 16.2% | 442 | 8.5% | 1.9 |
| No | Yes | 71 | 21.3% | 93 | 1.8% | 12 |
| No | No | 50 | 15.0% | 4652 | 89.1% | 0.2 |
| **Total** | | **333** | **100%** | **5223** | **100%** | |

[a] Data from Cicero et al. (2004).

NBA does not tell you as much if you already know that the NT is ≥3.5 mm. Even in chromosomally normal fetuses, enlarged NT is associated with NBA. Of normal (D−) fetuses with a negative NT (<3.5 mm), only 2.0% had NBA. Of normal (D−) fetuses with a positive NT (≥3.5 mm), 7.5% had NBA. A false-positive NT makes a false positive on the nasal bone examination more likely. Ontologically, narrowing of the nuchal stripe and ossification of the nasal bone both occur as the fetus develops.

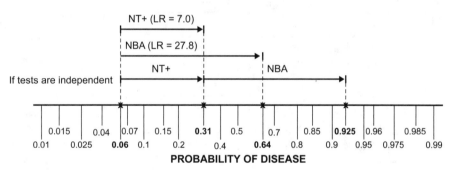

Figure 8.3    If the NT and nasal bone exams are independent, the LR of a combined positive result is the product of the LRs for a positive result on each test. On the log scale, multiplying LRs is the same as laying their arrows end-to-end.

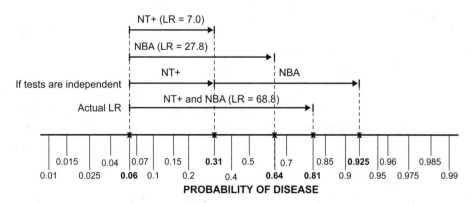

Figure 8.4    The LR associated with the combination of NT ≥3.5 mm (NT+) and NBA is less than the product of the LR for each result individually.

### Box 8.1: Spectrum bias in estimating the sensitivity of the nasal bone examination for fetal chromosomal abnormalities

Examination of the nasal bone is a noninvasive test used to determine which fetuses are at high enough risk to warrant chorionic villus sampling, which is a test for all chromosomal abnormalities, not just trisomy 21. Accurately estimating the nasal bone exam's sensitivity requires a clinically realistic group of chromosomally abnormal (D+) fetuses. The previously presented data from Table 8.1 on the sensitivity of the nasal bone examination are:

|            |     | D+  | D−    |
| ---------- | --- | --- | ----- |
| Nasal Bone | Yes | 229 | 129   |
| Absent     | No  | 104 | 5,094 |
| Total      |     | 333 | 5,223 |

Sensitivity = 229/333 = 69%.

The D+ group included only fetuses with trisomy 21 and excluded 295 fetuses with other chromosomal abnormalities, especially trisomy 18. If the purpose of the nasal bone exam is to determine when to get chorionic villus sampling, these 295 fetuses with chromosomal abnormalities other than trisomy 21 should be included in the D+ group. Of the 295, 95 (32%, not 69%) had NBA:

|            |     | D+              | D−    |
| ---------- | --- | --------------- | ----- |
| Nasal Bone | Yes | 229 + 95 = 324  | 129   |
| Absent     | No  | 104 + 200 = 304 | 5,094 |
| Total      |     | 333 + 295 = 628 | 5,223 |

Sensitivity = 324/628 = 52% (not 69%).

Including these 295 in the D+ group results in a sensitivity of 52%, not 69%, which constitutes a more clinically useful estimate of the sensitivity of NBA for chromosomal abnormalities.

Some chromosomally normal fetuses must develop more slowly than usual, resulting in both a positive NT and NBA.

### Spectrum bias

The example of combining the NT and nasal bone examinations also illustrates the issue of spectrum bias that we discussed in Chapter 5. Our example assumes that the only fetal condition at issue is trisomy 21. In fact, the data we presented excluded from the D+ group 295 fetuses with chromosomal abnormalities other than trisomy 21. This biased upward the sensitivity of each test individually and also exaggerated the accuracy of the two tests when used in combination. Box 8.1 shows numerically how this spectrum bias exaggerates the sensitivity of the nasal bone examination for chromosomal abnormalities.

## Combining the results of multiple dichotomous tests

We have demonstrated one way to handle the results of multiple tests: gather data on the LR for each possible combination of test results. For two dichotomous tests, as in our example above, there are four possible results ($+/+$, $+/-$, $-/+$, and $-/-$). For three such tests, there are eight possible results; for four tests, sixteen results; and so on. Even with large samples, you might not have enough data to calculate LRs for the uncommon result combinations.

Another approach is to lump together all discordant results, calculating one LR for this category, while calculating separate LRs for the concordant results (all positive or all negative). In the case of two dichotomous tests, there would be an LR for "positive–positive ($+/+$)," "negative–negative ($-/-$)," and "discordant ($+/-$ or $-/+$)." However, we saw in Chapter 3 that some tests are much more valuable when they are positive than when negative, or vice versa. A pathognomonic finding (specificity = 100%) should rule in disease when positive, regardless of other test results. Thus, if the pathognomonic finding is present and all the other tests are negative, it does not make sense to lump this together with other discordant results. Also, a single category for "discordant results" cannot accommodate multilevel or continuous tests.

A variant of the "lumping together" approach is to combine multiple tests into a decision rule that is considered positive if any one of the tests is positive. This approach has been used in the Ottawa Ankle Rule (Stiell et al. 1994) to determine which ankle-injury patients should get radiographs,[3] the NEXUS (National Emergency X-Ray Utilization Study) Rule (Hoffman et al. 1998, 2000) to determine which neck-injury patients should get cervical spine films,[4] and the San Francisco Syncope Rule (Quinn et al. 2004) to identify high-risk syncope patients requiring hospitalization.[5] This strategy clearly maximizes sensitivity, though at the expense of specificity. The main issue is deciding which of many candidate tests to include in the rule – a topic to which we will return.

## Recursive partitioning

Another approach is to use recursive partitioning to develop a fixed optimal sequence in which to do the multiple tests. "Recursive partitioning" (also called CART, for Classification and Regression Trees) is just what it sounds like – recursive meaning you do it over and over again, and partitioning meaning you divide up the data in different ways.

In our example of NT and examination for the nasal bone as tests for trisomy 21, which test should we do first? Figure 8.5 shows a tree of probabilities of trisomy 21 after each possible test result: (**A**) performing the nuchal translucency test first and (**B**) performing the nasal bone exam first. The nasal bone exam is better at discriminating between trisomy 21 and chromosomally normal fetuses. After a positive nasal bone

---

[3] Radiographs are recommended if the patient has tenderness of either malleolus, navicular, or base of the fifth metatarsal; or the patient is unable to bear weight for four steps both at the time of injury and the time of evaluation.

[4] Cervical spine films are recommended if the patient has any of the following: midline posterior cervical spine tenderness, alcohol or drug intoxication, abnormal alertness, focal neurologic deficit, or distracting painful injury.

[5] Hospitalization is recommended if the patient has shortness of breath, history of congestive heart failure, triage systolic blood pressure less than 90 mm Hg, hematocrit less than 30%, or abnormal electrocardiogram.

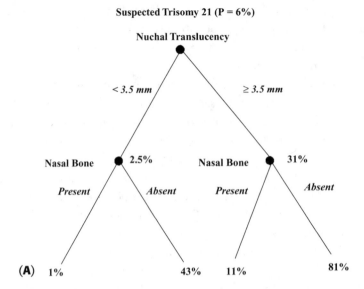

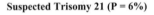

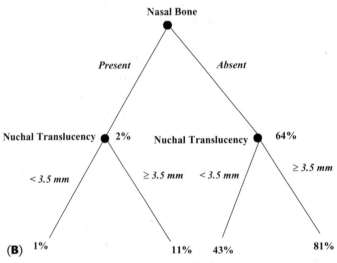

Figure 8.5 **(A)** Tree with branch-point probabilities of trisomy 21, assuming the NT test is performed first. **(B)** Tree with branch-point probabilities of trisomy 21 assuming the nasal bone exam is performed first.

exam (NBA), the probability of trisomy 21 is 64%; after a negative nasal bone exam (nasal bone present), the probability is 2%. This is as compared to 31% and 2.5% after positive and negative NTs, respectively. If your threshold probability ($P_{TT}$) for going on to chorionic villus sampling is 15%, you can stop after the nasal bone exam. After a positive nasal bone exam, a negative NT does not lower the probability of trisomy 21 below 15%, and after a negative nasal bone exam, a positive NT does not raise the probability of trisomy 21 above 15%. This suggests that you should do the nasal bone exam first.

For each sequence of tests, the LRs for the results of the second test are conditional on the result of the first test, the LR for the results of the third test are conditional on the results of the first and second tests, etc. At first, it would seem that you still have to work out the LRs for all possible combination of test results, but the algorithm is developed to "prune" branches of the tree and allow you to stop testing, or skip the next test(s) in the sequence. For example, after a negative result on a very sensitive test, you might stop testing – the probability has gotten so low that additional tests are not needed.

Whether to continue and do the NT test after the nasal bone exam depends on your actual threshold for chorionic villus sampling. We have seen that, if it is 15%, you can stop after the nasal bone exam. However, if it is 5% rather than 15% and the initial nasal bone exam is negative, you should continue with the NT test; a positive test will move the probability above the 5% threshold (Figs. 8.6A and 8.6B). If the initial nasal bone exam is positive, it does not make sense to do the NT test, because (at least as dichotomized here) the result cannot change your decision to proceed with chorionic villus sampling.

A classic example using recursive partitioning to develop a testing algorithm was developed by Goldman et al. to identify myocardial infarction in emergency department patients with chest pain (Goldman et al. 1988) (see Fig. 8.7). The percentages at each branch-point in Figure 8.7 represent the proportion of patients in that "partition" with acute myocardial infarction.

A much simpler example from the Pediatric Research in Office Settings Febrile Infant Study (Pantell et al. 2004) is shown in Figure 8.8. The percentages next to each branch-point in Figure 8.8 are the proportions of infants with bacteremia or meningitis.

Figures 8.5 through 8.8 display probabilities rather than LRs. We will return to this later, but if the LRs for a study like this are more generalizable than the actual probabilities, authors could publish just a subset of the LRs. Others could use these LRs with their own prior probabilities. For example, in the febrile infant example (Fig. 8.8), the only LRs related to temperature that would be needed would be those for $T \geq 38.6$ and $T < 38.6$ among infants who looked well and were at least 3.5 weeks old. This recursive partitioning algorithm ends up being a rule, like the Ottawa Ankle Rule and others mentioned above, that is considered positive if *any* of the individual tests is positive; that is, the infant is classified as "high risk" if he or she appears moderately ill, is $<3.5$ weeks old, or has a temperature $\geq 38.6°C$. This is a common, but by no means necessary, result of recursive partitioning algorithms; the chest pain algorithm in Figure 8.7 provides a counter-example.

Recursive partitioning handles continuous test results by selecting cut-offs to dichotomize the results. As we discussed in Chapter 4, selecting a fixed cut-off to dichotomize a test reduces the information to be gained from it, because a result just on the abnormal side of the cut-off is equated with a result that is maximally abnormal. However, with recursive partitioning, you are not necessarily done with a variable once you have dichotomized it. For example, an algorithm for predicting meningitis from CSF findings might first dichotomize the CSF WBC count

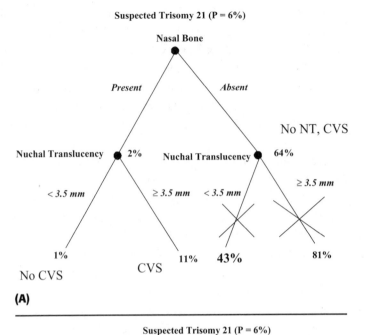

**(A)**

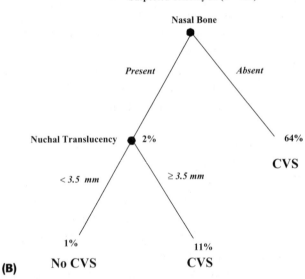

**(B)**

Figure 8.6    **(A)** If the probability threshold for chorionic villus sampling is 5% and the nasal bone is absent, a negative NT cannot change the decision to do chorionic villus sampling, so these branches in the tree may be pruned. **(B)** If the threshold probability for proceeding to chorionic villus sampling is 5%, the combination of nasal bone exam and NT becomes a two-test rule that is considered positive if either of the tests is positive.

(per mm$^3$) at 1,000; and then, if it was <1,000, dichotomize again at 100, where patients with CSF WBC count between 100 and 1,000 would be classified as high risk for bacterial meningitis if they had some other finding (e.g., low CSF glucose) as well.

Recursive partitioning software works by trying all different ways of splitting the data, and then selecting the way that leads to the least misclassification. The user is

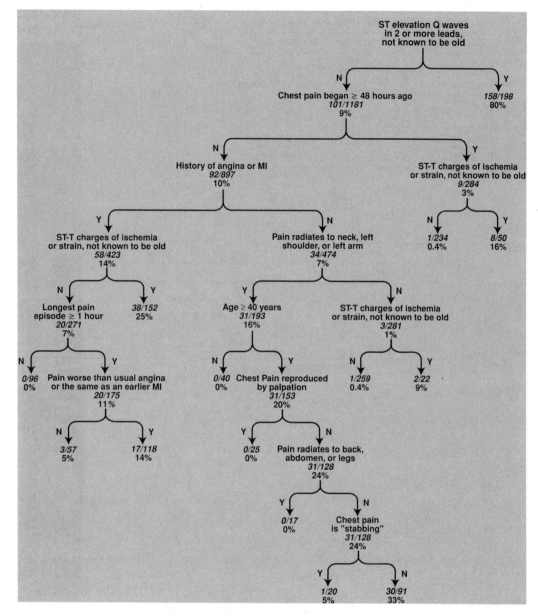

Figure 8.7　Recursive partitioning to predict the likelihood that a chest pain patient has myocardial infarction (Goldman et al. 1988; Lee et al. 1991).

allowed to specify the ratio of misclassification costs – that is, how much worse it is to have a false-negative than a false-positive result. For the febrile infant study example above (Fig. 8.8), the tree resulted from an analysis with the ratio of false-negative to false-positive misclassification costs set at 50:1.

Recursive partitioning does not assume that the risk of disease changes monotonically with a continuous test result. For example, in Chapter 4 we assumed that the probability of bacteremia increases as the peripheral WBC count increases, but this is not necessarily true in very young infants. A WBC count <5,000 has as high an

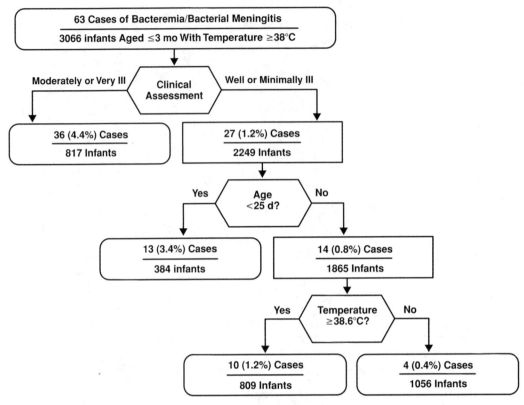

Figure 8.8    Recursive partitioning combining general appearance, age in weeks, and temperature to determine likelihood of bacteremia or bacterial meningitis in febrile infants <3 months old (Pantell et al. 2004). Used with permission.

LR for bacteremia as a WBC count between 25,000 and 30,000 (see Problem 4–5 for an illustration). However, if risk does change monotonically with a continuous test result, logistic regression (which we will discuss in the next section) provides a more efficient use of the data in predicting the risk of disease.

## Logistic regression

Partially because recursive partitioning deals less efficiently with continuous variables than with discrete variables, the most popular way to accommodate the results of multiple diagnostic tests where at least some results are continuous is multiple logistic regression modeling (Wasson et al. 1985; Laupacis et al. 1997; Katz 1999). In Chapter 3, we used odds instead of probabilities in Bayes's Theorem. Unlike probabilities, odds do not have an upper bound of 1, and pre-test odds can be multiplied by the LR of a test result to get post-test odds. Also in Chapter 3, we converted this multiplication into addition by replacing odds with their logarithms on the LR slide rule. Logistic regression takes advantage of these desirable properties of odds (compared with probabilities) and models the natural logarithm of the odds of disease [ln(odds)] as a linear function of the test results.

> **Box 8.2: How to calculate the OR for NBA in the diagnosis of trisomy 21**
>
> Here are the data on the nasal bone exam in fetuses with and without trisomy 21:
>
> |  |  | Trisomy 21 | | |
> |---|---|---|---|---|
> |  |  | **Yes** | **No** | **Odds** |
> | **NBA** | **Yes** | 229 | 129 | $229/129 = 1.775$ |
> |  | **No** | 104 | 5,094 | $104/5,094 = 0.020$ |
> |  | **Odds** | 229/104 | 129/5,094 | |
> |  |  | 2.202 | 0.025 | |
>
> The OR is
>
> $$\frac{\text{Odds of Disease in those with a Positive Test}}{\text{Odds of Disease in those with a Negative Test}} = \frac{\text{Odds}(D+|+)}{\text{Odds}(D+|-)} = \frac{1.775}{0.020} = 87$$
>
> Because of the symmetry of the odds ratio, this is the same as
>
> $$\frac{\text{Odds of a Positive Test in those with Disease}}{\text{Odds of a Positive Test in those without Disease}} = \frac{\text{Odds}(+|D+)}{\text{Odds}(+|D-)} = \frac{2.202}{0.025} = 87$$

## Odds ratios

The logistic regression coefficient for each test result is the natural logarithm of its multivariate odds ratio (OR). In Chapter 9, we will return to the OR in the context of quantifying the benefits of a treatment. (The OR is often used inappropriately to quantify treatment effects in randomized trials.) Here, we discuss how ORs are used to quantify the information provided by a positive test result or presence of a risk factor. ORs are easiest to understand when the test is dichotomous; in this case, the OR is the quotient of the odds of disease in those with a positive test divided by the odds of disease in those with a negative test:

$$\text{Odds Ratio} = \frac{\text{Odds of Disease in those with a Positive Test}}{\text{Odds of Disease in those with a Negative Test}}$$

In contrast with probabilities, odds work symmetrically so that this is also the quotient of the odds of a positive test in those with disease divided by the odds of a positive test in those without disease:

$$\text{Odds Ratio} = \frac{\text{Odds of a Positive Test in those with Disease}}{\text{Odds of a Positive Test in those without Disease}}$$

Box 8.2 shows the calculation of the OR for NBA in the diagnosis of trisomy 21.

The OR for a dichotomous test is also the LR of a positive result divided by the LR of a negative result. ORs and LRs are frequently confused. For test results, LRs are generally more appropriate to use than ORs, but when assessing risk factors with widely varying prevalences from population to population, the OR may be more useful, as shown in Box 8.3.

When the test is dichotomous, the farther the OR is from 1, the stronger the association between the test result and the disease. For continuous tests, the OR from logistic regression is the amount the odds of disease change per unit increase

**Box 8.3: Understanding the difference between ORs and LRs**

If we start with the prior probability of disease, P(D+), we can convert to prior odds, Odds(D+), and then multiply by the LR(+) or LR(−) to get the posterior odds:

Odds of disease given a positive test or exposure $= \text{Odds(D+|+)} = \text{Odds(D+)} \times \text{LR(+)}$

Odds of disease given a negative test or no exposure $= \text{Odds(D+|−)}$

$$= \text{Odds(D+)} \times \text{LR(−)}$$

The OR is the ratio of the posterior odds in those who test positive (or are exposed to a risk factor) to those who test negative (or are unexposed). Because the prior odds cancel out of that ratio, the OR is just LR(+)/LR(−).

$$\text{OR} = \text{Odds(D + |+)}/\text{Odds(D + |−)} = [\text{Odds(D+)} \times \text{LR(+)}]/[\text{Odds(D+)} \times \text{LR(−)}]$$
$$= \text{LR(+)}/\text{LR(−)}$$

If you want the odds of disease in a patient with a positive test result or exposure to a risk factor, you can either multiply the odds of disease *in the overall population* by the LR(+), or multiply the odds of disease *in the test-negative or unexposed population* by the OR. In other words, if you start with the overall odds of disease, you use the LR(+); if you start with the odds of disease in the test-negative or unexposed group, you use the OR. The only time the OR approximates the LR(+) is when the prevalence of a positive test or an exposure is so low that it doesn't significantly affect the population prevalence of disease. [In that case, the LR(−) will be very close to 1.]

The difference between ORs and LRs is illustrated in Figure 8.9. Consider a disease that has a strong risk factor, the prevalence of which varies widely in different populations. An example one of us has studied is UTIs in young febrile infant boys (Newman et al. 2002). The OR for UTI in uncircumcised boys, compared with circumcised boys, is about 10. What would be the LRs? The answer is that the LRs will depend on the proportion of the population that is circumcised. In Figure 8.9A, most of the boys in the population are circumcised. Therefore, the prior odds of UTI in a febrile boy will be low, and if he is circumcised (which we are calling being unexposed to the risk factor), the odds will not decline very much because they already start out low. On the other hand, if he is one of the few who is uncircumcised, the LR+ will be high and significantly increase his posterior odds.

Now consider the situation in a population where hardly any boys are circumcised (Fig. 8.9B). The prior odds start out much higher, reflecting this high prevalence of a strong risk factor for UTI. However, in this case, the odds change much more if the boy is circumcised than if he is not. Thus, for this type of clinical situation, LRs have the disadvantage that they are unlikely to be generalizable from one population to another. This is not the case for the sort of predictive factors that LRs were designed for: clinical tests, such as laboratory and imaging tests. For example, the prevalence of abnormality on laboratory tests (like the urinalysis) does not vary widely in populations as the prevalence of circumcision does. Hence, LRs for laboratory tests are more likely to be generalizable than LRs for risk factors or behaviors, the prevalence of which may vary widely across populations.

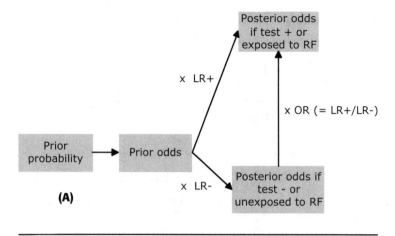

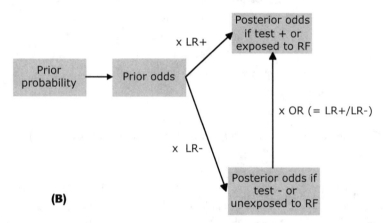

Figure 8.9    Relationship between prior odds, LRs (LR+ and LR−), posterior odds, and the OR. (**A**) Low prevalence of strong risk factor. (**B**) High prevalence of strong risk factor. The length of an LR arrow corresponds to the magnitude of the LR (actually the logarithm of the LR). The LR magnitudes change depending on the prevalence of the risk factor, whereas their ratio, the OR, remains the same.

in the test result. Thus, the OR for fever per degree will differ depending on whether the temperature is measured in Centigrade or Fahrenheit. (It will be farther from 1 for temperature measured in Centigrade.) If the units of measurement vary, it is not true that ORs farther from 1 always mean a stronger association with disease.

### Logistic regression modeling

We applied a logistic regression approach to the NT and nasal bone exam data, using NT ≥3.5 mm and NBA as dichotomous predictors of trisomy 21. The dataset included 5,556 records, one for each fetus evaluated. The variable for NT was valued "1" for NT ≥3.5 mm and "0" for <3.5 mm; the variable for NBA was similarly valued "1" if nasal bone absent or "0" if nasal bone present. The binary outcome variable for trisomy 21 was also coded in standard fashion. We entered the frequencies from Table 8.2 into our favorite statistical program (Stata). The results, as they might appear in a journal article, are shown in Table 8.3.

**Table 8.3.** Multivariate ORs resulting from a logistic regression model using fetal NT and NBA as dichotomous predictors of trisomy 21

|  | Multivariate OR for trisomy 21 | 95% CI for the OR |
|---|---|---|
| NT ≥ 3.5 mm | 8.7 | 6.3–11.8 |
| NBA | 53.0 | 38.7–72.7 |

The multivariate OR for NBA is much greater than the multivariate OR for NT. This allows us to say that, when both are available, NBA is a more important predictor of trisomy 21 than NT.

A multiple logistic regression model adjusts the OR associated with one dichotomous test for the fact that one or more additional tests are performed. Based on the data in Table 8.1, the univariate OR for NBA is 87.0 (calculated in Box 8.2) and the univariate OR for NT is 17.4. Because the two tests are not independent, the multivariate ORs are lower when both variables are included together than they are for each variable separately.

---

**Box 8.4: Advanced material on logistic regression: interaction terms and goodness of fit**

The logistic model presented in Table 8.3 does not include an interaction term. An "interaction term" is an additional term that distinguishes when both tests are positive from when only one or the other is positive. In the above model, the interaction term would be NT × NBA, which would equal "1" only if both tests were positive. Unless a logistic regression model includes interaction terms, the result of any given test changes the ln(odds) of disease by the same amount, regardless of how the other tests came out. For this reason, it is important to assess how well the logistic model fits the data – the so-called goodness of fit. The lack of an interaction term means our model for predicting trisomy 21 assumes that NBA has the same effect on the ln(odds) regardless of whether NT is ≥3.5 mm or <3.5 mm. As shown in the table below, this model fits the data reasonably well, and an interaction term is probably unnecessary.

**Comparison of Actual Probability of Trisomy 21 with Probability Predicted by the Logistic Regression Model Without an Interaction Term**

|  |  | Probability of Trisomy 21 | |
|---|---|---|---|
| Nuchal Translucency | Nasal Bone | Actual (%) | Predicted (%)[a] |
| ≥3.5 | Absent | 81 | 85 |
|  | Present | 11 | 10 |
| <3.5 | Absent | 43 | 39 |
|  | Present | 1 | 1 |

[a] Logistic regression model with no interaction term.

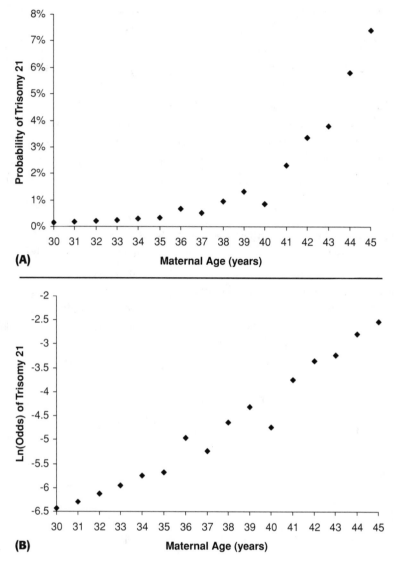

Figure 8.10 Probability of trisomy 21 as a function of maternal age (data from Snijders et al. 1999, Table 1). (**A**) Plot of probability versus maternal age. (**B**) Plot of ln(odds) versus maternal age.

### Logistic regression using the results of a single continuous test

So far in this chapter, we have violated the principle of Chapter 4 and discarded information by dichotomizing NT at 3.5 mm, calling an NT <3.5 mm "negative" and ≥3.5 mm "positive" for trisomy 21. In fact, an NT of 6 mm is much more suggestive of trisomy 21 than an NT of 3.5 mm. One of the main reasons to use logistic regression is to accommodate one or more continuous test results. To see why logistic regression models ln(odds) instead of probability, consider another predictor of trisomy 21: maternal age. Figure 8.10A shows the probability of trisomy 21 (at 16 weeks gestation) by maternal age. (Snijders 1999) Because probabilities are bounded by 0 and 1, the relationship between probability and a continuous variable, such as maternal age, is a distinctly nonlinear curve. If, instead of probability, we graph the ln(odds) as a function of maternal age, as in Figure 8.10B, we tend to get a simple linear relationship. This is why logistic regression models ln(odds) instead of probability as a linear function of test results.

As discussed in Chapter 4, we sometimes choose a cut-off value for a continuous test to trigger some action. In maternal–fetal medicine, the cut-off for obtaining a fetal karyotype by chorionic villus sampling or amniocentesis has been arbitrarily set at a 1 in 300 (0.33%) risk of trisomy 21. Based on logistic regression models used to fit data like those displayed in Figure 8.10, the maternal age cut-off should therefore be 35 years old.

### Logistic regression using the results of two continuous tests

The situation becomes more complex when logistic regression models use more than one continuous test to determine the patient's probability of disease. For example, a decision rule about proceeding to chorionic villus sampling might consider NT as well as maternal age. Now, we move from a single-variable logistic regression model to a multivariable model. The single cut-off value (35 years old) is replaced by a cut-off line or curve (Fig. 8.11). The line represents the NT cut-off at each maternal age. We expect this line to have a negative slope; the NT threshold should decrease as the maternal age increases.

For Figure 8.11, we defined high risk of trisomy 21 as probability greater than 1%. In a 21-year-old woman, a fetus with NT of 3 mm is considered low risk (<1%

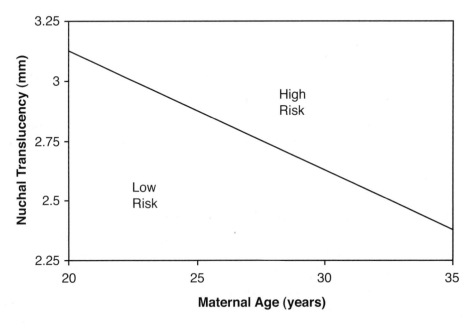

Figure 8.11 A hypothetical nomogram showing the combinations of maternal age and NT that identify fetuses at high risk for trisomy 21. In this nomogram, "high risk" is greater than 1% probability of trisomy 21 (Data abstracted from Nicolaides 2004, Figure 6, page 20).

probability of trisomy 21), but in a 34-year-old woman, a lower NT of 2.5 mm is considered high risk ($>1\%$ probability).

### Clinical decision rules developed using logistic regression

Like the rule of Goldman et al. for predicting myocardial infarction, developed using recursive partitioning, a famous example of a clinical decision rule developed using logistic regression is also for predicting myocardial infarction, as well as unstable angina. This is the Acute Coronary Ischemia–Time Insensitive Predictive Instrument (ACI-TIPI) (Selker et al. 1991, 1998). The predictors in this logistic model include sex, age, existence/importance of chest pain as a presenting symptom and multiple ECG findings (Table 8.4).

As an example, a 55-year-old man with chest pain as his major symptom and new Q waves on his ECG but no ST or T wave changes would have ln(odds) of acute coronary ischemia of $-3.93 + 1.23 + 0.88 + 0.71 + 0.67 - 0.43 + 0.62 = -0.25$, so the odds would be $e^{-0.25} = 0.78$ and the probability would be $0.78/1.78 = 44\%$. Although this is not practical for a clinician to calculate, the rule can be programmed into an ECG machine so that, if the technician enters a few items from the history, the estimated probability of acute coronary ischemia can be printed with the automated ECG analysis.

Another famous use of multiple logistic regression was the development of the PORT Pneumonia Score (Fine et al. 1997) to predict death in patients with

**Table 8.4.** Logistic regression coefficients from the ACI-TIPI model[a,b]

| Intercept | Coefficient | Multivariate OR |
|---|---|---|
| | −3.93 | |
| Presence of chest pain | 1.23 | 3.42 |
| Pain major symptom | 0.88 | 2.41 |
| Male sex | 0.71 | 2.03 |
| Age ≤40 | −1.44 | 0.24 |
| Age >50 | 0.67 | 1.95 |
| Male >50 years[c] | −0.43 | 0.65 |
| ST elevation | 1.314 | 3.72 |
| New Q waves | 0.62 | 1.86 |
| ST depression | 0.99 | 2.69 |
| T waves elevated | 1.095 | 2.99 |
| T waves inverted | 1.13 | 3.10 |
| T wave + ST changes[c] | −0.314 | 0.73 |

[a] From Selker et al. (1991).

[b] The multivariate OR is obtained by exponentiating the coefficients.

[c] This score includes two interaction terms. Male sex has an OR of 2.03 and age >50 years has an OR of 1.95. Without an interaction term, the OR for being both male and over 50 would be $2.03 \times 1.95 = 3.96$. The OR of 0.65 for being both male and over 50 indicates that 3.96 is too high and that $0.65 \times 3.96 = 2.57$ is a better estimate.

**Table 8.5.** Calculation of the PORT score to predict likelihood of death among patients with pneumonia

| Characteristic | Points assigned[a] |
|---|---|
| Demographic factor | +Age (years) |
| Age | |
| Sex | |
| Women | −10 |
| Nursing home resident | +10 |
| Coexisting illness | |
| Neoplastic disease | +30 |
| Liver disease | +20 |
| Congestive heart failure | +10 |
| Cerebrovascular disease | +10 |
| Renal disease | +10 |
| Physical-examination findings | |
| Altered mental status | +20 |
| Respiratory rate $\geq$30/min | +20 |
| Systolic blood pressure <90 mm Hg | +20 |
| Temperature <35°C or $\geq$40°C | +15 |
| Pulse $\geq$125/min | +10 |
| Laboratory and radiographic findings | |
| Arterial pH <7.35 | +30 |
| Blood urea nitrogen $\geq$30 mg/dL | +20 |
| Sodium <130 mEq/L | +20 |
| Glucose $\geq$250 mg/dL | +10 |
| Hematocrit <30% | +10 |
| Partial pressure of arterial oxygen <60 mm Hg | +10 |
| Pleural effusion | +10 |

[a] A total point score for a given patient is obtained by summing the patient's age in years (age − 10 for women) and the points for each applicable characteristic. The points assigned to each predictor variable were based on coefficients obtained from the logistic-regression model.

pneumonia. The authors used the coefficients from their logistic regression model to create the point scoring system shown in Tables 8.5 and 8.6.

## What happened to pre-test probability and misclassification costs? The clinician versus the decision rule

The output of the ACI-TIPI model as printed on the ECG header is a probability of acute coronary ischemia. Similarly, the recursive partitioning algorithms depicted in Figures 8.6 through 8.8 show disease probabilities next to the nodes. In Chapters 3 and 4, we always combined the test result with the pre-test likelihood of disease. In this chapter, we have estimated the probabilities from multivariable models assuming

**Table 8.6.** Mortality according to the PORT
score, excluding lowest risk "Class 1" patients[a]

| Score | 30-Day mortality |
| --- | --- |
| <71 | 0.6% |
| 71–90 | 2.8% |
| 91–130 | 8.2% |
| >130 | 29.2% |

[a] From Fine et al. (1997).

that our patients have a pre-test probability of disease that is the same as that in the sample used to develop the models. This is reasonable if the sample population is similar to our own or the model takes account of all the important variables that we would use to adjust our subjective pre-test probability estimate.

The clinician's advantage over a multivariable decision rule is the ability to adjust interpretation of test results based on the patient's pre-test probability of disease, if she knows that important variables have been left out of the model. The clinician's disadvantage is that this adjustment is done intuitively rather than mathematically, and without the benefit of the large dataset used to develop the decision rule.

The Ottawa Ankle Rules (Stiell et al. 1994) suggesting when radiographs can be deferred in patients with ankle injuries have been shown in a variety of settings to have high sensitivity for fracture while substantially reducing radiographs, relative to clinicians working without the benefit of the rules. This may be explained by the relative homogeneity (in terms of pre-test probability) of the population of patients with ankle injuries, or equivalently, by the rules' accounting for all the important predictors of finding a fracture on x-ray. It may be more difficult to account for all the important predictors of disease when the decision is whether to hospitalize a febrile child, or an adult with chest pain, syncope, or community-acquired pneumonia.

Clinical decision rules assume that the cost of failing to treat in the presence of disease and the cost of treatment in the absence of disease (B and C from Chapter 3) are the same from patient to patient. We have mentioned the clinician's ability to modify the decision threshold based on the pre-test probability of disease. But, the clinician also has the ability to adjust the decision threshold based on differing consequences of error. For example, failing to treat bacteremia in a 1-month-old has more serious consequences than failing to treat bacteremia in a 3-year-old; failing initially to treat bacteremia may also be worse if the family lives far from the hospital or has no home telephone. The above-mentioned risk threshold for fetal diagnostic procedures of 1 in 300 does not allow that failing to diagnose trisomy 21 may have different consequences for different women/couples/families. The ability to adjust for these differences is another potential advantage of the clinician over the decision rule.

## Selecting tests to include in a decision rule

Thus far, we have focused on how to combine the results of several tests, not on which tests to include in a clinical decision rule. We want to include those tests with the greatest ability to discriminate between D+ and D− individuals (at reasonable cost and risk). These are also the tests that we want to do first in a recursive partitioning algorithm. As an oversimplified example, if your "rule" for predicting fetal trisomy 21 can only consist of one sonographic screening test, it should clearly be examination of the nasal bone rather than NT (at least as dichotomized at 3.5 mm). There are always a number of candidate variables that may be important in determining the probability of disease. In developing a clinical decision rule, we have to choose just a few of these variables. This variable selection is best done based on biological understanding and the results of past studies. Often, however, research studies measure many predictor variables, and there is no strong basis for narrowing down the large number of candidate variables to the handful that provide the most predictive power. Stepwise multivariate models can help with this: they either start with a large number of variables in the model and remove the least statistically significant variables one at a time (backwards), or start with no predictor variables and add variables one at a time, each time adding the one that is most significant (forwards). The resulting models may be those that best predict outcome in the particular dataset from which they were derived, but they generally will do less well in other datasets, as discussed below.

### Importance of a derivation and a validation set

If you are allowed to choose combinations of tests and findings from a large number investigated, and then choose the cut-off that optimizes discrimination, you can often develop a prediction rule that works well in a specific sample (especially if the sample size is small). But this variable selection takes advantage of chance variations in the data that will no longer work to your advantage if you try to validate the prediction rule on a new dataset. As mentioned in Chapter 5, this is called "overfitting." For example, Oostenbrink et al. (2000) used four history variables, four laboratory variables, and ultrasound results to predict vesicoureteral reflux among 140 children (5 years and younger) who had their first UTI. Their final prediction rule had an AUROC of 0.78; at the cut-off they chose, it had 100% sensitivity and 38% specificity for Grade III or higher reflux, which was found in 28 subjects in their sample. When another group attempted to validate the rule on a similar group of 143 children, sensitivity and specificity at the same cut-off were only 93% and 13% respectively, neither clinically nor statistically significant (Leroy et al. 2006).[6]

The way to avoid (or at least quantify) overfitting is to develop a clinical prediction rule on one (generally randomly selected) group of patients, called the "derivation set" and then test it on a second group, called the "validation set." If overfitting occurred, the performance on the validation set will be substantially worse. If derivation and validation sets came from the same study, the investigator might be tempted to try again, tweaking the prediction rule so it performs better in the validation set. But, of course, this defeats the purpose of the validation set, and, in effect, makes the

---

[6] A quick shortcut: any time sensitivity and specificity sum to 1, the test is useless. In this case the sum is 1.06.

whole study a derivation set. (There is a subtle example in this chapter's Problem 2.) Finally, even if a prediction rule performs well in a validation set randomly selected from the study population, additional validation is helpful to determine how well it performs in different populations and different clinical settings.

## Summary of key points

1. When combining the results of multiple tests for a disease, it is only valid to multiply the LRs for the individual test results if the tests are independent.
2. Tests for the same disease are often nonindependent for three inter-related reasons:
   a) they measure the same pathophysiologic aspect of the disease;
   b) the diseased group is heterogeneous; and
   c) the nondiseased group is heterogeneous.
3. The ideal way to use results from multiple different tests would be to empirically define an LR for each possible combination of results. However, the number of possible combinations often makes this impossible.
4. The main two methods used to combine results of multiple tests are recursive partitioning and multivariable logistic regression.
5. Developing a decision rule for combining multiple tests often involves variable selection – that is, choosing which tests to include in the rule.
6. The choice of variables when deriving a decision rule is particularly subject to chance variations in the sample (derivation) dataset, and therefore, validation of the rule in a separate, independent population is important.

## References

Cicero, S., G. Rembouskos, et al. (2004). "Likelihood ratio for trisomy 21 in fetuses with absent nasal bone at the 11–14-week scan." *Ultrasound Obstet Gynecol* **23**(3): 218–23.

Fine, M. J., T. E. Auble, et al. (1997). "A prediction rule to identify low-risk patients with community-acquired pneumonia [see comments]." *N Engl J Med* **336**(4): 243–50.

Goldman, L., E. F. Cook, et al. (1988). "A computer protocol to predict myocardial infarction in emergency department patients with chest pain." *N Engl J Med* **318**(13): 797–803.

Hoffman, J. R., A. B. Wolfson, et al. (1998). "Selective cervical spine radiography in blunt trauma: methodology of the National Emergency X-Radiography Utilization Study (NEXUS) [see comments]." *Ann Emerg Med* **32**(4): 461–9.

Hoffman, J. R., W. R. Mower, et al. (2000). "Validity of a set of clinical criteria to rule out injury to the cervical spine in patients with blunt trauma. National Emergency X-Radiography Utilization Study Group." *N Engl J Med* **343**(2): 94–9.

Katz, M. H. (1999). *Multivariable Analysis: A Practical Guide for Clinicians.* Cambridge, Cambridge University Press.

Laupacis, A., N. Sekar, et al. (1997). "Clinical prediction rules. A review and suggested modifications of methodological standards." *JAMA* **277**(6): 488–94.

Lee, T. H., G. Juarez, et al. (1991). "Ruling out acute myocardial infarction. A prospective multicenter validation of a 12-hour strategy for patients at low risk." *N Engl J Med* **324**(18): 1239–46.

Leroy, S., E. Marc, et al. (2006). "Prediction of vesicoureteral reflux after a first febrile urinary tract infection in children: validation of a clinical decision rule." *Arch Dis Child* **91**(3): 241–4.

Newman, T. B., J. A. Bernzweig, et al. (2002). "Urine testing and urinary tract infections in febrile infants seen in office settings: the Pediatric Research in Office Settings' Febrile Infant Study." *Arch Pediatr Adolesc Med* **156**(1): 44–54.

Nicolaides, K. H. (2004). *The 11–13+6 Weeks Scan.* London, Fetal Medicine Foundation.

Oostenbrink, R., A. J. Van Der Heijden, et al. (2000). "Prediction of vesico-ureteric reflux in childhood urinary tract infection: a multivariate approach." *Acta Paediatr* **89**(7): 806–10.

Pantell, R. H., T. B. Newman, et al. (2004). "Management and outcomes of care of fever in early infancy." *JAMA* **291**(10): 1203–12.

Quinn, J. V., I. G. Stiell, et al. (2004). "Derivation of the San Francisco Syncope Rule to predict patients with short-term serious outcomes." *Ann Emerg Med* **43**(2): 224–32.

Selker, H. P., J. L. Griffith, et al. (1991). "A tool for judging coronary care unit admission appropriateness, valid for both real-time and retrospective use. A time-insensitive predictive instrument (TIPI) for acute cardiac ischemia: a multicenter study." *Med Care* **29**(7): 610–27. [For corrected coefficients, see http://medg.lcs.mit.edu/cardiac/tipicoef.htm.]

Selker, H. P., J. R. Beshansky, et al. (1998). "Use of the acute cardiac ischemia time-insensitive predictive instrument (ACI-TIPI) to assist with triage of patients with chest pain or other symptoms suggestive of acute cardiac ischemia. A multicenter, controlled clinical trial." *Ann Intern Med* **129**(11): 845–55.

Snijders, R. J., K. Sundberg, et al. (1999). "Maternal age- and gestation-specific risk for trisomy 21." *Ultrasound Obstet Gynecol* **13**(3): 167–70.

Stiell, I. G., R. D. McKnight, et al. (1994). "Implementation of the Ottawa ankle rules." *JAMA* **271**(11): 827–32.

Wasson, J. H., H. C. Sox, et al. (1985). "Clinical prediction rules. Applications and methodological standards." *N Engl J Med* **313**(13): 793–9.

## Chapter 8 Problems: multiple tests

1. Kaiser et al. (2002) performed a randomized study to evaluate CT and US as diagnostic tools for acute appendicitis in children. A total of 600 children with high clinical suspicion for acute appendicitis were enrolled; 283 were randomized to undergo US imaging only, and 317 children had both US and CT imaging (US was always done prior to CT scan).

   a) Use the results summarized in the Table below to create two 2 × 2 tables to calculate the positive LRs for CT and US results alone.

   Comparison of imaging findings with outcomes of patients who underwent both US and CT

   | | Concordant results (n = 267) | | Discordant results (n = 50) | |
   |---|---|---|---|---|
   | Outcome | US and CT positive | US and CT negative | US positive, CT negative | US negative, CT positive |
   | Appendicitis | 100 | 2 | 2 | 31 |
   | No appendicitis | 3 | 162 | 8 | 9 |

   *Note:* Data are numbers of patients, out of a total of 317 patients. Negative = findings were negative for appendicitis, positive = findings were positive for appendicitis. From Kaiser et al. (2002).

b) If your patient's prior probability of acute appendicitis was 10%, what would be the posterior probability, given positive (both) US and CT scan results? Assume that the two tests are independent.

c) Now create a 4 × 2 table like Table 8.2 and calculate the LRs for each possible US and CT result combination. Recalculate the posterior probability for a patient with a prior probability of 10% and positive results on both tests.

d) Are the two tests independent? Please explain how you know and suggest a possible biologic reason for your answer.

2. Kawasaki disease is an acute febrile illness in children of unknown cause that includes a rash, conjunctivitis, inflammation of mucous membranes, adenopathy, and swelling of hands and feet. Affected children are treated with intravenous immune globulin (IVIG) to prevent coronary artery aneurysms, the most serious complication of the disease. Using data from the intervention groups of two randomized controlled trials of IVIG, Beiser et al. (1998) developed an instrument to predict which children with Kawasaki disease would develop coronary artery aneurysms. The predictive instrument they developed is shown below (from Beiser et al. 1998. Used by permission.):

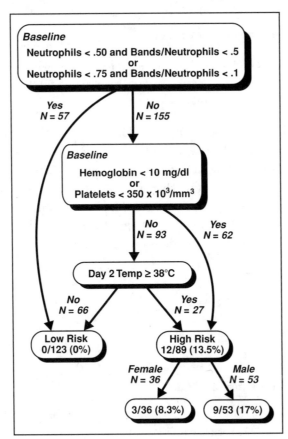

Neutrophils (also known as polymorphonuclear leukocytes) are one kind of WBC. Bands are immature neutrophils. "Neutrophils <0.5" means that, based on the WBC count differential, <50% of the white cells are neutrophils. "Bands/neutrophils <.5" means that, of all the neutrophils, fewer than 50% are bands.

a) What type of analysis do you think the investigators did to come up with this figure?

b) Assume you are treating a child like those included in the study. His initial CBC shows a hemoglobin of 11.2 g/dL, 600,000 platelets, and 13,000 WBCs/mm³, with 8,000 (61.5%) neutrophils of which 1,000 (1,000/8,000 = 12.5%) are bands. On day 2 of the illness, his temperature is 38.1°C. Would you classify him as high or low risk?

c) Now imagine the same patient, only this time he only has 5,000 neutrophils/mm³. He therefore is at low risk, regardless of his temperature on day 2. How does this help you manage your patient? For example, does this mean you don't need to treat him with IVIG?

d) In a study such as this, it is important that the clinical prediction rule be validated on a group of patients separate from the group used to derive it. The abstract of the study states:

"The instrument was validated in 3 test data sets . . . [it] performed similarly in the 3 test data sets; no patient in any data set classified as low risk developed coronary artery abnormalities."

However, the "Methods" section states:

"We developed many such [sequential classification] processes, each using a different combination of risk factors . . . Instruments that performed well on the development data set were validated using each of the 3 test data sets."

Is there a problem here? If so, what is it and how would it affect the results?

3. Based on results reported by Lee and Harper (1998), we simulated a dataset of 8,756 well-appearing, febrile children, 3 to 36 months of age, with no obvious source of infection (Kohn and Newman 2001). Using logistic regression, we developed two prototype decision rules combining temperature and WBC count to determine the need for antibiotic treatment. The figure below (from Kohn and Newman 2001) presents these two decision rules.

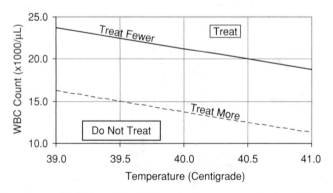

One rule ("treat more") prompts treatment when the odds of bacteremia are only 1:100; the other rule ("treat fewer") requires odds that are four times as high (1:25) before recommending treatment. In other words, the "treat more"

rule assumes that failing to treat a bacteremic child is 100 times worse than unnecessarily treating a child who is not bacteremic. The "treat fewer" rule assumes that such a false negative is only 25 times as bad as a false positive.

a) Assume that you agree with the "treat fewer" rule, that is, that your threshold odds for treatment are 1:25. Would you treat a 5-month-old boy with a fever of 39.5°C and a WBC count of $20 \times 10^3/\mu L$ if his prior probability was similar to that in the study from which the figure above was derived?

b) What if the fever was 41°C and the WBC count still 20,000/$\mu L$?

c) Explain why the slope of the line is negative (downward).

d) Explain why the "treat more" line is lower than the "treat fewer" line.

4. Goldman Prediction of Need for ICU.

Goldman et al. (1996) used recursive partitioning with a derivation dataset of 10,682 patients to divide emergency department chest pain patients into four risk groups: high, moderate, low, and very low. "Risk" refers to the risk of a major event (such as cardiac arrest, complete heart block, or cardiogenic shock) requiring intensive care.

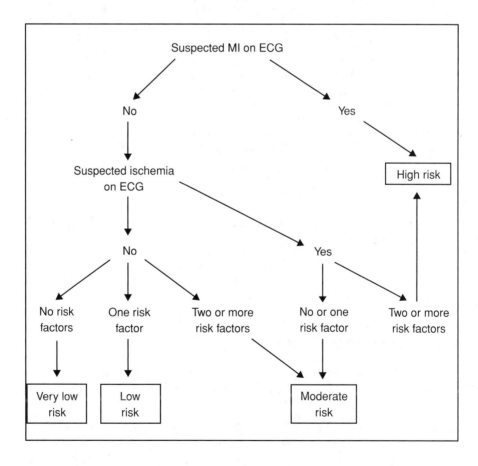

Myocardial infarction (MI) was suspected on the ECG if it showed ST-segment elevation of 1 mm or more or pathologic Q waves in two or more leads, and these findings were not known to be old. Ischemia was suspected if the ECG showed

ST-segment depression of 1 mm or more or T-wave inversion in two or more leads, and these findings were not known to be old. Risk factors included systolic blood pressure below 110 mm Hg, rales heard above the bases bilaterally on physical examination, and known unstable ischemic heart disease, defined as a worsening of previously stable angina, the new onset of postinfarction angina or angina after a coronary-revascularization procedure, or pain that was the same as that associated with a prior MI. The difference between each adjacent pair of risk groups was significant ($P < 0.001$).

a) A 67-year-old man presents to the Emergency Department with chest pain that he reports is "just like when I had my heart attack two years ago." His BP is 140/80 mm Hg, lungs are clear, and ECG is unchanged from one done in the cardiologist's office 6 weeks ago. What is his risk group?

b) The data (from the derivation dataset) on risks in each of the four risk groups are given in this table:

| Risk | Major Event | No Major Event | Total |
|---|---|---|---|
| High | 222 | 812 | 1,034 |
| Moderate | 158 | 1,791 | 1,949 |
| Low | 55 | 1,456 | 1,511 |
| Very Low | 48 | 6,140 | 6,188 |
| Total | 483 | 10,199 | 10,682 |

What is the overall risk of a major event in this population?

c) Assume that this system of risk stratification is reliable and that your population of chest pain patients has the same baseline risk of "major events" and is otherwise similar to Goldman's derivation set. What is your patient's risk?

d) As it turns out, the validation set for this risk stratification system had a different overall prevalence of major events. It was 168/4,676 or 3.6%. The LRs, however, were consistent between derivation and validation. If your population risk (prior probability) is more like the validation set, what would be the risk for a high-risk patient?

## References for problem set

Beiser, A. S., M. Takahashi, et al. (1998). "A predictive instrument for coronary artery aneurysms in Kawasaki disease. US Multicenter Kawasaki Disease Study Group." *Am J Cardiol* **81**(9): 1116–20.

Goldman, L., E. F. Cook, et al. (1996). "Prediction of the need for intensive care in patients who come to the emergency departments with acute chest pain." *N Engl J Med* **334**(23): 1498–504.

Kaiser, S., B. Frenckner, et al. (2002). "Suspected appendicitis in children: US and CT–a prospective randomized study." *Radiology* **223**(3): 633–8.

Kohn, M. A., and M. P. Newman (2001). "What white blood cell count should prompt antibiotic treatment in a febrile child? Tutorial on the importance of disease likelihood to the interpretation of diagnostic tests." *Med Decis Making* **21**(6): 479–89.

Lee, G. M., and M. B. Harper (1998). "Risk of bacteremia for febrile young children in the post-Haemophilus influenzae type b era." *Arch Pediatr Adolesc Med* **152**(7): 624–8.

# Quantifying treatment effects using randomized trials

## Introduction

As we noted in the Preface and Chapter 1, because the purpose of doing diagnostic tests is often to decide whether or how to treat the patient, we may need to quantify the effects of treatment to decide whether to do a test. For example, if the treatment for a disease provides a dramatic benefit, we should have a lower threshold for testing for that disease than if the treatment is of marginal or unknown efficacy. In this chapter, we discuss how to quantify the effects of treatments using the results of randomized trials. In Chapter 10, we will extend the discussion to observational studies of treatment efficacy.

In a randomized trial, study participants are randomly assigned to treatment groups, and the groups are compared to determine which had better outcomes. We begin by briefly reviewing the reasons to do randomized trials, then discuss their critical appraisal. Our approach is somewhat eclectic. Our goal is to highlight issues most important for obtaining and interpreting estimates of treatment effects, not to review the entire topic of randomized trials, and our selection is based partly on issues that seem to have received insufficient attention elsewhere.

We conclude this chapter with a discussion of calculating the treatment cost per bad outcome prevented, a rough step forward in the process of quantifying risks and benefits of treatments.

## Why do randomized trials?

The main reason to randomize is to estimate the effect of an intervention without confounding. "Confounding" in this context is the distortion of the estimated treatment effect by extraneous factors associated with the receipt of treatment and causally related to the outcome.[1] This distortion can occur in either direction. Confounding can make a treatment look better than it really is if factors associated with receiving treatment have a favorable effect on outcome. This can happen if, for example, the treatment is more likely to be received by people who are wealthier, better educated, or have better health habits or access to other beneficial treatments. Confounding can make a treatment look worse than it really is if the treatment is more likely to be given to people with a worse prognosis, for example, those who have a particular disease or for whom disease is more severe.

In Chapter 10, we will discuss ways to address the problem of confounding in observational studies of treatments. In this chapter, we discuss randomized trials, which minimize the possibility of confounding as a source of error. Randomization reduces the problem of confounding by creating treatment and control groups likely to be similar with respect to all confounders, both measured and unmeasured, known and unknown. Of course, even with proper randomization, it is possible that the two groups will be different with regard to certain confounders. If the groups do have significant chance asymmetries in important measured confounders, it is possible to control for these by using multivariable analysis or stratification. Most of the time, however, multivariable analyses are not needed.

## Critical appraisal of randomized trials

Before we turn to quantitatively estimating the effects of treatments, we review some issues in the design, conduct, and analysis of randomized trials that can affect the validity of these estimates.

### Design and conduct

#### Blinding

"Blinding," or masking, means keeping the treatment allocation secret. It can be done at three levels: the patient, the care provider, and the person assessing outcome. Blinding the patient prevents differences between groups due to the placebo effect. It is particularly important for subjective outcomes, like pain. Blinding patients in the control group keeps them from finding out that they are not getting active treatment and procuring it outside the study. Blinding the patient as well as the care provider helps avoid differences in co-interventions – that is, other interventions or changes in treatment such as additional care or medications. Finally, blinding the person responsible for outcome ascertainment is important to prevent observer bias. Again, this is most important for subjective outcomes. Thus, blinding the person responsible for outcome ascertainment would not be very important when total mortality is the outcome, but might be important for cause-specific mortality, which, as discussed in Chapter 6, depends on a more subjective process: assigning a cause of death.

---

[1] Terminology for this is not uniform. Some authors refer to this as selection bias. We prefer to refer to it as confounding because many of the methods used to deal with the problem are used to control confounding.

## Surrogate outcomes

It is important to distinguish between clinical outcomes the patient can perceive and surrogate outcomes. A "surrogate outcome" is one that is presumed to be associated with the outcome of interest, but is more easily measurable, or occurs more quickly and therefore is more convenient to use in a study. Examples include using changes in levels of risk factors for disease (e.g., blood pressure or bone density) rather than in the development of the disease itself (stroke or fractures), or changes in markers of disease activity or severity (e.g., viral load, hemoglobin A1c) rather than changes in morbidity or mortality from the disease. There are multiple examples of treatments that make the surrogate outcome better but have no effect (or harmful effects) on clinical outcomes of interest (Guyatt et al. 2008). As a general rule, you should be skeptical of studies where the only way the investigators could tell who benefited from an intervention was by doing tests.

## Composite endpoints

In some trials, several possible bad outcomes are grouped together into a composite endpoint. If this composite endpoint combines outcomes of varying importance, it may find a lower risk in the treatment group due entirely to a difference in the risk of a less important outcome. For example, a study (Waksman et al. 2002) of an intervention for blocked coronary artery bypass grafts showed improvement in a composite endpoint of death, myocardial infarction, and revascularization of the target vessel. However, death or myocardial infarction contributed only 5 of the 22 outcome events in the intervention group and 6 of the 43 events in the control group. Thus, there was no evidence that the intervention affected the more important outcomes of death or myocardial infarction – just revascularization. It is even possible for the treatment group to have more of the most important outcomes but sufficiently fewer minor outcomes to mask the increased risk of treatment or even make the composite treatment effect favourable. For example, in the Action to Control Cardiovascular Risk in Diabetes (ACCORD) trial of aggressive control of blood glucose in adults with diabetes (target hemoglobin A-1c level <6% vs 7−7.9%), the prespecified primary outcome was a composite outcome consisting of nonfatal MI, nonfatal stroke or cardiovascular death. (ACCORD Study Group, 2008). After a mean of 3.5 years of follow up there was a nonsignificant reduction in the risk of the primary outcome. But this negative result masked a statistically significant 1% absolute *increase* ($P = 0.04$) in total mortality that in the composite outcome was balanced by a 1% decrease ($P = 0.004$) in nonfatal myocardial infarction.

This sort of troubling discrepancy between fatal and nonfatal outcomes has been observed in other cardiovascular trials as well. A review (Ferreira-Gonzalez et al. 2007) of 114 randomized trials of cardiovascular interventions that used composite endpoints found that only 68% of the studies reported results for each component of the primary composite endpoint and that outcomes of greater importance to the patient (such as death) were associated with smaller relative treatment effects than less important outcomes.

Loss to follow-up

Loss to follow-up poses one of the most serious threats to the validity of randomized trials. A good rule to follow is: "once randomized, always analyzed." However, especially in long-term trials, it is possible to lose track of some study participants and, consequently, not know their outcomes. These losses to follow-up can reduce the power to find a difference simply by reducing the effective sample size, and they can introduce bias in either direction, especially if the reasons for losses to follow-up differ between the treatment groups.

For example, if the patients in the treatment group are lost to follow-up because of some negative effect of the treatment, or the patients in the control group are lost to follow-up because they have recovered from their illnesses, the study will be biased in favor of the treatment. As we described in Chapter 7, a sensitivity analysis can explore the maximum potential bias due to loss to follow-up, with a "worst-case" scenario that assumes poor outcomes for all losses to follow-up in the treatment group and good outcomes for all losses to follow-up in the control group. If a favorable effect of treatment persists, you can be confident that it is not an artifact due to losses to follow-up. More often, this approach will eliminate the treatment benefit or make treatment appear harmful and other approaches will be needed, such as seeking evidence of differences in prognostic factors between subjects lost to follow-up in the two groups.

## Analysis

Intention-to-treat, as-treated, and per-protocol analyses

When analyzing results in a randomized trial, the groups compared should be based on the treatment assigned rather than the treatment received. This is sometimes called an "intention-to-treat," as opposed to an "as-treated" analysis, because subjects are analyzed according to the intended treatment. An intention-to-treat analysis is important because patients who complete a course of treatment often have different (usually better) prognoses than patients who do not. For example, in a randomized comparison of coronary artery bypass graft surgery versus medical therapy for stable angina pectoris, some of the patients randomized to surgery became too ill to receive the operation and were treated medically instead (ECSSG 1979). If the results of this trial were analyzed on an "as-treated" basis, those patients too ill to receive surgery would be included in the medical treatment group, which would move patients with the worse prognoses from surgery to medical treatment and bias the results in favor of surgery (Hollis and Campbell 1999).

Between intention-to-treat and as-treated analyses are "per-protocol analyses," in which only those who were treated according to the protocol are analyzed. Although not as obviously biased as an as-treated analysis, a per-protocol analysis is still susceptible to bias, because patients treated according to the protocol are likely to be different from those who are not. A per-protocol analysis in the study of coronary artery bypass graft versus medical therapy would still have excluded patients with worse prognoses from the surgical group (because those patients did not receive the protocol treatment), but it would not have included them in the medical group. This still would have biased the results in favor of surgery, because the sickest patients would have been removed from that group (Hollis and Campbell 1999).

Dealing with this sort of crossover between groups using intention-to-treat analyses does have a disadvantage. The greater the number of subjects not treated according to the protocol, the less power the study will have, and the more the measure of effect size will be biased toward no effect. Thus, intention-to-treat analysis does not prevent bias; it just ensures that the bias is in a known direction (toward the null).

### Subgroup analyses

The focus of a randomized study is the comparison of the *overall* groups to which subjects are randomized, not comparisons of subgroups. Beware of studies that find no overall difference between treatment and control but highlight a treatment effect in one or another subgroup. If the authors looked at enough subgroups, they were bound to find a treatment effect in one of them. If the overall result is negative and one subgroup did better with treatment, then another subgroup probably did worse.

A classic illustration of the perils of subgroup analysis appeared in the publication of the ISIS-2 (Second International Study of Infarct Survival) results (ISIS-2 1988). This was a randomized trial of intravenous streptokinase, oral aspirin, both, or neither among 17,187 cases of suspected acute myocardial infarction. For the purposes of this discussion, the important overall result was that aspirin therapy (1 month of 160 mg/day) reduced cardiovascular mortality from 11.8% to 9.4% (P < 0.00001). There is no questioning this overall result in this well-done, randomized, blinded trial. The authors went on to discuss the results of aspirin therapy within several subgroups (diabetics, patients $\geq 70$ years old, patients with hypertension, a history of prior myocardial infarctions, etc.). They then cautioned readers about these subgroup analyses. To make this point, they divided the study population by astrological sign and showed that Geminis and Libras randomized to aspirin had 11.1% cardiovascular mortality, whereas those randomized to placebo only had 10.2% mortality (P = NS). Of course, given the overall positive effect of aspirin in the study, the patients with the other astrological signs had much lower mortality in the aspirin than in the placebo group (9.0% vs. 12.1%, P < 0.00001). Quoting from the paper:

> It is, of course, clear that the best estimate of the real size of the treatment effect in each astrological subgroup is given not by the results in that subgroup alone but by the overall results in all subgroups combined.

The ultimate message is to be wary of subgroup analyses, especially those without a strong biological basis.[2]

### Multiple comparisons

Unless there is a breakdown in either the randomization or the blinding, the only way to come up with a falsely positive result in a randomized double-blind trial

---

[2] We will see in Chapter 11 that the infinitesimally small pre-study probability that astrological sign affects response to aspirin, combined with weak evidence in favor of such an effect, results in a still negligible likelihood of a real effect.

(analyzed according to intention-to-treat) is by chance. The P-value provides only a rough indication of the likelihood of chance as a basis for the association. (We will discuss P-values in Chapter 11.) One of the most common causes for a falsely positive randomized double-blind trial result is that the investigators looked at multiple different outcomes in multiple different groups of patients in multiple different ways.

### Between-groups versus within-groups comparisons

One would think, having gone to all of the trouble of randomizing the subjects, that investigators would then compare the groups according to group assignment – that is, compare outcomes *between* groups. However, this is not always the case. Sometimes in a randomized trial, investigators will focus on within-group comparisons.

For example, a 2003 study (Nissen et al. 2003) randomized patients with acute coronary syndrome to receive either recombinant ApoA-I Milano or placebo. The authors reported in the abstract that atheroma volume decreased significantly in the treatment group ($P = 0.02$) but not in the control group ($P = 0.97$). However, the P-value for the difference between the two groups (reported in a footnote) was 0.29. Focusing on the within-group changes (in this surrogate outcome) suggested stronger evidence of benefit than the study provided.

### Direction of biases in randomized blinded trials

If randomization and blinding are done properly, follow-up is reasonably complete, and an intention-to-treat analysis is done, most other problems, such as poor adherence to treatment and random error in the measurement of the outcome variable, will make it harder to find statistically significant differences between the two groups, even if they exist (i.e., the trial will be falsely negative).

The tendency of poorly done studies to be biased toward finding no effect is a particular problem with equivalency trials, where a drug is judged to be effective if it is not demonstrably worse than a drug of known efficacy. In the case of equivalency trials, the normal motivation of investigators to do a trial very carefully in order to maximize the probability of finding a difference between groups is missing. This presents a difficult problem for regulatory agencies. If a treatment is known to be effective, it may not be ethical to randomize people to placebo. But if the investigators' goal for a trial is to demonstrate equivalence, it is easy to do a sloppy job in multiple subtle ways and increase the likelihood of obtaining the desired result.

## Quantifying treatment effects

### Continuous outcome variables

Many randomized trials have continuous outcome variables. For example, in Chapter 3, we estimated the benefit of treatment of influenza with oseltamivir as a reduction in the duration of illness by about one day. It is actually about 32 hours (Treanor et al. 2000). Aside from duration of illness, other examples of good continuous outcome variables are changes in symptom scores, weight, visual acuity, or pain level, because these are not surrogate outcomes but outcomes that the patient can perceive.

**Table 9.1.** Measures of effect size from a randomized trial summarized in a 2 × 2 table

|  | Bad outcome | No bad outcome | Totals |
|---|---|---|---|
| Treatment | a | b | **a + b** |
| Control | c | d | **c + d** |

$R_T$ = Risk in Treatment Group = $a/(a + b)$

$R_C$ = Risk in Control Group = Baseline Risk = $c/(c + d)$

$RR = R_T/R_c = \dfrac{a/(a + b)}{c/(c + d)}$

$RRR = 1 - RR$

$ARR = -\text{Risk Difference} = -(R_T - R_C) = R_C - R_T = c/(c + d) - a/(a + b)$

$NNT = 1/ARR$

$OR = ad/bc$ (generally should not be used for clinical trials)

The magnitude of differences between groups will depend on the units of measurement. When continuous outcomes are measured on an unfamiliar scale (e.g., a newly created symptom score), they are sometimes standardized by dividing the difference between groups by the standard deviation of the measurement.

### Dichotomous outcome variables

For dichotomous outcomes, such as death or recurrence of cancer, the treatment effect in a randomized trial can be measured with the risk ratio or relative risk (RR), relative risk reduction (RRR), the absolute risk reduction (ARR), and its inverse, the number needed to treat (NNT). The odds ratio (OR), as discussed below, is overused for measuring treatment effects in randomized trials. These measures are defined in Table 9.1.

A helpful (but by no means universal) convention is to put outcomes in columns and predictors in rows, with the "Bad Outcome" column on the left and the "Treatment" row on the top. When this convention is followed, an RR < 1 means the treatment is beneficial – that is, that it decreases bad outcomes. In contrast, an RR > 1 means the treatment is harmful in some way, as is commonly the case when the bad outcome is a side effect. Box 9.1 gives a specific example, calculating RR, RRR, ARR, and NNT for a randomized blinded trial to prevent breast cancer recurrence in postmenopausal women.

### Relative versus absolute measures of treatment effect

As was the case in the article cited in Box 9.1, the RRR is the most commonly reported summary measure of treatment effect. To truly understand the effectiveness of the treatment, however, not only relative measures like the RRR and RR, but also absolute measures (ARR and NNT) that account for the baseline risk should be considered. When the baseline risk is low (i.e., the outcome is rare), absolute risks are especially important to report, in order to give a realistic estimate of the likelihood of a treatment benefit for an individual patient. For example, in the letrozole study (Box 9.1), saying that the drug reduces risk of recurrence by 2.2% (from 5.1% to

**Box 9.1: Letrozole and breast cancer recurrence**

A front page headline in the *San Francisco Chronicle* (October 10, 2003) read: "Drug cuts risk of breast-cancer relapse. Findings so promising, study halted so scientists could release news" (Russell 2003). The article reported on a randomized double-blind trial of the aromatase inhibitor letrozole to prevent breast cancer recurrence after tamoxifen therapy in postmenopausal women. For the purposes of this chapter, the key quote from the newspaper story is the following:

The trial was interrupted almost $2^1/_2$ years after it began. Researchers had scheduled a midpoint peek at the data, and found letrozole was apparently working far better than expected. The women who took it had **43 percent** fewer recurrences of their breast cancer compared to those assigned in the study to take a placebo, or dummy pill.

    This letrozole study (Goss et al. 2003) was properly randomized and blinded, used an intention-to-treat analysis, and had minimal losses to follow-up. The trial originally planned to follow subjects for 5 years but was stopped after a median follow-up of 2.4 years. We will use the results to illustrate how to calculate the various measures of treatment effect: RR, RRR, ARR, and NNT:

|           | Recurrence | No Recurrence | **Total** |
|-----------|-----------|---------------|-----------|
| Letrozole | 75        | 2500          | **2575**  |
| Placebo   | 132       | 2450          | **2582**  |

Risk(Letrozole) = 75/2575 = 2.9%

Risk(Placebo) = Baseline Risk = 132/2582 = 5.1%

**RR** = Relative Risk or Risk Ratio = (2.9%)/(5.1%) = 0.57

**RRR** = Relative Risk Reduction = 1 − RR = 1 − 0.57 = 43%

**ARR** = Absolute Risk Reduction = − Risk Difference

$$= -(2.9\% - 5.1\%) = 2.2\% \text{ (over 2.4 years)}$$

**NNT** = Number Needed to Treat = 1/ARR = 1/2.2% = 45. This means that we need to treat 45 women with letrozole for an average of 2.4 years to prevent one additional recurrence of breast cancer.

**Treatment Cost per Bad Outcome Prevented:** The dose of letrozole is 2.5 mg/day. The cost of 30 pills (2.5 mg) is about $266,[3] so the cost of 2.5 years (30 months) of therapy is 30 months × $266/month = $7980. Because we have to treat 45 women to prevent one breast cancer recurrence, the treatment cost per breast cancer recurrence prevented is about 45 × $7980 = $359,100.

2.9%) sounds less impressive than saying that it reduces risk of recurrence by 43%. From the ARR of 2.2%, we can obtain the NNT of 45. What if the absolute recurrence rate in the control group were 1%? Then, the same 43% RRR would translate to an ARR of 0.43% and the NNT would be 1/0.57% = 175.

---

[3] (www.drugstore.com, 1/7/08).

Inflating the apparent effect size by using the odds ratio

The OR (Table 9.1) is another measure of treatment effect that is sometimes reported. However, it is generally not necessary or desirable to report the OR as a measure of effect size in a randomized controlled trial. The OR is an appropriate measure of association for case–control studies and a natural output of observational studies that use logistic regression to control for confounding. However, the RR has a much more natural and intuitive interpretation than the OR. Perhaps the reason that investigators sometimes use OR to report treatment effects in randomized controlled trials is that the OR is always farther from 1 than the RR. This can make results seem much more impressive than they are, especially when the outcome is relatively common. For example, in a randomized trial of varenicline to support smoking cessation, the 13- to 24-week abstinence rate was 70.5% with varenicline, compared with 49.6% with placebo (Tonstad et al. 2006). The authors reported the OR of 2.48, which is more impressive than the RR of 1.42. (They also did not follow the convention of putting the bad outcome, resumption of smoking, on the top.)

### Treatment cost per bad outcome prevented

In Chapter 1, we presented the following clinical scenario.

> **Clinical Scenario: Flu Prophylaxis**
>
> It is the flu season, and your patient is a 14-year-old girl with fever, myalgias, cough, and sore throat persisting for 1 day. Her mother has seen a commercial for Tamiflu® (oseltamivir) and asks you about prescribing it for the whole family so they don't catch the flu. Other family members in the household are the child's parents, her two younger brothers, and her maternal grandparents (in their 70s). They are currently well, but none has had the flu shot this year.
>
> You are considering testing the patient with a rapid bedside test for influenza A and B.

Welliver et al. (2001) addressed the issue of prophylactic oseltamivir in household contacts of patients with the flu. Their study was a randomized blinded trial of oseltamivir (Tamiflu®; 75 mg/day for 5 days) to prevent influenza in the household contacts of patients with flu-like symptoms during the 1998–1999 flu season. The results were stratified by whether the index case had laboratory-proven influenza (415 subjects) or not (540 subjects). This study was properly randomized and blinded, used an intention-to-treat analysis, and had minimal losses to follow-up.

The results of oseltamivir prophylaxis in household contacts of index cases with laboratory-proven influenza are shown in Table 9.2.

When the index case had laboratory-proven influenza, the baseline risk of the family contacts getting symptomatic influenza in the placebo group was 12.6%. The oseltamivir prophylaxis reduced this risk to 1.4%, an RRR of 89%.

The results of prophylaxis when the index cases did not have influenza suggested a nearly identical RRR, but a much lower baseline risk of getting symptomatic influenza (Table 9.3). In these family contacts of a flu-negative index case, the baseline risk of influenza was only 3.1%. The prophylaxis reduced this risk to a risk of 0.4%, again an RRR of 89%.

**Table 9.2.** Results of oseltamivir prophylaxis in household contacts of patients with laboratory proven influenza

| Index case flu+ | Household contacts | | | Risk |
| | Flu | No flu | Total | |
| --- | --- | --- | --- | --- |
| Oseltamivir | 3 | 206 | **209** | 3/209 = 1.4% |
| Placebo | 26 | 180 | **206** | 26/206 = 12.6% |
| **Total** | **29** | **386** | **415** | |

RR: 1.4%/12.6% = 0.114
RRR: 1 − RR = 89%
ARR: 12.6% − 1.4% = 11.2%
NNT[4]: 1/ARR = 9

If the RRRs were reported without the baseline risks, we would have no way of knowing how much better it is to treat a household contact when the index case is positive than when the index case is negative; the RRR was 89% in both groups.

In the letrozole example in Box 9.1, we introduced the idea of multiplying the NNT by the treatment cost ($C_{treat}$) to get the treatment cost of preventing one bad outcome:

NNT = Number Needed to Treat to Prevent One Bad Outcome

$C_{treat}$ = Cost of One Treatment

NNT × $C_{treat}$ = Treatment Cost/Bad Outcome Prevented

The ratio of treatment costs to bad outcomes prevented is a "cost effectiveness ratio." It is not *the* cost effectiveness ratio, because there are other ways to calculate a ratio of costs to outcomes prevented (see Box 9.2). Tamiflu® costs about $85 for ten

**Table 9.3.** Results of oseltamivir prophylaxis in household contacts of index cases who did not have influenza

| Index case flu− | Household contacts | | | Risk |
| | Flu | No flu | Total | |
| --- | --- | --- | --- | --- |
| Oseltamivir | 1 | 283 | **284** | 1/284 = 0.4% |
| Placebo | 8 | 248 | **256** | 8/256 = 3.1% |
| **Total** | **9** | **531** | **540** | |

RR: 0.4%/3.1% = 0.113
RRR: 1 − RR = 89%
ARR: 3.1% − 0.4% = 2.8%
NNT: 1/ARR = 36

---

[4] Strictly speaking, when the outcome prevented is an infectious disease, the number needed to treat should be decreased to account for the decreased transmission beyond the first-level contact. If $\alpha$ is the probability that one individual will pass the disease to another, the "discount factor" is $(1 - \alpha)$. We ignore the issue of second- and higher-generation infections because we want this discussion to apply to bad outcomes other than infectious diseases.

> **Box 9.2: Treatment cost per bad outcome prevented vs. traditional cost effectiveness analysis and cost benefit analysis**
>
> Multiplying the NNT by the treatment cost does not consider the dollar costs associated with the bad outcome that is prevented by the treatment. Thus, what we are calculating is the treatment cost of preventing one bad outcome along with all dollar costs associated with that bad outcome:
>
> $C_{treat}$ = Cost of One Treatment
>
> $C_{outcome}$ = Cost of One Bad Outcome
>
> $$NNT \times C_{treat} = \frac{\text{Treatment Cost}}{\text{Bad Outcome Prevented (including its costs)}}$$
>
> Because it is often much easier to estimate treatment cost ($C_{treat}$) than the costs associated with a bad outcome ($C_{outcome}$), we prefer to leave these outcome costs in the denominator. If, however, we are willing to estimate the bad outcome's costs, we can subtract these costs from the numerator and more closely approximate the cost effectiveness ratio that would result from a traditional cost effectiveness analysis.
>
> $$(NNT \times C_{treat}) - C_{outcome} = \frac{\text{Treatment Cost} - C_{outcome}}{\text{Bad Outcome Prevented}}$$
>
> In our example of flu prophylaxis, suppose the dollar costs of a case of the flu amount to $400. (This would include all of the dollar costs we can easily count,[5] including missed work, ibuprofen for myalgias and fever, some chance of a doctor visit, etc., but not the discomfort of having the flu.) Our original treatment cost per flu case prevented was $405. Now, because each flu case is associated with $400 in costs, the new cost effectiveness ratio is $405 − $400 = $5 per flu case prevented. Considering the costs of a bad outcome along with treatment costs to prevent the bad outcome leads to a lower total cost per bad outcome prevented. For the rest of this chapter, we will lump the costs associated with a bad outcome along with the bad outcome itself in the denominator.
>
> Once we account for all of the financial costs, we are left with the cost to prevent the discomfort of the flu. Theoretically, we could assign a dollar value to that, too. Then we could do a cost–benefit analysis, in which we simply add up all of the costs and benefits and see if we come out ahead. For example, if we assign a dollar value of $440 for the discomfort of having the flu, then we could say we spend a net $5 on medication and get $440 worth of relief of suffering in return, so we would come out $435 ahead for each case of the flu we prevent. (Of course, we might do even better with the influenza vaccine!)

75-mg pills.[6] We assume that a prophylactic course (5 pills) would cost about $45. With this treatment cost ($C_{treat}$), we can calculate the cost of preventing a case of influenza if the index case is influenza-positive (Flu+) or influenza-negative (Flu−).

Index Case Flu+:

NNT = 9 (Treat 9 household contacts, prevent 1 flu case.)

NNT × $C_{treat}$ = 9 × $45 = $405/flu case prevented

---

[5] Something that we can't easily count, but probably should be considered, is the possibility of contributing to the development of resistance to oseltamivir.

[6] www.drugstore.com 1/7/08.

Index Case Flu−:

NNT = 36 (Treat 36 household contacts, prevent 1 flu case.)

NNT × $C_{treat}$ = 36 × \$45 = \$1620/flu case prevented

The RRR associated with treating the contacts of Flu− index cases is the same as for contacts of Flu+ index cases. However, the baseline risk of contracting influenza is four times lower, so the absolute benefit is four times lower, and the cost per flu case prevented is four times higher. In fact, for the rest of this discussion, we will assume that the benefit of treating the household contacts of Flu− patients is negligible. In Chapter 1, we discussed the definition of disease and the assumption that nondiseased patients would not benefit from treatment. In this case, the "disease" is being the household contact of a Flu+ index case. While the "nondiseased" contacts of a Flu− case would, in fact, benefit slightly, this benefit can be ignored with minimal loss of accuracy.

## Uncertainty about whether the patient has the disease

When we do not know whether our patient has the disease (D+) and will benefit from treatment, we must adjust our NNT upward (again assuming no benefit to treating D− patients). The adjusted NNT (NNT*) is the original number needed to treat (calculated only using D+ patients) divided by the probability (P) of disease.

NNT = Number Needed to Treat to prevent one bad outcome assuming that all
        those treated are D+

P = Probability of D+

NNT* = Adjusted Number Needed to Treat = NNT/P

In our flu prophylaxis example, we do not know if our 14-year-old patient actually has influenza or some other viral illness. The prevalence of laboratory-proven influenza in the oseltamivir prophylaxis study (Welliver et al. 2001) was about 45%. Assuming that this is the prevalence of influenza in our population, the expected ARR is only 45% as large, so the NNT will be 1/0.45 times as high[7]:

NNT if index case Flu+ = 9.

Probability of flu = P = 0.45

ARR* = 0.45 × ARR

NNT* = NNT/P = 9/0.45 = 20

NNT* × $C_{treat}$ = Treatment Cost/Bad Outcome Prevented

Cost/Case Prevented = 20 × \$45 = \$900

Now suppose we decide that it is worth no more than \$1080 in treatment costs to prevent a case of the flu (and its associated costs). Because each patient we treat costs

---

[7] More generally, the ARR will be a weighted average of the ARR in those in whom the index case does and does not have the flu. In this case, it would be ARR = P × 11.2% + (1 − P) × 2.8%

$45, we can say that if the NNT* is more than $1080/$45 = 24, then it would not be worth treating. So now the question is: at what probability of influenza in the index case $P_{TT}$ will the NNT* be no more than 24? Again, neglecting the small benefit from treating influenza-negative index patients, that probability will be when NNT* = NNT/$P_{TT}$ (see above), so it will be when $P_{TT}$ = NNT/NNT* = 9/24 = 0.375. Thus, if you treat household contacts when the index case's probability of the flu is 37.5% or higher, you will not spend more than $1080 per case of flu prevented. Now, assume that you can test for the flu. In Chapter 3, we discussed how to use $P_{TT}$ and the test characteristics [LR(+) and LR(−)] to calculate lower and upper probabilities where a testing strategy could make sense.[8]

### "Number needed to harm"

To this point we have only considered the trade-off between the dollar costs of treatment and the effectiveness of treatment in preventing bad outcomes. Treatments are often associated with undesired effects that should also be balanced against the reduced risk of the primary outcome. Undesired effects of treatment can be evaluated using the same kind of 2 × 2 table as desired effects. In our flu prophylaxis example, oseltamivir was more frequently associated with nausea than was placebo (Table 9.4).

The RR for a side effect like nausea is greater than one (RR = 2.1), and because the risk of the bad outcome is higher in the treatment group than in the control group, the ARR is negative. Because we prefer dealing with positive numbers, we calculate an absolute risk increase (ARI = −ARR), rather than an ARR. The number needed to harm (NNH)[9] is defined as 1/ARI, so it is actually the number of patients treated for each one harmed. In this case, the NNH is 35, so for every 35 patients treated, we will cause one additional case of nausea.

In some cases, especially when a treatment is associated with severe or common side effects, we might be interested in quantifying the trade-off between side effects and primary outcome prevention, rather than the trade-off between dollar costs

**Table 9.4.** Association of oseltamivir prophylaxis with nausea

|  | Household contacts | | | |
| --- | --- | --- | --- | --- |
|  | Nausea | No nausea | **Total** | Risk |
| Oseltamivir | 27 | 467 | **494** | 27/494 = 5.5% |
| Placebo | 12 | 449 | **461** | 12/461 = 2.6% |

RR: 5.5%/2.6% = 2.10

ARR: 2.6% − 5.5% = −2.9%

ARI: 5.5% − 2.6% = 2.9%

NNH: 1/ARI = 35

---

[8] In terms of Chapter 3, net benefit B of treating a household contact of a flu+ individual is the expected benefit of treatment less the cost of treatment: 1/9 × $1080 − $45 = $75. The cost C of treating a household contact of a flu− individual (who we assume will not benefit) is $45. The threshold odds are C/B = $45/$75 = 0.6, and the threshold probability is 0.6/(1 + 0.6) = 0.375. Since you would use the test on the index case to guide treatment on 6 individuals, the testing cost T is the cost of testing the index case divided by 6.

[9] "Number Needed to Harm" is an established term that really means "Number Needed to Treat to Cause Harm in One."

and outcome prevention. For example, we might be more interested in the trade-off between the nausea associated with oseltamivir treatment and the reduced likelihood of the flu. We can then calculate the number of "harms" per primary outcome prevented. This is simply the ARI for the undesired effect divided by the ARR for the primary outcome, or equivalently, the NNT divided by the NNH:

"Harms"/Bad Outcome Prevented = ARI/ARR = NNT/NNH.
In the case of flu prophylaxis,

Cases of Nausea/Flu Case Prevented = ARI/ARR = NNT/NNH = 9/35 ~ 1/4

This means that we cause one-fourth of a case of nausea for each case of the flu that we prevent, or one case of nausea caused for every four cases of the flu prevented. This is an attractive trade-off because a case of the flu is typically much worse than an episode of medication-induced nausea. The ratio of side effects caused per primary outcome prevented is a cost effectiveness ratio in which the costs are measured in side effects caused instead of dollars spent.

For the nausea associated with oseltamivir prophylaxis and for most other side effects of treatment, the NNH should not be adjusted for the likelihood of disease, as there is no reason to believe that oseltamivir is less likely to cause nausea in household contacts of Flu− patients than in those of Flu+ patients.

## Summary of key points

1. In a randomized blinded trial of a treatment, the purpose of the randomization is to ensure that, at baseline, the groups are similar with respect to confounders, both known and unknown.
2. The purpose of the blinding is to prevent differential co-interventions and biased outcome assessment.
3. In order to preserve the value of randomization, the study should compare the randomized groups in an intention-to-treat analysis and minimize losses to follow-up.
4. Use caution with studies using surrogate outcomes or relying on subgroup analysis to show a treatment effect.
5. When the outcome of a randomized blinded trial is dichotomous, such as death or recurrence of cancer, one assesses the treatment effect by comparing the outcome risk in the treatment and the control groups. The ratio of these risks is the risk ratio; the difference between them is the absolute risk reduction.
6. The inverse of the absolute risk reduction is the number needed to treat to prevent one outcome.
7. The treatment cost per bad outcome prevented is simply the number needed to treat times the cost of treatment.
8. In the case of side effects, the risk of the undesired outcome is higher in the treatment than the control group; the risk difference is the absolute risk increase, and its inverse is the number needed to harm.
9. Using the results of randomized blinded trials to balance the effectiveness of treatment in preventing undesired outcomes with the costs and risks of

unnecessary treatment helps determine the treatment threshold – that is, the likelihood of disease at which treatment is indicated.

10. This treatment threshold probability can, in turn, be used with test characteristics to determine when a diagnostic test might be helpful in guiding treatment decisions.

## References

Accord Study Group (2008). "Effects of intensive glucose lowering in type 2 diabetes." *N Engl J Med* **358**(24): 2630–3.

ECSSG (1979). "Coronary-artery bypass surgery in stable angina pectoris: Survival at two years. European Coronary Surgery Study Group." *Lancet* **1**(8122): 889–93.

Ferreira-Gonzalez, I., J. W. Busse, et al. (2007). "Problems with use of composite end points in cardiovascular trials: systematic review of randomised controlled trials." *Br Med J* **334**(7597): 786.

Goss, P. E., J. N. Ingle, et al. (2003). "A randomized trial of letrozole in postmenopausal women after five years of tamoxifen therapy for early-stage breast cancer." *N Engl J Med* **349**(19): 1793–802.

Guyatt, G., D. Rennie, et al. (2008). *Users' guides to the Medical Literature: A Manual for Evidence-Based Clinical Practice.* 2nd ed. Chicago, IL, AMA Press: 119–130.

Hollis, S., and F. Campbell (1999). "What is meant by intention to treat analysis? Survey of published randomised controlled trials." *Br Med J* **319**(7211): 670–4.

Hulley, S. B., S. R. Cummings, et al. (2007). *Designing Clinical Research: An Epidemiologic Approach.* 3rd Ed. Philadelphia, PA, Lippincott Williams & Wilkins.

ISIS-2 (1988). "Randomised trial of intravenous streptokinase, oral aspirin, both, or neither among 17,187 cases of suspected acute myocardial infarction: ISIS-2. ISIS-2 (Second International Study of Infarct Survival) Collaborative Group." *Lancet* **2**(8607): 349–60.

Nissen, S. E., T. Tsunoda, et al. (2003). "Effect of recombinant ApoA-I Milano on coronary atherosclerosis in patients with acute coronary syndromes: a randomized controlled trial." *JAMA* **290**(17): 2292–300.

Russell, S. (2003). Drug cuts risk of breast-cancer relapse. *Chronicle.* San Francisco, CA. Oct 10, Page l.

Tonstad, S., P. Tonnesen, et al. (2006). "Effect of maintenance therapy with varenicline on smoking cessation: a randomized controlled trial." *JAMA* **296**(1): 64–71.

Treanor, J. J., F. G. Hayden, et al. (2000). "Efficacy and safety of the oral neuraminidase inhibitor oseltamivir in treating acute influenza: a randomized controlled trial. US Oral Neuraminidase Study Group." *JAMA* **283**(8): 1016–24.

Waksman, R., A. E. Ajani, et al. (2002). "Intravascular gamma radiation for in-stent restenosis in saphenous-vein bypass grafts." *N Engl J Med* **346**(16): 1194–9.

Welliver, R., A. S. Monto, et al. (2001). "Effectiveness of oseltamivir in preventing influenza in household contacts: a randomized controlled trial." *JAMA* **285**(6): 748–54.

## Chapter 9 Problems: quantifying the treatment effects

1. Otitis media with effusion (OME) is common in infants and young children. The basic problem is that the eustachian tube does not work well, and the kids get fluid and negative pressure in the middle ear, which can cause mild to moderate conductive hearing loss and an increased risk of acute (purulent) otitis media (ear infection).

A controversial clinical trial (Mandel et al. 1987) found that, in children who had OME for 3 months, resolution rates at 4 weeks were about 30% with the antibiotic amoxicillin (with or without an antihistamine/decongestant) and about 14% with placebo.

a) Using the conventions suggested in the chapter (RR is the risk of something bad in the treatment group relative to the control group), what are the RR, RRR, ARR, and NNT to prevent one persistent effusion?

b) Why are the RRR and ARR so similar in this case?

The reason why the study was so controversial is that one of the investigators (Erdem Cantekin) so disagreed with the other investigators that he published an alternative report on the same study in *JAMA* (Cantekin et al. 1990, 1991; Rennie 1991) after the other investigators reported the results in the *New England Journal of Medicine*. One of Cantekin's main points was that blinding was suspect and no benefit was apparent when the outcome was assessed objectively (by tympanometry). After excluding 43 children (13.3% of the placebo group and 7.4% of amoxicillin group; $P = 0.122$) who had developed acute otitis media during the follow-up period, he came up with the following numbers (simplified from his Table 3):

| Outcome Measure | Amoxicillin (%) | Placebo (%) | Difference (%) | P |
|---|---|---|---|---|
| Normal by otoscopy | 35.2 | 19.2 | 16.0 | 0.004 |
| Normal by algorithm (defined in protocol) | 25.6 | 13.9 | 11.7 | 0.027 |
| Normal by tympanometry | 17.8 | 10.0 | 7.8 | 0.121 |
| Normal by hearing test | 21.9 | 18.0 | 3.9 | 0.611 |
| Hearing improved >10 dB | 31.5 | 32.5 | −1.0 | 0.311 |

c) Do you agree with the decision to exclude children who developed acute otitis during the follow-up period? What effect might this have had on the results tabulated above?

d) Do you agree with Cantekin's conclusion that amoxicillin was not effective, based on the results for the most objective outcome measurement (tympanometry)?

2. Children with bacterial meningitis can suffer brain damage or hearing loss, referred to respectively as neurologic or audiologic sequelae. Odio et al. (1991) did a randomized blinded trial of the corticosteroid dexamethasone to prevent neurologic or audiologic sequelae in 99 infants and children with bacterial meningitis. From the "Results" section of their abstract:

At follow-up examination, 7 of the . . . 51 dexamethasone-treated children (14 percent) and 18 of 48 . . . controls (38 percent) had one or more neurologic or audiologic sequelae ($P = 0.007$); the relative risk of sequelae for a child receiving placebo as compared with a child receiving dexamethasone was 3.8 (95 percent confidence interval, 1.3 to 11.5) . . .

a) The risk of sequelae was lower in the dexamethasone group (14%) than in the control group (38%). In other words, the dexamethasone was beneficial. Why is the reported RR greater than 1?
b) Even allowing for part (a), the reported RR is incorrect. Calculate the correct RR.
c) How did the authors get the wrong number?

3. Patients with chronic hepatitis who have the "e" antigen of the hepatitis B virus in their blood stream (HBeAg), tend to suffer worse liver damage. Patients with chronic hepatitis are also commonly treated with interferon alfa. Read the following abstract with this question in mind: Does treatment with interferon alfa improve clinical outcome in this group of patients?"

---

Long-Term Follow-Up of HBeAg-Positive Patients Treated with Interferon Alfa for Chronic Hepatitis B (Niederau et al. 1996)

**Background** In patients with chronic hepatitis B, treatment with interferon alfa and the consequent loss of hepatitis B e antigen (HBeAg) from the blood leads to a reduction in inflammatory activity, but the clinical benefits of this treatment have not been established. **We evaluated whether HBeAg seroconversion induced by interferon alfa improves clinical outcome.** [Emphasis added]

**Methods** We studied prospectively a cohort of 103 patients treated with interferon alfa for chronic hepatitis B; the mean ($\pm$SD) follow-up was $50.0 \pm 19.8$ months. Fifty-three untreated patients served as controls.

**Results** After treatment with interferon alfa, 53 of 103 patients no longer had detectable HBeAg or hepatitis B virus DNA, although only 10 patients became seronegative for hepatitis B surface antigen (HBsAg) . . . Of the 53 untreated patients, only 7 spontaneously eliminated HBeAg . . . and all remained positive for HBsAg ($P < 0.001$ for the comparison with the treated patients, by the proportional-hazards model). During follow-up, 6 of the 103 treated patients died of liver failure, and 2 needed liver transplantation; all 8 were persistently positive for HBeAg. In another eight treated patients, complications of cirrhosis developed; all but one of these patients remained positive for HBeAg. Overall survival and survival without clinical complications were significantly longer in patients who were seronegative for HBeAg after therapy with interferon alfa than in those who remained seropositive ($P = 0.004$ and $P = 0.018$, respectively). In a regression analysis, clearance of HBeAg was the strongest predictor of survival. Of the 53 untreated patients, 13 had severe complications (including 4 deaths and 1 need for liver transplantation); all 13 continued to be HBeAg-positive. **Conclusions** In patients with chronic hepatitis B infection, the clearance of HBeAg after treatment with interferon alfa is associated with improved clinical outcomes.

    a) The treatment group had 103 patients, and the control group had 53 patients. How were patients assigned to these groups?

    b) Create a 2 × 2 table comparing the composite outcome of liver transplant or death from liver failure in the treated and untreated patients. Lay out the 2 × 2 table according to the conventions suggested in the chapter and calculate the risk (of the composite outcome) in the control group, $R_C$, and the risk in the treatment group, $R_T$. Also calculate the RR.

    c) Is the conclusion of the abstract correct? Discuss.

4. An abstract of a trial of intranasal lidocaine (a local anesthetic) for treatment of migraine headaches (Maizels 1996) is excerpted below:

> OBJECTIVE: To evaluate the effectiveness of intranasal lidocaine for treatment of acute migraine headache.
>
> DESIGN: Prospective, randomized, double-blind, placebo-controlled trial.
>
> SETTING: Community urgent care department.
>
> PATIENTS: A total of 81 patients (67 women and 14 men; median age, 42 years; range, 19–68 years) with a chief complaint of headache who fulfilled criteria of the International Headache Society for migraine participated . . .
>
> INTERVENTION: Patients were randomized in a 2:1 ratio to receive a 4% solution of intranasal lidocaine or saline placebo, respectively.
>
> MAIN OUTCOME MEASURES: The primary outcome measure was at least 50% reduction of headache within 15 minutes after treatment . . .
>
> RESULTS: Of 53 patients who received intranasal lidocaine 29 (55%) had at least a 50% reduction of headache compared with 6 (21%) of 28 controls (P = .004)
>
> CONCLUSIONS: Intranasal lidocaine provides rapid relief of headache in approximately 55% of ambulatory patients with migraine . . .

    a) Is the main outcome variable in this study subjective or objective?

    b) Intranasal administration of 4% lidocaine might feel different to the patient than administration of saline. What problem could this cause?

    c) Do you agree with the conclusion that: "Intranasal lidocaine provides rapid relief of headache in approximately 55% of ambulatory patients with migraine?" Why or why not?

5. In the chapter, we learned from the ISIS-2 Study (ISIS-2 1988) that aspirin therapy (1 month of 160 mg/day) in patients with acute myocardial infarction (AMI) reduced 30-day cardiovascular mortality from 11.8% in the placebo group to 9.4% in the aspirin group (P < 0.00001).

    a) What is the ARR?

    b) How many AMI patients need to be treated with aspirin for 30 days to prevent one death?

c) A 120-pill bottle of 81-mg aspirin tablets costs about $5.00. Considering only the cost of the treatment drug, use this to calculate the cost per bad outcome prevented for aspirin therapy of AMI. (Be careful, you only need 60 aspirin pills to treat 1 patient for 30 days.)

ISIS-2 and other studies also showed that, when added to aspirin, thrombolysis with streptokinase reduced mortality even further. The GUSTO Study (GUSTO 1993) compared thrombolysis using tissue plasminogen activator (tPA) with thrombolysis using streptokinase (SK) in reducing the 30-day mortality of patients with AMI receiving aspirin. This study showed a 14% RRR in the tPA-treated patients. Controversy exists because other large studies found no difference in 30-day mortality. Also, only the subgroup of American (not European) patients showed a benefit, and it was not a blinded study. However, for this problem, assume that the 14% RRR is real. The 30-day mortality risk in the SK group was 7.3%.

d) What was the 30-day mortality risk in the tPA group?

e) What was the ARR associated with tPA (vs. SK)?

f) How many patients need to be treated with tPA instead of SK to prevent one death?

g) The cost of tPA is about $3,400 per course of treatment, and the cost of SK is about $560 (Peacock et al. 2007). What is the approximate treatment drug cost per death prevented by using tPA instead of SK?

6. A randomized, double-blind, multi-center trial of tegaserod (Zelnorm®) for chronic constipation in 1,264 patients (Kamm et al. 2005) reported response rates of 40.2% with tegaserod 6 mg twice a day, compared with 26.7% with placebo ($P = 0.0059$). (A 2-mg dose was less effective.) The primary outcome was an increase of at least 1 complete spontaneous bowel movement (CSBM) per week over a 4-week period, compared with a 2-week baseline period.

a) If we consider those who did not respond to be treatment failures, what are the RR, RRR, and ARR (for treatment failure) for tegaserod 6 mg twice a day in this study?

b) What is the approximate NNT (with 6 mg Zelnorm twice a day for 4 weeks) for each patient that responds by having at least one CSBM per week?

c) Before it was taken off the market for causing heart attacks, Zelnorm® cost about $180 for 60 pills (http://www.drugstore.com, accessed 11/9/06). What is the cost of a week of treatment at the dose above per patient that responds?

d) The endpoint of this study was an increase of ≥1 CSBM. If each of the responders actually has two additional CSBM per week, what is the approximate cost of Zelnorm® per CSBM?

## References for problem set

Cantekin, E. I., T. W. McGuire, et al. (1990). "Biomedical information, peer review, and conflict of interest as they influence public health." *JAMA* **263**(10): 1427–30.

Cantekin, E. I., T. W. McGuire, et al. (1991). "Antimicrobial therapy for otitis media with effusion ('secretory' otitis media)." *JAMA* **266**(23): 3309–17.

GUSTO (1993). "An international randomized trial comparing four thrombolytic strategies for acute myocardial infarction. The GUSTO investigators." *N Engl J Med* **329**(10): 673–82.

ISIS-2 (1988). "Randomised trial of intravenous streptokinase, oral aspirin, both, or neither among 17,187 cases of suspected acute myocardial infarction: ISIS-2. ISIS-2 (Second International Study of Infarct Survival) Collaborative Group." *Lancet* **2**(8607): 349–60.

Kamm, M. A., S. Muller-Lissner, et al. (2005). "Tegaserod for the treatment of chronic constipation: a randomized, double-blind, placebo-controlled multinational study." *Am J Gastroenterol* **100**(2): 362–72.

Maizels, M., B. Scott, et al. (1996). "Intranasal lidocaine for treatment of migraine: a randomized, double-blind, controlled trial." *JAMA* **276**(4): 319–21.

Mandel, E. M., H. E. Rockette, et al. (1987). "Efficacy of amoxicillin with and without decongestant-antihistamine for otitis media with effusion in children. Results of a double-blind, randomized trial." *N Engl J Med* **316**(8): 432–7.

Niederau, C., T. Heintges, et al. (1996). "Long-term follow-up of HBeAg-positive patients treated with interferon alfa for chronic hepatitis B." *N Engl J Med* **334**(22): 1422–7.

Odio, C. M., I. Faingezicht, et al. (1991). "The beneficial effects of early dexamethasone administration in infants and children with bacterial meningitis." *N Engl J Med* **324**(22): 1525–31.

Peacock, W. F., J. E. Hollander, et al. (2007). "Reperfusion strategies in the emergency treatment of ST-segment elevation myocardial infarction." *Am J Emerg Med* **25**(3): 353–66.

Rennie, D. (1991). "The Cantekin affair." *JAMA* **266**(23): 3333–7.

# Alternatives to randomized trials for estimating treatment effects

## Introduction

We said in Chapter 9 that randomized blinded trials are the best way of determining treatment effects because they minimize the potential for confounding, co-interventions, and bias, thus maximizing the strength of causal inference. However, sometimes observational studies can be attractive alternatives to randomized trials, because they may be more feasible, ethical, or elegant. Of course the issue of inferring causality from observational studies is a major topic in classical risk factor epidemiology. In this chapter, we focus on observational studies of treatment effects rather than risk factors, describing methods of reducing or assessing confounding that are particularly applicable to such studies.

## Confounding by indication

We discussed in Chapter 9 that confounding refers to the distortion of the effect of variable A on the outcome C by a third variable B, which is both associated with A and a cause of C. We focus on treatments that are supposed to be beneficial, that is, to have an RR < 1 for a bad outcome. One type of confounding makes treatments appear better than they really are – for example, finding a beneficial treatment effect when, in truth, the treatment either has no effect or causes harm. In this situation, a confounder is associated with receiving the treatment and reduces the risk of a bad outcome (Fig. 10.1).

An example is use of vitamin E to prevent cardiovascular disease. Multiple observational studies suggested a protective effect, but randomized trials have found no benefit (Eidelman et al. 2004), suggesting that some other factors (e.g., better diet, exercise, or health awareness) are the true cause of the lower risk of cardiovascular disease among users of vitamin E (Fig. 10.2).

Alternatively, when a confounder that is associated with receiving the treatment increases the risk of a bad outcome, it can mask or reduce the apparent benefit of the

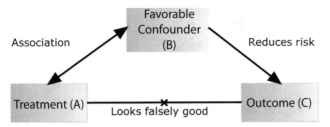

**Figure 10.1** Confounder is the true cause of improved outcomes making the treatment look more effective than it really is.

treatment[1] (Katz 1999). For example, if only the sickest people get the treatment in question, the treatment may look harmful even when it actually helps. This effect is often called "confounding by indication," because often those in whom the treatment is most indicated are those at highest risk of the bad outcome that the treatment is designed to prevent.

An example of confounding by indication is diuretic treatment of hypertension in diabetics. It is now clear that treating hypertensive diabetics with diuretics reduces their risk of cardiovascular mortality (Turnbull et al. 2005). However, a cohort study (Warram et al. 1991) appeared to show that diuretics increased the risk of cardiovascular mortality in hypertensive diabetics compared with leaving the hypertension untreated. The confounder was the severity of cardiovascular disease. The patients with more severe disease were more likely to be treated with diuretics, and they were also more likely to die of their cardiovascular disease (Fig. 10.3).

Confounding by indication can be controlled the same way as any other type of confounding. However, thinking about confounding by indication takes some getting used to, because in classical risk-factor epidemiology, investigators are usually looking for factors that increase, rather than decrease, risk. In epidemiologic studies, protective factors that decrease risk tend not to be selectively present in those otherwise at higher risk, as happens when treatments are given to people at higher risk of the outcome. Thus, suppression is more likely to be an issue in studies of treatments than in studies of naturally occurring risk factors.

## Instrumental variables

When we discussed the "Intention to Treat" principle in Chapter 9, we acknowledged that, in randomized controlled trials, there might be an imperfect relationship between the predictor variable of interest (e.g., actual receipt of medication) and the predictor variable analyzed (group assignment). We stressed that, to maintain the strength of causal inference provided by randomization, it is important to analyze by group assignment – that is, people assigned to take the medication should be compared with people assigned to placebo, rather than comparing people who took the medication with those who did not. However, if this analysis results in

---

[1] This type of confounding is sometimes referred to as *suppression* and the confounder is referred to as a *suppressor*. (Katz 1999)

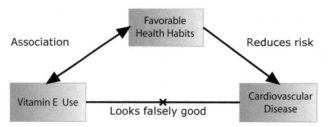

Figure 10.2 Confounding: Vitamin E seemed to reduce the risk of cardiovascular disease when presumably it is only associated with other factors that reduce risk.

significant misclassification of exposure (e.g., because some people assigned to the drug do not take it and/or some assigned to placebo obtain the active drug), power will be reduced and the estimate of effect size will be biased toward the null. Although the loss of power may be overcome by increasing the sample size, additional data and assumptions will generally be necessary to estimate how much the estimate of treatment effectiveness might have been biased toward no effect by crossover between groups.

Instrumental variables use this same type of logic. The idea is that, instead of the investigator randomly assigning subjects to a treatment group, which is then (strongly) associated with treatment but not otherwise associated with outcome, the investigator identifies some other variable that is associated with the treatment of interest and thought not to be (independently) associated with the outcome. The outcome is then determined in relation to this "instrumental variable," instead of to group assignment. For example, the instrumental variable could be related to a time or place that is associated with the receipt of the treatment, but is thought not to relate independently to the outcome. The expected bias toward the null that may occur from misclassification of exposure is overcome with a combination of a large sample size and calculations to estimate the effect of the imperfect relationship between the instrumental variable and the predictor of interest.

The concepts here are somewhat abstract, so the easiest way to explain and understand instrumental variables may be with some examples. A study one of us helped design used an instrumental variable to study delayed effects of military service during the Vietnam-era on mortality (Hearst et al. 1986). The exposure of interest in this case was military service. The outcome variable for the study was

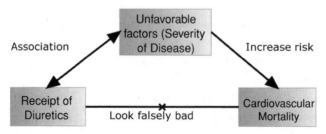

Figure 10.3 Confounding by indication. The favorable effect of diuretics on cardiovascular disease mortality is masked by the association between unfavorable factors and receipt of diuretics.

mortality, as determined from electronic death certificate registries from California and Pennsylvania that included the date of birth of the decedent and the cause of death. Although mortality rates in Vietnam veterans could easily be compared with those in nonveterans, the inference that differences in mortality after the period of service were *caused by* the military service would be weak, because men who served differed in many ways from those who did not – military service was not randomly assigned. However, for several years beginning in December 1969, annual draft lotteries were held, and 19-year-old men were randomly assigned a number from 1 to 366 based on their birth dates. Beginning in January each of the following years, men were drafted starting with the lowest lottery numbers, until a sufficient number of men had been drafted for that year. Thus, the instrumental variable chosen for this study was *eligibility* for the draft, as determined by whether a man's birth date corresponded to a draft lottery number above or below the highest number called for his year of birth (e.g., #195 for men born in 1950). Draft eligibility seemed to be a good instrumental variable, because it was associated with the predictor of interest, military service, but not independently associated with the outcome, mortality.

As it turned out, draft eligibility was a poor marker for actual military service. Only 25.6% of men whose birth dates made them eligible for the draft actually served, compared with 9.3% of men whose birth dates made them exempt. Nonetheless, the large sample size enabled the study to find statistically significantly higher mortality among draft-eligible men in the years following the period of possible military service, with observed relative risks of 1.13 for suicide (P = 0.005), 1.08 for motor vehicle accidents (P = 0.03), and 1.04 for all-cause mortality (P = 0.03).

These results, analogous to an "intention to treat" analysis of a randomized trial in which there was considerable crossover between groups, provide strong evidence of causality. However, the RRs using the instrumental variable are biased toward the null if the true cause of the mortality differences was military service, not eligibility for the draft. Therefore, the investigators algebraically calculated what the RR for military service would need to be in order to produce the association found between the instrumental variable of draft eligibility and mortality. If all of the excess risk among draft-eligible men was due to military service (a hypothesis that could not be tested with this design) RRs would need to be 1.86 for suicide, 1.53 for motor vehicle accidents, and 1.25 for total mortality.[2]

As in the previous example, instrumental variables analyses are often done with large databases, in order to overcome the bias toward no effect caused by a loose relationship between the instrumental variable and the predictor variable of interest. Another example of this is a study by Bell and Redelmeier (2001), who tested the hypothesis that reduced staffing might increase hospital mortality in Ontario hospitals. The predictor variable of interest was staffing levels, but the investigators were concerned that staffing level could vary with (and hence be confounded by) disease

---

[2] The calculation requires an assumption that the observed risks in eligible and exempt men are each a weighted average of risks among those who did and did not serve, and that these risks are the same in eligible and exempt men. This RR applies only to those who served *as a result* of having a low lottery number. There is no way of telling the effects of service on those who would have served regardless.

severity. The authors chose admission day of the week as the instrumental variable because staffing varied by day of the week, but the researchers did not believe disease severity (and/or mortality) was likely to vary by admission day for the diagnoses they studied. The assumption was that any differences in mortality by day of the week (beyond those explainable by other measured variables, such as age, race, and sex) could be attributed to staffing differences. In this design, the analysis is not of the relationship between predictor variable and outcome (patients per nurse and mortality) but rather between the instrumental variable (day of the week) and the outcome. The authors found significantly higher mortality during weekends, when staffing was lower, for 3 prospectively identified conditions they thought would be sensitive to staffing levels (ruptured abdominal aortic aneurysms, acute epiglottitis, and pulmonary embolism), but no differences for 3 control conditions (acute myocardial infarction, acute intracerebral hemorrhage, and acute hip fracture). In fact, weekend admissions were also associated with significantly higher mortality rates for 23 of the top 100 causes of death and not associated with lower mortality for any.

For some treatments, such as procedures for which good evidence about benefits, risks, or indications is lacking, there is considerable variation in the extent to which the treatments are used. This may reflect variation in the level of illness of patients being treated, as well as variable expertise with the treatments in different places. If both the treatment method and outcome are available in large electronic databases, an instrumental variable can be the proportion of patients receiving a particular treatment at the hospital at which each individual patient was seen. The hope is that the proportion of patients receiving the treatment will be associated with the treatment received but not otherwise associated with the outcome.

For example, Johnston (2000) noted marked variation among academic medical centers in the use of coiling (an endovascular procedure done by interventional neuroradiologists) and clipping (an operation done by neurosurgeons), two procedures used to treat cerebral aneurysms. A direct comparison (Johnston et al. 1999) of mortality following these two procedures suggested higher mortality from clipping (2.3% vs. 0.4%), but because patients were not randomly assigned, confounding by indication was possible (if the sicker patients were being treated with the clipping procedure). Estimating that the overall mortality risk (adjusted for age, sex, and comorbidity of the patients) should be similar across academic medical centers, Johnston used the proportion of patients with aneurysms treated by coiling as an instrumental variable. This variable was associated with the predictor but assumed not to be independently associated with mortality. Therefore, if coiling were superior to clipping, after adjusting for baseline differences, mortality should be lower in hospitals that do more coiling. This is, in fact, what he found: hospitals that did more coiling had lower adjusted mortality rates; the overall adjusted risk ratio per 10% increase in the proportion of cases treated by coiling was 0.91 for ruptured and 0.84 for unruptured aneurysms.[3]

---

[3] The author used a multivariate technique called Generalized Estimating Equations, which accounts for clustering of observations within hospitals, to obtain these risk ratios.

## Measurement of unrelated variables to estimate confounding or bias

Clinical trials, natural experiments, and studies using instrumental variables all are designed with a goal of minimizing or controlling confounding. An alternative approach is not to control confounding, but to make measurements that provide an indication of its importance. There are two directions from which these measurements can be made. The first is to measure another outcome that would be affected by the unmeasured confounder of concern but not by the treatment. If the treatment seems to affect this second outcome, confounding is likely to be a problem. The second is to measure another predictor variable in addition to the treatment of interest that is not felt to have a causal effect on the outcome but which should be associated with the unmeasured confounder. If confounding has an important effect on the relationship between the treatment and the outcome, it should also affect the relationship between the second predictor and the outcome. Concrete examples of these two methods should help clarify the abstract discussion above.

### Measuring another outcome

Selby et al. (1992) provide an excellent example of measuring a second outcome, subject to the same potential confounders as the outcome of interest, in order to show absence of confounding. They did a case–control study of screening sigmoidoscopy to prevent colon cancer death. The colon cancer deaths were divided into those caused by cancers that likely were and were not within reach of the sigmoidoscope. The cancers not within reach of the sigmoidoscope were the second outcome; they were presumably associated with the same confounders as those within reach of the scope, but not associated with the predictor. Although the authors used logistic regression to adjust for relevant covariables, the particularly elegant and convincing aspect of the study is their demonstration that sigmoidoscopy conferred protection against deaths from colon cancers that were within reach of the sigmoidoscope (adjusted OR = 0.41; 95% CI 0.25 to 0.69), but not from those that were beyond the reach of the sigmoidoscope (OR = 0.96; 95% CI 0.61 to 1.50). If unmeasured confounders were responsible for the apparent protective effect of sigmoidoscopy, it seems likely that they would have led to apparent protection from cancers both within and beyond the reach of the sigmoidoscope.

This strategy has also been used to study factors like income and access to ambulatory care. For example, Booth and Hux (2003) studied diabetic emergencies in Ontario. They found a clear inverse association between income level (estimated from neighborhood of residence) and admissions and emergency department visits for hyper- or hypoglycemia. However, admission rates for hip fracture and appendicitis, the control conditions (second outcomes) subject to the same potential confounders but thought not likely to be sensitive to ambulatory care, did not differ. Another example (Cook and Campbell 1979, pp. 218–21) comes from a study of an intervention aimed at reducing drunk driving in Britain. A crackdown using "breathalyzers" to estimate alcohol levels in pubs was associated with an abrupt drop in motor vehicle accidents on weekend nights when pubs were open. However, there was no change in the second outcome: accident rates occurring during hours when pubs were closed. If the decrease occurred because of a temporal trend rather than the breathalyzer intervention, the accident rate should have dropped generally, not just when the pubs were open.

### Measuring another predictor

The second approach, measuring other predictors in addition to the treatment of interest, is illustrated by a study of calcium channel blockers (CCBs) as a possible cause of myocardial infarction (MI; Psaty et al. 1995). The authors noted a progressive increase in risk of MI with increasing doses of CCBs: the adjusted OR increased from 1.13 for low dose to 1.42 for medium dose and 1.81 for high dose use. Of course one would expect that those treated with higher doses would have worse hypertension and be at higher risk, thus confounding by indication would be a major concern. However, the dose–response relationship went in the opposite direction for beta blockers – higher doses of beta blockers were associated with decreased risk of MI. Beta blockers were studied as a second predictor with a similar relationship to the confounders of interest (severity of disease) but not related to MI. The adjusted OR for beta blocker use decreased from 1.00 (reference) to 0.88 to 0.73 with increasing dose. If confounding by indication were the cause of the dose–response relationship between CCBs and MI, we might expect something similar for beta blockers, the opposite of what was observed.[4]

This strategy is clearly not a panacea, however. In both the Health Professionals study (Rimm et al. 1993) and the Nurses' Health Study (Stampfer et al. 1993), taking at least 400 I.U. of vitamin E daily was associated with a reduced risk of coronary heart disease, even after adjusting for all known confounders. Of course, people who take vitamin E are different from people who do not – for example, they might be more health conscious. But if that were the case, one would expect a favorable outcome in people taking a multivitamin pill or vitamin C as well, behaviors that are also associated with being health conscious. However, this was not observed. The lack of an association of the outcome with a covariable that one would expect to suffer from the same confounding as the treatment of interest suggested causality strongly enough that one of us (TBN) started to take supplemental vitamin E. Unfortunately, as mentioned above, subsequent evidence from randomized trials suggests vitamin E is of no benefit, and may even be harmful (Eidelman et al. 2004; Miller et al. 2005).

## Propensity scores

A relatively new approach to controlling confounding in observational studies of treatment efficacy is the use of propensity scores. In order for a variable to be a confounder, it has to be associated with both treatment and outcome. The usual approach to using multivariate analysis to control for confounding is to create a

---

[4] This does not prove that CCBs cause MI. If CCBs were entirely inert, but were prescribed in increasing doses for those at higher risk of MI, while beta-blockers were effective at reducing risk, we could see results like these. But one could argue that taking an inert medicine, rather than something that works, is a cause of MI.

model that includes the treatment variable and other predictors of outcome (the potential confounders). If the model fits, the coefficient for the treatment will reflect its independent contribution to the outcome.

For example, the equation for the *logistic* model can be written as:

$$\ln\left[\frac{P(Y)}{(1-P(Y))}\right] = a + b_1X_1 + b_2X_2 + \cdots + b_kX_k$$

where

"P(Y)" is the probability of the outcome Y,

"$\ln\left[\dfrac{P(Y)}{(1-P(Y))}\right]$" is the log-odds of the outcome,

"a" is a constant (the intercept, related to the overall probability of the outcome),

"$X_i$" are the different predictor variables associated with outcome, including the predictor variable of interest as well as the potential confounders. For example, the variable of interest to you might be $X_2$ (the treatment you are studying) and the rest would be confounders.

"$b_i$" are coefficients (equal to the logarithm of the odds ratio if "$X_i$" is dichotomous) associated with each predictor.

"k" is the number of predictor variables.

One limitation of this approach is that, if there are many potential confounders, there may not be enough outcomes in the dataset to be able to estimate their coefficients with much precision. There's a rule-of-thumb: you would like to see at least 10 outcomes for each predictor variable. (By "outcome" we mean 10 instances of the thing you are trying to predict, e.g., deaths.) Imagine there are 1,000 patients, of whom 300 received the treatment of interest, but only 30 died. With only 30 outcomes, it will be difficult to control for confounding by more than 2 other variables aside from the treatment variable – the dataset just does not have enough outcomes to do this well.

Enter propensity scores. The idea of propensity scores is that, instead of controlling for all possible predictors of outcome, investigators instead control for predictors of the treatment. This is done by creating a model to estimate the predicted probability of treatment (or propensity to be treated). Subjects are then either matched or stratified on this propensity score, and the risks of the outcome in people who actually were or were not treated within each stratum are compared. Thus, continuing the notation above, if $X_2$ is the treatment of interest, the model for the propensity score would look like this:

$$\ln\left[\frac{P(X_2)}{1-P(X_2)}\right] = a + b_1X_1 + b_3X_3 + \cdots + b_jX_j$$

Note that the difference is that the probability we are trying to predict is not the probability of outcome [P(Y)], it is probability of treatment, $P(X_2)$. The number of predictors of treatment may be different than the number of predictors of outcome, so we end up with j instead of k − 1 variables. In fact, because the model being created to estimate $P(X_2)$ does not have to work in any dataset except the one being analyzed,

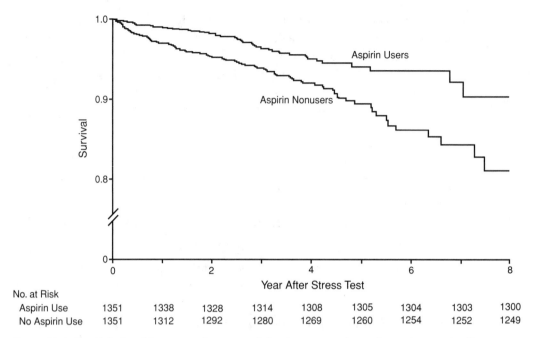

Figure 10.4   Survival of aspirin users and nonusers following stress echocardiography, matched by propensity score for aspirin use. (From Gum et al. 2001; used with permission.)

the investigator can include several predictor variables, interactions, and quadratic terms, without worrying about how the model might work on another data set.

Now the investigator can stratify on this $P(X_2)$ variable (e.g., in quintiles of "propensity for treatment") and compare the risk of outcome in those who actually were and were not treated within these quintiles of subjects, each of whom had approximately the same propensity to be treated. Alternatively, the investigator can match subjects who were and were not treated by their value of $P(X_2)$ and compare outcomes between matched subjects.

For example, Gum et al. (2001) prospectively studied total mortality of 6,174 consecutive adults undergoing stress echocardiography, 2,310 of whom (37%) were taking aspirin. In unadjusted analyses, mortality did not differ between users and nonusers of aspirin – 4.5% in each group. Multivariable analysis, however, suggested a mortality benefit. This was confirmed by matching subjects by propensity scores and then comparing survival in the two groups (Fig. 10.4).

Note that the figure is based on only 1,351 subjects in each group. This is because only 1,351 of the 2310 subjects who received aspirin had a "match," – that is, had someone with the same propensity to receive aspirin but did not receive it – in the control group. This is not unexpected in observational studies such as this one. When the treatment is not randomized, the average propensity to receive aspirin will be higher in the group that received it than in the group that did not, which may make it difficult to match all treated subjects to untreated subjects. This loss of subjects affects both power (which was still more than adequate in this study) and generalizability. For example, the results of this study are only generalizable to patients whose propensity to receive aspirin was in a range where there was overlap between those who did and did not receive it. But this makes sense. If there are some

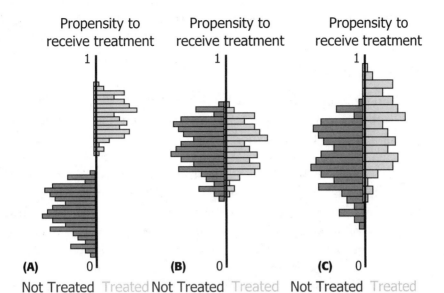

Figure 10.5 (**A**) Propensity scores do not overlap; treated and untreated groups are not comparable. A propensity analysis cannot be done and any comparison between groups is hazardous. (**B**) Propensity distributions are nearly identical. A propensity analysis is not necessary as groups are already matched or treatment was randomly assigned. (**C**) Good overlap in propensity scores; the subjects in the overlapping parts of the distribution can be studied. (Figure courtesy of Thomas Love; Case Western Reserve University Center for Health Research and Policy.)

people who absolutely should get aspirin and some who should not, their propensities will be close to 1 and 0, respectively; they will not have a match and hence will not be included in the matched results. Think of this exclusion of subjects with propensity scores near 0 or 1 as analogous to exclusion criteria in a clinical trial. If there are some persons for whom either drug or placebo is known to be contraindicated, then you neither can nor should study the difference between drug and placebo in those patients. In fact, this is another advantage of a propensity analysis: if there is little overlap between the propensity scores of those who were and were not treated, it means that those treated appear to be very different from those not treated, in terms of their indication for the treatment, and that trying to adjust for this with multivariate analysis may require questionable extrapolations beyond the data.

A propensity score analysis requires that scores overlap between a substantial portion of the treated and untreated groups. If the model predicts treatment too well, only a few subjects in the treated and untreated groups will have the same propensity score (Fig. 10.5A). For this reason, one should avoid including in a propensity score factors that are associated with receiving treatment but unlikely to cause the outcome, such as day of week or geographical location. (Note that these same factors make good instrumental variables!) On the other hand, if the propensity score distributions in the treated and untreated groups are nearly identical, there is no point in doing a propensity score analysis (Fig. 10.5B).

Propensity score analysis in an observational study of a treatment helps to separate out the effects of the treatment itself from other factors associated both with receiving the treatment and with the outcome. However, propensity score analysis is not helpful if the goal is to identify or to quantify the effects of these other confounding factors.

## Summary

1. Although randomized blinded trials are the best way to establish causal relationships between treatments and outcomes, it is sometimes possible, by thinking creatively, to design observational studies that provide strong evidence of causality.

2. One approach is to identify an instrumental variable that is associated with treatment but not independently related to the outcome. Comparing outcomes between groups based on values of the instrumental variable is then similar to an intention-to-treat analysis of a randomized trial with substantial crossover between the treatment and control groups. The direction of the treatment effect is correct, but the magnitude of the effect is diminished.

3. Another approach is to test for the possibility of confounding by measuring a second outcome that is causally associated with the confounder but not the treatment. If no association exists between treatment and this second outcome, confounding is less likely to be a problem.

4. Similarly, one can identify additional predictors (other than the treatment) that are associated with the confounder but have no effect on the outcome. If these additional predictors are not found to be associated with the outcome, confounding is again less likely to be a problem.

5. Finally, one can model the propensity to receive treatment and compare outcomes of subjects with similar treatment propensities.

## References

Bell, C. M., and D. A. Redelmeier (2001). "Mortality among patients admitted to hospitals on weekends as compared with weekdays." *N Engl J Med* **345**(9): 663–8.

Booth, G. L., and J. E. Hux (2003). "Relationship between avoidable hospitalizations for diabetes mellitus and income level." *Arch Intern Med* **163**(1): 101–6.

Cook, T. D., and D. T. Campbell (1979). *Quasi-Experimentation: Design & Analysis Issues for Field Settings.* Chicago, IL, Rand McNally College Pub. Co.

Eidelman, R. S., D. Hollar, et al. (2004). "Randomized trials of vitamin E in the treatment and prevention of cardiovascular disease." *Arch Intern Med* **164**(14): 1552–6.

Gum, P. A., M. Thamilarasan, et al. (2001). "Aspirin use and all-cause mortality among patients being evaluated for known or suspected coronary artery disease: a propensity analysis." *JAMA* **286**(10): 1187–94.

Hearst, N., T. B. Newman, et al. (1986). "Delayed effects of the military draft on mortality. A randomized natural experiment." *N Engl J Med* **314**(10): 620–4.

Johnston, S. C. (2000). "Effect of endovascular services and hospital volume on cerebral aneurysm treatment outcomes." *Stroke* **31**(1): 111–7.

Johnston, S. C., R. A. Dudley, et al. (1999). "Surgical and endovascular treatment of unruptured cerebral aneurysms at university hospitals." *Neurology* **52**(9): 1799–805.

Katz, M. H. (1999). *Multivariable Analysis: A Practical Guide for Clinicians.* Cambridge, Cambridge University Press.

Miller, E. R., 3rd, R. Pastor-Barriuso, et al. (2005). "Meta-analysis: high-dosage vitamin E supplementation may increase all-cause mortality." *Ann Intern Med* **142**(1): 37–46.

Psaty, B. M., S. R. Heckbert, et al. (1995). "The risk of myocardial infarction associated with antihypertensive drug therapies." *JAMA* **274**(8): 620–5.

Rimm, E. B., M. J. Stampfer, et al. (1993). "Vitamin E consumption and the risk of coronary heart disease in men." *N Engl J Med* **328**(20): 1450–6.

Selby, J. V., G. D. Friedman, et al. (1992). "A case-control study of screening sigmoidoscopy and mortality from colorectal cancer." *N Engl J Med* **326**(10): 653–7.

Stampfer, M. J., C. H. Hennekens, et al. (1993). "Vitamin E consumption and the risk of coronary disease in women." *N Engl J Med* **328**(20): 1444–9.

Turnbull, F., B. Neal, et al. (2005). "Effects of different blood pressure-lowering regimens on major cardiovascular events in individuals with and without diabetes mellitus: results of prospectively designed overviews of randomized trials." *Arch Intern Med* **165**(12): 1410–9.

Warram, J. H., L. M. Laffel, et al. (1991). "Excess mortality associated with diuretic therapy in diabetes mellitus." *Arch Intern Med* **151**(7): 1350–6.

## Chapter 10 Problems

1. Thimerosal, a mercury-containing preservative, was removed in 2001 from vaccines routinely given to infants because of concern that the total mercury dose, added up over all recommended vaccines, exceeded the U.S. Environmental Protection Agency safety limit. There are many lawsuits pending in which plaintiffs claim that autism or other neurodevelopmental problems occurred in their children because of exposure to mercury in thimerosal.

   Imagine that you have access to an enormous database that includes electronic records of several million health plan members from 1990 to the present, that diagnoses of autism are recorded in the database, but that, like everywhere else, definitions may have been unstable over time. You know that Rh Immune Globulin (Rhogam®), which is given during pregnancy to most Rh-negative women who get good prenatal care, had 25 μg of mercury (as thimerosal) per dose until 2001, and you are interested in possible toxic effects of this amount of mercury on the fetus. Assume that you have plenty of subjects and accurate data on who got Rhogam and on blood types, and that some mothers in your health plan miss a lot of prenatal visits, and might not get Rhogam for that reason.

   Design a study to take advantage of these facts in order to assess the impact of this dose of mercury on the risk of autism. What groups would you compare to have the greatest strength of causal inference?

2. You plan to use a large clinical database to perform a retrospective cohort study to investigate whether screening digital rectal examinations (DRE) by primary care providers prevent deaths from prostate cancer.
   a) What would be your main *predictor variable?*
   b) Your outcome variable will be prostate cancer death rates in different groups, so the numerators will be men who died of prostate cancer. What should the denominators of those rates be?
   c) What could you do to address the problem of confounding (or selection bias)?

3. There is some evidence that regular use of nonsteroidal antiinflammatory drugs (NSAIDS) for arthritis may reduce the risk of colon cancer. You wish to design a

study to see whether occasional ibuprofen use reduces colon cancer risk. Explain why you might want to ask about acetaminophen use and how you would use the answers to such questions.

4. Consider a cohort study (Nichol et al. 2003) that estimated the effect of flu vaccination on mortality during the 1998–1999 and 1999–2000 flu seasons. The study population included almost 300,000 subjects at least 65 years old, of whom about 58% were vaccinated. Among vaccinated and unvaccinated subjects, 1.2% and 2.0%, respectively, died during the flu season.

   a) What confounder(s) could make flu vaccine appear less effective than it really is?

   b) What confounder or bias might have biased the results in the opposite direction?

   c) Using multivariable analysis to adjust for potential confounder(s), the authors estimated an RR of about 0.5, an ARR ≈1.0% and an NNT ≈100 for all-cause mortality.

      Since it is hard to believe that half of deaths could be prevented by the flu vaccine, you are concerned that there are potential unmeasured and unmeasurable confounders. Without doing a whole other study, how could you test the question of whether the flu vaccination's apparent effect in reducing mortality during the flu season was actually due to unmeasured factors that were associated with flu vaccination?

5. Lindenauer et al. (2004) reported that perioperative use of lipid-lowering agents may decrease mortality following cardiac surgery by about 30% to 40%. They controlled for confounding by creating a propensity score.

   a) Describe in words what the propensity score for this study was.

   b) Figure 1 from that paper (reprinted below) shows that mortality was lower among users of lipid-lowering drugs in all but the first quintile of propensity.

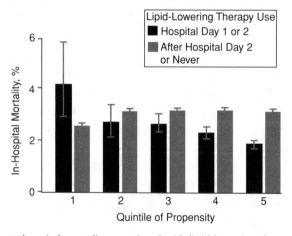

In-hospital mortality associated with lipid-lowering therapy in propensity-based quintiles. Error bars indicate 95% confidence intervals. Seventeen patients (0.002%) were excluded from multivariable analysis due to missing data; therefore, among 780,574 patients, mean lipid-lowering therapy use per quintile of propensity was 0.5% (quintile 1, n = 156,114), 1.9% (quintile 2, n = 156,115), 9.8% (quintile 3, n = 156,115), 10.9% (quintile 4, n = 156,115), and 31.3% (quintile 5, n = 156,115). From Lindenauer et al. (2004). Used with permission.

   i) Why are the error bars for the mortality estimate for the left-most column of the graph so much longer than those for the other columns?

  ii) It appears that, for subjects in the lowest propensity quintile, use of lipid lowering drugs on hospital day 1 or 2 appeared to be harmful rather than beneficial. Assume for this question that there is no random error and no confounding – that is, that the results in the figure are accurate and causal. What implication does this have for promoting increased use of such drugs to reduce perioperative mortality after noncardiac surgery?

## References for problem set

Lindenauer, P. K., P. Pekow, et al. (2004). "Lipid-lowering therapy and in-hospital mortality following major noncardiac surgery." *JAMA* **291**(17): 2092–9.

Nichol, K. L., J. Nordin, et al. (2003). "Influenza vaccination and reduction in hospitalizations for cardiac disease and stroke among the elderly." *N Engl J Med* **348**(14): 1322–32.

# Understanding P-values and confidence intervals

## Introduction

In the previous two chapters, we discussed using the results of randomized trials and observational studies to estimate treatment effects. We were primarily interested in measures of effect size and in problems with design (in randomized trials) and confounding (in observational studies) that could bias effect estimates. We did not spend much time considering the precision of our effect estimates or whether the apparent treatment effects could be a result of chance. The statistics used to help us with these questions – P-values and confidence intervals – are the subject of this chapter.

No area in epidemiology and statistics is so widely misunderstood and mistaught. We cover a more sophisticated understanding of P-values and confidence intervals in this text because 1) it is right, 2) it is important, and 3) we think you can handle it. After all, you have survived three chapters (3, 4, and 8) on using the results of diagnostic tests and Bayes's Theorem to update a patient's probability of disease. So now you are poised to gain a Bayesian understanding of P-values and confidence intervals as well. We will give you a taste in this chapter; those wishing to explore these ideas in greater depth are encouraged to read an excellent series of articles on this topic by Steven Goodman. (Goodman 1999a; Goodman 1999b; Goodman 2001)

## Background: the null hypothesis, test statistics, and P-values

Before we can talk about what P-values and confidence intervals mean, we need to review classical statistical significance testing. The basic process is as follows:

1. State an appropriate "null hypothesis" ($H_0$), a hypothesis of "no effect," the exact phrasing of which depends on the type of variables and the relationship between them that you wish to investigate. The null hypothesis will be something like: "there is no difference between the means in the two groups" or "the

response rates do not differ" or "there is no linear association between variables A and B."

2. Choose $\alpha$, the maximum probability of a Type 1 error that you are willing to tolerate. A "Type 1" error is when you reject the null hypothesis when it is true – that is, conclude that the difference you observed was not due to chance, when in fact it was. (A "Type 2" error is failing to reject the null hypothesis when it is false – that is, concluding that the difference could be due to chance when in fact it is not. The maximum probability of a Type 2 error is $\beta$.)

3. Use the results of the study to calculate the value of a "test statistic" with a known distribution if the null hypothesis is true. Examples are a t statistic, $\chi^2$ statistic, or a regression coefficient divided by its standard error. The test statistic you use depends on the design of the study and the type of variables evaluated.

4. Use that test statistic to calculate a P-value. Classically, if the P-value is less than $\alpha$, you reject the null hypothesis; however, authors of clinical research articles rarely explicitly reject or fail to reject the null hypothesis. More commonly, they will simply report the P-value and consider the result "statistically significant" if P is less than 0.05, otherwise not.

## What do P-values really mean?

Unfortunately, the first thing we have to do is help you unlearn some of what you may have learned from other sources. There is no debate about whether the common misunderstanding of the meaning of P-values and confidence intervals is correct. The debate is entirely pedagogical. Does it matter? Is it worth the time it takes to explain what they actually mean? Can you understand the correct meaning of P-values and confidence intervals?

It is an issue one of us (TBN) has debated with some other teachers of evidence-based medicine. Their view is that it does not matter much if people misunderstand this material, because for most people, misunderstanding the correct interpretation of the P-value will not lead to huge misinterpretations of the literature. On the other hand, there are some issues that arise in nearly every research study (like whether it makes a difference if hypotheses are stated in advance, and whether you need to adjust for multiple comparisons) that simply do not make sense if you misunderstand the meaning of the P-value. To those teachers and students who insist that one can get along just fine not really understanding what P-values mean, we would point out that you also can get along fairly well believing that the sun revolves around the earth. It is much more satisfying, however, to learn (and teach) what is right. So here are correct and incorrect definitions of the P-value.

**Correct Definition:** A P-value is the probability of observing a value of the test statistic at least as extreme as that observed in the study, if in fact the null hypothesis is true.

**Incorrect Definition:** A P-value is the probability that the null hypothesis is true (i.e., that there is no difference between the groups, no relationship between the variables, etc.), given the results of the study. That is, if P = 0.05, there is a 5%

probability that the observed departure from the null hypothesis occurred by chance and a 95% probability that it did not and the observed difference is real.

The difference between the two definitions above may seem subtle, but it is important. An analogy with diagnostic testing can help make it clearer.

## Using your understanding of diagnostic tests to understand P-values

### Introduction to Bayesian thinking: false-positive confusion

Remember the specious argument from Chapter 3, when we addressed what we called "false-positive" and "false-negative" confusion? Box 3.3 (about the need always to do a urine culture after a negative urinalysis) and Problem 3.3 (about the need always to culture the throat after a negative rapid test) were about false negatives. Recall that the faulty logic went something like this:

1. The sensitivity is 90%.
2. Therefore, the false negative rate is 10%.
3. Therefore, if the test is negative, there is a 10% chance that it is a false negative.

But, in fact, statement 3 was false, because in statement 2, "false negative" refers to $(1 -$ Sensitivity), and in statement 3 it refers to $(1 -$ Negative Predictive Value).

For this chapter, it is false-positive confusion that is most relevant. In the diagnostic testing setting, the false-positive confusion goes something like this:

1. The specificity of a test is 95%.
2. Therefore, the false-positive rate is 5%.
3. Therefore, if a patient has a positive result, there's a 5% chance that it is a false-positive and the patient does not have the disease.
4. Therefore, if a patient has a positive result, there is a 95% chance that he does have the disease.

Once again, the problem is with statement 3 in which the probability of a positive result given no disease was converted into the probability of no disease given a positive result. That is, in the standard $2 \times 2$ table (Fig. 11.1), the usage of the term "false-positive rate" in statements 1 and 2 was $b/(b + d) = 1-$ Specificity. This corresponds to going vertically in the $2 \times 2$ table.

Then, in statement 3, we switched and started going horizontally, and the "false-positive rate" changed to $b/(a + b) = 1-$ Positive Predictive Value (Fig. 11.2).

The "false-positive rate" that goes horizontally $(1 -$ Positive Predictive Value) is more clinically relevant once you get a positive result; it is the probability that

Figure 11.1 When "false positive rate" refers to 1 – specificity or $b/(b + d)$, we are looking at the vertical "No Disease" column in the standard $2 \times 2$ table for a diagnostic test.

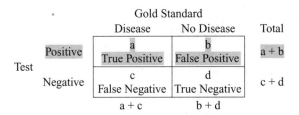

Figure 11.2  When "false positive rate" refers to 1 − Positive Predictive Value or b/(a + b), we are looking at the horizontal "Test Positive" row of the standard 2 × 2 table for a diagnostic test.

your patient still does not have the disease, despite that positive result. However, we learned that it cannot be calculated from just (sensitivity and) specificity, because it depends on the prior probability of the disease.

Now consider the following argument:

1. We set $\alpha$, the probability of a Type 1 error, at 5%.
2. Therefore, the probability of falsely concluding there is a difference, when in fact none exists, is 5%.
3. Therefore, if the P-value for our study is less than 0.05 and we reject the null hypothesis, the chance that we will be wrong is 5%.
4. Therefore, if the P-value is less than 0.05, there is at least a 95% chance that the difference between groups is not due to chance.

Can you see that this is exactly the same fallacy? Once again, the problem is with statement 3, although the ambiguity of statement 2 contributed to the problem. Statement 3 confuses the probability of the results given the null hypothesis with the probability of the null hypothesis given the results.

The key is that the P-value is a conditional probability; it is calculated assuming that the null hypothesis is true. In this way, it is like 1 − Specificity, which is calculated conditional on not having the disease. 1 − Specificity is the probability of testing positive if you do not have the disease, whereas the P-value is the probability of observing an effect (or, to be more precise, a value of the test statistic) at least as extreme as that observed in the study if the null hypothesis were true.[1]

This analogy between diagnostic and statistical tests can be visualized with a 2 × 2 table, similar to the ones we used for diagnostic tests (Fig. 11.3).

Just as was the case with diagnostic tests, what you really want is to go horizontally in this table – that is, what you want to know is the probability that there truly is a difference between groups, given the study results. But when you calculate a P-value, you are going vertically. That is, you assume the null hypothesis is true in order to calculate the P-value.

---

[1] For any one research question, there are many possible null hypotheses, and hence many test statistics that can be calculated. For example, there are test statistics to compare means, ranks, and standard deviations between groups, and they will not always give the same P-value. Note that it is also possible to calculate distributions of test statistics and P-values under assumptions other than the null hypothesis. For example, in an equivalency study, one might want to test the hypothesis that drug A is inferior to drug B by a specified amount. This is like calculating test characteristics for disease A vs. disease B, as opposed to Disease A present and absent. For example, "specificity" could be how often the test is negative in people with disease B rather than in everyone who does not have Disease A.

| | | TRUTH | |
| | | Difference | No Difference |
| Study | Positive | Power $(1-\beta)$ | $\alpha$ |
| | Negative | $\beta$ | $1 - \alpha$ |

Figure 11.3 The analogy between diagnostic and statistical tests can be visualized with a 2 × 2 table, similar to the one we used for diagnostic tests. Power $(1 - \beta)$ is analogous to sensitivity and $\alpha$ is analogous to 1 − Specificity.

We can summarize the Bayesian understanding of P-values exactly as we did when discussing diagnostic tests:

What you thought before + New information = What you think now

The new information, in this case, is the result of the study. The P-value is a measure of how consistent the result of the study is with the null hypothesis. However, it is not the posterior probability of the null hypothesis, because you cannot obtain a posterior probability without a prior probability.

## Extending the analogy

The analogy between diagnostic tests and research studies can provide a lot of help understanding other aspects of P-values, too. A full analogy, adapted from an article Warren Browner and TBN wrote in 1987 (Browner and Newman 1987) is shown in Table 11.1.

**Table 11.1.** The analogy between diagnostic tests and research studies

| Diagnostic test | Research study |
| --- | --- |
| Absence of Disease | Truth of null hypothesis |
| Presence of disease | Null hypothesis is false (e.g., real difference between groups exists) |
| Severity of disease in the diseased group | Magnitude of the true difference between groups |
| Cutoff for distinguishing positive and negative results | Alpha |
| Test result | P-value |
| Negative result (test within normal limits) | P-value exceeds alpha |
| Positive result | P-value less than alpha |
| Sensitivity | Power |
| False positive rate (1 − specificity) | Alpha |
| Prior probability of disease (of a given severity) | Prior probability of a difference between groups (of a given magnitude) |
| Posterior probability of disease, given test result | Posterior probability of a difference between groups, given study results |

We can think of a research study as a diagnostic test to detect a difference (or association) between groups. Just as a sensitive test is more likely to find disease when it is present, a study with plenty of power (i.e., large sample size) is more likely to find a difference when it is present. In Chapter 5, we learned that many diseases are not homogenous, and that sensitivity would be expected to increase with the severity of disease. The analogy for research studies is that large differences between groups (i.e., strong associations) are easier to identify than small ones. Just as sensitivity depends on the severity of disease you wish to detect, power depends on the magnitude of the difference between groups you wish to detect; bigger differences, like more severe disease, are easier to find.[2]

When one does formal hypothesis testing for a research study, one compares the P-value from a study with a previously defined cut-off ($\alpha$) for determining whether to reject the null hypothesis. This is analogous to deciding whether a test result falls within the "Normal Range." Note that the more sure you want to be that a test is abnormal before labeling it as such, the wider your normal range will be. Similarly, the more sure you want to be that a P-value is inconsistent with the null hypothesis, the lower the alpha you will require.

Of course, simply comparing a P-value to alpha and reporting that it is lower (e.g., "P < 0.05") discards information. A P-value of 0.001 provides stronger evidence against the null hypothesis than a P-value of 0.049. This is similar to the point we made in Chapter 4, that dichotomizing WBC counts at 15,000 throws away information; a WBC count of 28,000 provides stronger evidence of bacteremia than a WBC count of 16,000.

### Intentionally ordered tests and hypotheses stated in advance

If after a history and physical examination, you suspect a particular disease, and order a diagnostic test to confirm your hypothesis, a positive result is quite believable. This is because the disease you were testing for had a high prior probability. The posterior probability of disease depends only on the prior probability and the test result, however, not on whether you were smart enough to entertain the diagnosis in advance. Thus, the fact that a test was ordered by the third-year medical student with no particular suspicion of the disease does not mean the attending physician needs to assign a low prior probability when interpreting the result, if the history and physical examination immediately suggested the correct diagnosis to the attending.

Similarly, when testing research hypotheses, it is generally true that hypotheses stated in advance have higher prior probabilities than hypothesis arrived at after examining the data. But whether or not a hypothesis was stated in advance is not what is important. All that matters is the prior probability of the hypothesis being tested. Thus, if, after the data have been collected, some other study suggests a particular hypothesis, that hypothesis can be tested and will have a reasonable prior

---

[2] The analogy is not perfect, because for truly dichotomous disease states we need not specify a severity or stage of disease when estimating sensitivity, whereas we always must specify the magnitude of the difference we wish to detect when estimating power. This is because the degree of departure from the null hypothesis is not dichotomous.

probability, even if it was not stated in advance of the data collection. This happens in clinical medicine as well. A finding that the clinician either initially did not pay much attention to or dismissed as a red herring can suddenly provide evidence in favor of a disease when other findings pointing to that previously unconsidered disease become available.

## Multiple hypotheses and multiple tests

It is well known that, if you look for enough different associations, either by selecting from multiple predictor and outcome variables or by restricting attention to various subgroups, it is easy to find statistically significant associations. The usual explanation for this is that, if there is a 5% chance of making a Type 1 error testing a single hypothesis, then if you test two (independent) hypotheses, the chance of such an error with either one would be closer to 10%; and if you test enough hypotheses, your chances of finding one or more with $P < 0.05$ approaches one. To address this issue, the Bonferroni correction is sometimes applied. The Bonferroni correction says that, if you want to test k different hypotheses and maintain a particular value for $\alpha$, the Type 1 error rate for your whole study, you should use $\alpha / k$ as the Type 1 error rate for each individual hypothesis tested. Thus, if you wanted to test 2 hypotheses, you would require $P < 0.025$ before rejecting the null hypothesis; for 5 hypotheses, you would require $P < 0.01$, and so on.

The Bonferroni correction is overly conservative, because it does not account for the possibility that more than one of the null hypotheses can be falsely rejected.[3] There are less conservative methods (such as the Holm, Student–Newman–Keuls or the Tukey tests) for adjusting the Type I error rate of each individual comparison when you are doing multiple comparisons (Glantz 2002). However, any adjustment to $\alpha$ for individual comparisons based on the overall $\alpha$ is problematic to apply. If you have collected your data and start running analyses, do you have to start counting every P-value your statistics package calculated as one of your hypotheses and reduce your value of $\alpha$ for individual comparisons accordingly? Must your level of $\alpha$ be forever affected? What if your colleague is running analyses as well? Do her hypothesis tests count against your $\alpha$? If the drug you are studying is associated with a bothersome side effect (e.g., cardiac arrhythmias), can you render the result not statistically significant by testing enough additional hypotheses about other side effects?

The problem with multiple hypothesis testing is that most of the multiple hypotheses have low prior probabilities. This is similar to the difference between a test that is intentionally ordered and one that pops up as abnormal on a twenty-test chemistry

---

[3] To understand this, you need to understand the following probability theorem:

$$P(A \text{ or } B) = P(A) + P(B) - P(A \& B)$$

It makes sense to subtract P(A & B) because otherwise the probability gets counted twice. (Try drawing a Venn diagram to see this.) With the Bonferroni correction, event A is rejection of null hypothesis A and event B is rejection of null hypothesis B. $P(A) = P(B) = \alpha$, so $P(A \text{ or } B) = P(A) + P(B) - P(A \& B) = \alpha + \alpha - P(A \& B) = 2\alpha - P(A \& B)$. Of course, it is possible to falsely reject 2 different null hypotheses, so $P(A \& B) > 0$. Therefore, the probability of falsely rejecting either of the null hypotheses must be less than $2\alpha$.

panel. The interpretation of a particular statistical hypothesis test does not depend on how many other hypotheses were tested in the same study, just as the interpretation of a serum sodium level does not depend on whether you ordered an alkaline phosphatase on the same specimen. If clinical laboratories believed in the Bonferroni correction, they would widen the normal range of laboratory tests depending on how many tests were done on the same specimen. That being said, statistical approaches to avoid making too much of small P-values in the face of multiple comparisons are probably reasonable, because estimation of prior probabilities of hypotheses is a difficult and subjective process. But it is important to remember that, despite the aura of objectivity around statistical adjustment for multiple comparisons, no amount of statistical manipulation can ever get you a posterior probability without including some estimate of the prior probability. All of these methods basically aim to limit the probability of one or more Type 1 errors under the assumption that all of the null hypotheses are true.

### Bias and laboratory error

Up to this point, when considering whether an observed difference between groups was real, we have been primarily concerned about chance as an alternative explanation for the study findings. However, another possible explanation could be bias: the results did not occur by chance, yet there may not be any real difference between groups. Bias in research studies is analogous to laboratory error. For example, in a patient reported to have an elevated potassium level, the specimen may have hemolyzed, and the true potassium level might be within the normal range. In fact, the patient could be hypokalemic; laboratory error can cause false-negative as well as false-positive results. Similarly, bias can hide real associations in addition to creating spurious ones.

### Alternative diagnoses and confounding

An abnormal laboratory finding may not be due to a laboratory error, but still may not be due to the disease you are testing for; some other disease might be responsible. Similarly, a difference between groups (in an observational study) may not be due to chance, but still may not be due to a causal relationship; a third, confounding factor might be responsible. Thus, just as diagnosis requires a lot more than determining whether results of tests are normal, interpreting clinical research requires much more than ruling out chance and bias as the basis for associations.

## Confidence intervals

There is no direct analogy between interpretation of results of diagnostic tests and of confidence intervals for research studies. Nonetheless, because confidence intervals are even more widely misunderstood than P-values, we review their meaning here.

The temptation is to say that there is a 95% probability that the true value of the parameter you are trying to estimate (e.g., the relative risk) lies within the 95% confidence interval (CI). As we have seen with P-values above, this is not the case, because this is a statement of posterior probability, which you cannot make without knowing the prior probability.[4] It turns out it is easier to say what confidence intervals do not mean than what they do mean. Confidence intervals do *not* indicate a range with a 95% probability of including the true value. What do they mean? We think a nonquantitative definition works best: *the confidence interval indicates a range of values consistent with what was observed in the study.*[5] The higher the "level of confidence" (e.g., 99% vs. 95%), the wider the interval will be, corresponding to a looser definition of "consistent." Of course, by chance alone, the true value might not be consistent with what was observed in the study, because the study happened to give the wrong answer.

The pedagogical debate we mentioned earlier, related to whether to try to give the correct interpretation of P-values, applies even more to confidence intervals, which are a bit harder to understand. For example, Douglas Altman, a bright light in the field of statistics and medicine, has written (Sackett et al. 2000; Guyatt et al. 2002):

A strictly correct definition of a 95% CI is, somewhat opaquely, that 95% of such intervals will contain the true population value. Little is lost by the less pure interpretation of the CI as the range of values within which we can be 95% sure that the population value lies.

We disagree. We think a lot is lost by the less pure interpretation, because different hypotheses have a wide range of prior probabilities. Therefore, the interpretation of the CI as the range of values within which we can be 95% sure that the population value lies is, in many cases, not even close.

Here is a simple example showing that the commonly used interpretation of the CI is wrong:

Picture a randomized trial, comparing Treatment A with Treatment B, that only has ten subjects per group. Four in each group die. The RR for mortality is 1.0 with a 95% CI of 0.34 to 2.9. You might believe that there is only a 5% chance that the true value is outside that CI, because it is fairly wide. But the 40% CI is a bit more narrow (0.75 to 1.33). Is there a 40% chance that it contains the true value? If so, there must be a 60% chance that the true value is outside that 40% CI – that is, that the true RR is <0.75 or >1.33. In other words, there is a 60% chance that Treatment A either lowers mortality by 25% or increases it by 33%! But your study provided no information to suggest this was the case. How can a study that shows no difference between groups lead to a probability of 60% that there is at least a 25% difference in either direction?[6]

Let us just try to understand the strictly correct definition of the 95% CI. The idea that 95% of such intervals include the population value refers to a process, not to a particular interval. If we performed the study 100 times, we would expect that the 95% CIs of 95% of the studies would include the true value. But if we only did

---

[4] Statisticians get around the fact that confidence intervals don't mean what it seems like they should by creating their own definition of the word "confidence." This definition makes the statement that you can be 95% *confident* that the true value lies within the 95% *confidence* interval both true and tautologous.

[5] Another definition of the 95% confidence interval is *the range of hypotheses that would NOT have been rejected by this study at the 5% significance level ($\alpha = 0.05$)*. More generally, the $(1 - \alpha)$ confidence interval is the range of hypotheses that would not have been rejected at significance level $\alpha$.

[6] The answer is that the posterior probability that the true RR is <0.75 or >1.33 could be 60% only if the prior probability were more than that. Given no additional information about treatments A and B, there is no reason to presume that this is the case.

the study once, other information (i.e., a low prior probability of the result) might suggest that the 95% CI that we happened to get might not include the true value. In that case, the probability that the true value is within that study's 95% CI could be very different from 95%.

To understand this idea of a "process," imagine that you have a bag filled with nineteen oranges and one grapefruit. The process of selecting one piece of fruit at random from the bag has a 95% chance of drawing an orange. If I tell you I have selected a piece of fruit, but give you no additional information, you will say that there is a 95% probability that I have an orange. However, if I tell you that it feels quite large for an orange, the probability that it is an orange decreases significantly. As with oranges versus grapefruits, in medicine, you usually have some prior information about the particular quantity you are trying to estimate. If the 95% CI that you obtained from your study seems as unlikely as a grapefruit-sized orange, then the probability that the interval contains the true parameter value is substantially less than 95%.

Again, we can summarize the Bayesian understanding of confidence intervals similarly to that of P-values and diagnostic tests:

> What you thought before + New information = What you think now

The "new information" in this case is the result of the study. The 95% CI is a range of parameter values consistent with the parameter estimate from the study, but it does not have a 95% probability of containing the true parameter value, because you cannot obtain posterior probability without prior probability.

## Understanding and reporting negative studies: P-values, power, and confidence intervals

There is a trend toward eschewing P-values in favor of confidence intervals, the latter being felt to be more informative. Confidence intervals are, in fact, more informative; although, it isn't really a fair comparison, because confidence intervals have two numbers and the P-value is only one number. Confidence intervals are particularly useful for negative studies – they let you see how big an effect could have been missed.

Consider the reporting and interpretation of negative studies as a progression from the most elementary to the most sophisticated. We can present this the way Sackett et al. (1991) have presented interpretation of diagnostic tests, using a progression of colored karate belts.

We will use as an example a study of treatment of febrile infants with oral amoxicillin to prevent complications (like meningitis or infected joints or bones) of bacteremia (bacteria in the blood). The study included children 3–36 months old with fevers of at least 39°C (Jaffe et al. 1987). The authors reported that 27 of the 955 children in the study were bacteremic and that complications occurred in 2 of 19

(10.5%) bacteremic infants treated with amoxicillin compared with 1 of 8 (12.5%) bacteremic infants treated with placebo, a difference that was not statistically significant (P = 0.9). Note that there were more than twice as many bacteremic children in the amoxicillin group (N = 19) as in the placebo group (N = 8), presumably due to bad luck (P = 0.07), although a problem with the randomization is also possible.

### White belt

The white belt just involves looking at the P-value to see whether it is ≥0.05 (or whatever alpha was chosen). Thus, a white belt reader would look at the study above and conclude, "amoxicillin doesn't work," because the P-value is far from significant. Many doctors and investigators have a white belt.

### Yellow belt

The yellow belt involves considering not only the P-value, but also the power of the study. (Recall that the power is $1 - \beta$, the probability that the null hypothesis will be rejected, given that a true difference of a specified magnitude exists.) The power of a study is often included with a sample size calculation in the "Methods" section of a paper. In fact, some reviewers and editors insist on this, although in fact (as discussed below), it is not of much use to readers. The basic idea is that a negative study is not convincing if it was underpowered.

The study cited above was, in fact, underpowered. The authors state in the discussion that the power to detect a fourfold difference between groups in the odds of complications was only 24%. The authors' conclusion that their "data do not support routine use of standard doses of amoxicillin . . ." is certainly reasonable, but that conclusion would also be true if they had studied 2 rather than 955 patients.

### Green belt

The green belt is to examine the 95% CI for the RR or OR. In this case, the authors did present a 95% CI for the OR for complications.[7] The point estimate of the OR was 1.2 with a 95% CI of 0.02 to 30.4. (This is actually the ratio of the odds of complications in the placebo group to the odds of complications in the amoxicillin group; they did not follow the convention of putting the odds in the active treatment group on top.) This tells you explicitly the range of values consistent with the study. One of us (TBN) was surprised that a negative study published in the *New England Journal of Medicine* would have such a wide confidence interval for its major outcome, and (with Dr. Robert Pantell) wrote a letter to the editor (Newman and Pantell 1988). The letter pointed out that a confidence interval for the OR that ranges from 0.02 to 30.4 suggests that the study provided virtually no information on the research question. True enough, but not the whole answer. Too bad we didn't have a brown belt! Read on.

---

[7] Why they presented the OR, and not the RR is not clear, as this was a randomized trial. It is especially puzzling because the 95% CI for the RR is quite a bit narrower! They also presented the risk difference (12.5% − 10.5% = 2%) and its confidence interval (−15% to +32%).

**Blue belt**

The blue belt does not apply to all studies, but does in this example. The key is to make sure that you do an intention-to-treat analysis. The analysis done by the authors compared complications *only among bacteremic patients*! But, as discussed in Chapter 9, the analysis should include all subjects randomized. At the time the amoxicillin was given, there was no way to know which children were bacteremic and which were not. Thus, benefits, risks, and costs might occur in nonbacteremic patients, and need to be compared between the entire amoxicillin group and the entire placebo group. The correct RR (keeping, for comparison purposes, the placebo group on top) is the ratio of 1/448 (the risk of complications in the placebo group) to 2/507 (the risk of complications in the amoxicillin group), which equals 0.57 with a 95% CI of 0.05 to 6.2.[8]

**Brown belt**

The confidence interval for the RR calculated in the "Blue belt" section is fine, but for making clinical decisions, it is really the absolute risk reduction (ARR), not the RR, that determines the balance of risks and benefits and hence clinical decisions. The brown belt involves calculating the (correct) ARR and its 95% CI. The ARR in this case was −0.17%. (Because the point estimate was an increase in risk with amoxicillin, the risk reduction is negative.) The 95% CI for the ARR goes from −0.9% to +0.5%. That is, the upper limit of the 95% CI for the benefit of amoxicillin in this study is an absolute reduction in risk of complications of 0.5%. This, in turn, means that the lowest number needed to treat consistent with this study would be 1/0.5% = 200. If we are pretty sure that a NNT of 200 is too high, then the study makes us confident that we should not routinely treat febrile infants with amoxicillin.

If we are trying to use the study results to help with a clinical decision about a treatment, the ARR and its confidence interval are most useful. However, the relative risk reduction (RRR) tends to be more generalizable than the ARR. Thus, for patients at higher risk of bacteremia and/or complications, the NNT could easily be lower and whether they might benefit from treatment remains unknown.

Looking at the 95% CI for the ARR is a good idea for positive studies as well. The whole P-value and hypothesis-testing system is designed to determine the consistency of the data with an effect size of zero. But ruling out an effect size of zero is not as useful as ruling out an effect size that would be too small to warrant treatment. Thus, we could be fairly certain that a treatment has some small beneficial effect but still uncertain about whether to prescribe it. If a 95% CI not only excludes no effect, but also excludes benefits that are clinically trivial (i.e., that would lead to an NNT that is much too high), the study provides much stronger evidence of a clinically meaningful effect.

---

[8] Note that the direction of the effect, albeit totally explicable by chance, is now in favor of placebo; the placebo group had a lower risk of complications than the amoxicillin group.

> KEY POINT: The most important thing to look for when a study of a possible treatment shows no difference between groups is the confidence interval for the ARR, to see whether a clinically significant benefit (or risk) is consistent with the study results.
>
> For a positive study, we want to look at the 95% CI for the ARR to see whether a clinically insignificant effect is consistent with the results.

### Black belt

This one doesn't exist yet. We're saving it just in case we get more insights!

### Once the study is completed, why are confidence intervals so much better than power?

When investigators set out to design a study, one of the things they need to do is estimate the required sample size. This generally involves making some guesses or assumptions about how the variables they wish to measure are distributed and the magnitude of the difference they hope to detect. Sometimes these assumptions turn out to be wrong. For example, perhaps when the investigators of the study of amoxicillin described above did their sample size calculation, they estimated that they would have many more bacteremic patients than they found. Once the study is done, however, it really doesn't matter what the investigators *thought* they were going to find when they designed the study. What they actually did find is what determines how informative the study is. This is much better expressed using a 95% CI, which incorporates evidence generated by the study. The power calculation, done before the results of the study were available, was based on less information.

For a negative study, the confidence interval is particularly useful when there is a trend in the data. For example, a little known result from the International Reflux Study in Children, a study of medical versus surgical treatment of vesicoureteral reflux, (reflux of urine from the bladder up the ureter to the kidney; Weiss et al. 1992) is the "within-groups" relationship between pyelonephritis (kidney infections) and renal scarring. Standard teaching is that scarring in children with reflux is due to infection – that is, to reflux of infected urine into the kidney. But in that study, children with one or more episodes of acute pyelonephritis were *less* likely to develop renal scarring: RR = 0.28; 95% CI = 0.07 to 1.14. The fact that the point estimate is far below one and that the upper limit of the 95% CI only goes to 1.14 is much more informative than just a statement that the results were not statistically significant. This study may not have had power to detect a doubling of the risk of scarring with infection, but because of how the results came out, it suggests that an effect of that magnitude is highly unlikely.[9]

---

[9] If you're really paying attention, you might argue that the prior probability that the relative risk would be less than 1 was very small, and we'd have to agree. That's why we said we can be pretty sure the risk is not *doubled*, rather than just saying we can be pretty sure it's within the 95% CI. You might also ask why we present the RR and its confidence interval, rather than the ARR. The reason is that the RR is better for assessing causality (the goal here), while the ARR is better for clinical decision making.

## Useful shortcut: confidence intervals for small numerators

A situation that arises frequently in clinical research is that you observe either no instances of the outcome (called "events" in probability lingo) or a very small number of them. Years ago, Hanley and Lippman–Hand (1983) wrote a classic paper about zero numerators, called "If Nothing Goes Wrong, Is Everything All Right?". They described the "Rule of Three," which states that, if you observe zero events out of N trials (e.g., no deaths in N = 100 people on a drug), then the upper limit of the 95% CI for the true event rate is about 3/N (Box 11.1).

**Example:** A new drug is given to 60 people. It seems to work, and has no serious adverse effects. The authors conclude it is "safe and effective." The upper limit for the 95% CI for any serious adverse effect is about 3/60, or 5%.

---

**Box 11.1: Derivation of the Rule of Three**

If p is the probability of an event, x is the number of events, and N is the number of trials, your goal is to find the value of p such that $P(x = 0) = 0.05$.

$$P(x = 0) = (1 - p)^N = 0.05$$

$$N \ln(1 - p) = \ln(0.05)$$

MacLaurin Series Expansion:

$$\ln(1 - p) = -p - p^2/2 - p^3/3 - p^4/4 - \cdots \approx -p, \text{ for small } p$$

$$N(-p) \approx \ln(0.05)$$

$$Np \approx \ln(20)$$

$$Np \approx 2.996$$

$$p \approx 3/N$$

(The "3" in the "Rule of 3" comes from the natural logarithm of 20, which is 3, or equivalently, from the natural logarithm of 1/20, which is −3.)

---

The "Rule of Three" for 0 numerators has analogs for slightly higher numerators, too (Newman 1995). Basically, for numerators of 0, 1, 2, 3, and 4, the numerator for the upper limit of the 95% CI is somewhere around 3, 5, 7, 9, and 10, respectively (Table 11.2). These numbers are not exact, but they are close enough, and a whole lot easier to do in your head or on your calculator than exact confidence intervals.

It is easier to illustrate this shortcut with examples than to explain it.

1. Three deaths are observed in 500 patients on a new drug. What is the upper limit of the 95% CI for the death rate?

   The short cut for 3 is to use 9 as the numerator for the upper limit of the 95% CI. So it would be ~9/500, or 1.8%. (The exact binomial answer is 1.74%.)

**Table 11.2.** Extension of the "Rule of 3" for 0
numerators to numerators up to 4

| Observed numerator | Approximate numerator for upper limit of 95% CI |
|---|---|
| 0 | 3 |
| 1 | 5 |
| 2 | 7 |
| 3 | 9 |
| 4 | 10 |

2. One case of HIV is found among 101 household contacts. What is the upper limit of the 95% CI for the risk of HIV among contacts?

   For a numerator of 1, you use 5. So the upper limit of the 95% CI is $\sim 5/101 = 5\%$. (The exact binomial answer is 5.4%.)

3. A laboratory test done on 50 patients with disease is found to be 98% sensitive. What is the lower limit of the 95% CI for sensitivity?

   a) First you need to figure out that there must have been 49/50 ($= 0.98 \times 50$) positive tests.

   b) Therefore, the false-negative rate was 1/50.

   c) The upper limit of the 95% CI for false-negative rate of 1/50 is about 5/50, or 10%.

   d) Therefore, lower limit of 95% CI for sensitivity is $100\% - 10\% = 90\%$. (Exact binomial answer is 89.4%.)

## Summary of key points

1. P-values are sometimes misinterpreted as the probability that the null hypothesis (e.g., of no difference between groups) is true. But because P-values are calculated conditional on the null hypothesis, they cannot provide the probability that it is true.

2. Confidence intervals provide a range of values consistent with results of the study, but it is not true that a 95% CI from a study has a 95% probability of containing the true value of the parameter being studied.

3. 95% CI for negative studies are more useful than power, because they include information obtained from the study results

4. In negative studies, look at the confidence interval for the absolute risk reduction (ARR), to see whether a clinically significant benefit (or risk) is consistent with the study results.

5. The 95% CIs of the ARR for positive studies are most convincing when they not only exclude a null effect, but also exclude effects too small to be clinically meaningful.

6. The "Rule of 3" for 0 numerators can be used to estimate the upper limit of the 95% CI for studies with no events. The rule can be extended to a "Rule of 3, 5, 7, 9, and 10" for numerators of 0, 1, 2, 3, and 4.

## References

Browner, W. S., and T. B. Newman (1987). "Are all significant P values created equal? The analogy between diagnostic tests and clinical research." *JAMA* **257**(18): 2459–63.

Glantz, S. A. (2002). *Primer of Biostatistics*. New York, NY, McGraw-Hill, Medical Pub. Div.

Goodman, S. N. (1999a). "Toward evidence-based medical statistics. 1: The P value fallacy." *Ann Intern Med* **130**(12): 995–1004.

Goodman, S. N. (1999b). "Toward evidence-based medical statistics. 2: The Bayes factor." *Ann Intern Med* **130**(12): 1005–13.

Goodman, S. N. (2001). "Of P-values and Bayes: a modest proposal." *Epidemiology* **12**(3): 295–7.

Guyatt, G., D. Rennie, et al. (2002). *Users' Guides to the Medical Literature: Essentials of Evidence-Based Clinical Practice*. Chicago, IL, AMA Press.

Hanley, J. A., and A. Lippman-Hand (1983). "If nothing goes wrong, is everything all right? Interpreting zero numerators." *JAMA* **249**(13): 1743–5.

Jaffe, D. M., R. R. Tanz, et al. (1987). "Antibiotic administration to treat possible occult bacteremia in febrile children." *N Engl J Med* **317**(19): 1175–80.

Newman, T. B. (1995). "If almost nothing goes wrong, is almost everything all right? Interpreting small numerators." *JAMA* **274**(13): 1013.

Newman, T. B., and R. H. Pantell (1988). "Occult bacteremia in febrile children." *N Engl J Med* **318**(20): 1338–9.

Sackett, D. L., R. B. Haynes, et al. (1991). *Clinical Epidemiology: A Basic Science for Clinical Medicine*. Boston, MA, Little Brown.

Sackett, D. L., R. B. Haynes, et al. (2000). Evidence-Based Medicine: How to practice and teach EBM, 2nd Ed. Edinburgh: Churchill Livingstone: 233.

Weiss, R., J. Duckett, et al. (1992). "Results of a randomized clinical trial of medical versus surgical management of infants and children with grades III and IV primary vesicoureteral reflux (United States). The International Reflux Study in Children." *J Urol* **148**(5 Pt 2): 1667–73.

## Chapter 11 Problems

1. Evaluate each of the following statements about statistical inference as true or false. Briefly explain your answer.
    a) If the P-value = 0.05, then there is a 95% probability that the results did not occur by chance.
    b) The null hypothesis generally states that there is a difference between the groups.
    c) If the P-value is sufficiently high, the null hypothesis is not rejected.
    d) The 95% CI is the range of values with a 95% probability of containing the true (population) value.

2. You may have been told or observed that, when a test is ordered as part of a chemistry panel of 20 tests, an abnormal result is more likely to be false positive than when the test is ordered by itself. Is this correct? Why?

3. A randomized trial from Italy (Veronesi et al. 2003) compared sentinel-node biopsy (just removing one underarm lymph node to see if it has cancer in it) with routine axillary dissection (opening up the armpit and trying to remove all of the nodes) in 516 women with primary breast cancer tumors ≤2 cm in diameter.

They found significantly less swelling, pain, scarring, and numbness or tingling in the women in the sentinel-node group. There also were fewer unfavorable events and deaths in that group, as shown in the table below:

|  | Axillary Dissection | Sentinel-Node Biopsy |
| --- | --- | --- |
| Number of subjects | 257 | 259 |
| Adverse events other than death (metastases, recurrences, etc.) | 21 | 13 |
| Deaths | 6 | 2 |

The authors' conclusion was: "Sentinel-node biopsy is a safe and accurate method of screening the axillary nodes for metastasis in women with a small breast cancer."

a) The point estimate for the death rate in the sentinel-node biopsy group was $2/259 = 0.77\%$. Use the shortcut in the chapter to estimate the upper limit of the 95 % CI for this estimate.

An accompanying editorial, however, was critical of the Italian study because of its small sample size (Krag and Ashikaga 2003). It cited two other trials in process as having appropriate sample sizes: one with power to detect about a 2% (absolute) difference in survival and the other with power to detect a 5% difference. As the editorialists put it:

> The era in which randomized clinical trials are dominated by a single institution – an approach that was perhaps justifiable in the past – is now over, since virtually no single institution can enroll enough patients to allow detection of small differences between two study groups...
>
> The conclusion that sentinel-node surgery does not result in reduced survival and therefore that it is a safe procedure, equivalent to axillary dissection, must await the completion of larger clinical trials with sufficient power.

Assume that, as suggested by the editorialists, a $\geq 2\%$ absolute difference in total mortality would be clinically significant. Partial output from Stata (csi command) to compare total mortality in the two groups is shown below. (The sentinel-node group is considered "exposed" and "cases" are deaths.)

**csi 2 6 257 251**

|  | Exposed | Unexposed | Total |  |
| --- | --- | --- | --- | --- |
| Cases | 2 | 6 | 8 |  |
| Noncases | 257 | 251 | 508 |  |
| Total | 259 | 257 | 516 |  |
| Risk | .007722 | .0233463 | .0155039 |  |
|  | Point estimate |  | [95% CI] |  |
| Risk difference | −0.0156243 |  | −0.0369425 | .0056939 |
| Risk ratio | 0.3307593 |  | 0.0673847 | 1.623539 |
|  | $\chi^2(1) = 2.06$ |  | $Pr > \chi^2 = 0.1509$ |  |

b) Based on the 95% CI, is a clinically significant ($\geq 2\%$) increase in mortality with sentinel-node biopsy consistent with the findings?

c) Imagine that you went through your answer to part (b) with the editorialists, and they remained skeptical. How would you explain their continued skepticism in Bayesian terms?

4. A case–control study (Foxman and Frerichs 1985) of urinary tract infections (UTIs) among female college students found that, among women who had sexual intercourse less than once a week, diaphragm use (compared with oral contraceptive use) was associated with increased odds of UTI (OR = 7.0; 95% CI 0.04 to 625).

a) Based on this result, what can you say about the posterior probability of the hypothesis that diaphragm use causes UTI in these women?

b) Why do you think the confidence interval is so wide?

5. A Glaxo–Smith–Kline-funded study compared the antidepressants paroxetine and imipramine with placebo in a randomized, double-blind study in adolescents with major depression (Keller et al. 2001). The "Results" section of that paper states:

> Serious adverse effects occurred in 11 [of 93] patients in the paroxetine group, 5 [of 95] in the imipramine group, and 2 [of 87] in the placebo group . . . The serious adverse effects in the paroxetine group consisted of headache during discontinuation taper (1 patient) and various psychiatric events (10 patients) . . . Of the 11 patients, only headache (1 patient) was considered by the treating investigator to be related to paroxetine.

The "Discussion" states:

> Because these serious adverse events were judged by the investigators to be related to treatment in only 4 patients (Paroxetine, 1; imipramine, 2; placebo, 1), causality cannot be determined conclusively.

The last sentence of the abstract is:

> CONCLUSIONS: Paroxetine is generally well tolerated and effective for major depression in adolescents.

Although no P-values for adverse events are presented in the paper, we calculated the P-value for serious adverse events, comparing paroxetine with placebo, and it is 0.014 (two-tailed).

a) The calculation above entirely ignores the fact that there was an imipramine group. If that group is included, the investigators would want to make three comparisons: paroxetine vs. imipramine, paroxetine vs. placebo, and imipramine vs. placebo. Using the Bonferroni correction for testing these three hypotheses at $\alpha = 0.05$, a P-value of $0.05/3 = 0.0133$ would be required to reject the null hypothesis, and results above would not be statistically significant. Do you think the Bonferroni correction is appropriate in this case? Why or why not?

    b) The authors indicate that the treating physicians generally did not attribute adverse effects in the paroxetine group to paroxetine, and for this reason "causality cannot be determined conclusively." Do you agree? Explain.

6. We have talked about the analogy between diagnostic tests to identify a disease and clinical research studies to identify a causal relationship between predictor and outcome. What is the expected effect of the Bonferroni correction used to adjust for multiple hypothesis testing on the *sensitivity* and *specificity* of a research study for identifying a causal relationship?

## References for problem set

Foxman, B., and R. R. Frerichs (1985). "Epidemiology of urinary tract infection: I. Diaphragm use and sexual intercourse." *Am J Public Health* **75**(11): 1308–13.

Keller, M. B., N. D. Ryan, et al. (2001). "Efficacy of paroxetine in the treatment of adolescent major depression: a randomized, controlled trial." *J Am Acad Child Adolesc Psychiatry* **40**(7): 762–72.

Krag, D., and T. Ashikaga (2003). "The design of trials comparing sentinel-node surgery and axillary resection." *N Engl J Med* **349**(6): 603–5.

Veronesi, U., G. Paganelli, et al. (2003). "A randomized comparison of sentinel-node biopsy with routine axillary dissection in breast cancer." *N Engl J Med* **349**(6): 546–53.

# Challenges for evidence-based diagnosis

## Introduction

We wrestled for a long time with the question of whether to include the term "evidence-based" in the title of this book. Although both of us are firm believers in the principles and goals of evidence-based medicine (EBM), we also knew that the term "evidence-based" would be viewed negatively by some potential readers (Grahame-Smith 1995; Lancet 1995; Healy 2006). We decided to keep "evidence-based" in the title and use this chapter to directly address some of the criticisms of EBM, many of which we believe have merit. We also recognize that, as elegant and satisfying as evidence-based diagnosis is, there are some very real barriers to applying it in a clinical setting. These barriers are the second topic of this chapter. Finally, we end the book with some thoughts on the future of evidence-based diagnosis and why it will be increasingly important.

## Criticisms of evidence-based medicine

### 1. EBM overvalues randomized blinded trials and denigrates other forms of evidence, including clinical experience

EBM is frequently misrepresented as requiring randomized blinded trials (or better yet, a systematic review of such trials) to prove that a treatment is useful. This has been humorously illustrated in a "systematic review" of "Parachute Use to Prevent Death and Major Trauma Related to Gravitational Challenge" (Smith and Pell 2003). The authors found no controlled trials of parachute use for the "gravitationally challenged" (people jumping out of airplanes) and concluded that "everyone might benefit if the most radical protagonists of evidence based medicine organised and participated in a double blind, randomised, placebo controlled, crossover trial of the parachute."

We admit this criticism finds some resonance with us, which was one of the reasons for including Chapter 10 ("Alternatives to Randomized Trials") in this book.

However, the solution is not to dismiss EBM; rather, it is to help its users to understand better the strengths and limitations of different types of evidence. Although we favor healthy skepticism about results of observational studies, particularly studies of treatments, EBM should not and does not require randomized blinded trials to prove the effectiveness of every treatment. We do not require randomized trials to prove that people with myopia see better with glasses, that electric shock works for ventricular fibrillation, or that antibiotics help patients with bacterial pneumonia (Gorman 2007). However, most treatments are not as obviously effective as wearing glasses. Often, the effectiveness of a treatment is doubtful enough to justify a randomized controlled trial. In this case, the results of a properly done trial will generally trump the observational results.

## 2. Evidence-based treatment recommendations tend toward the nihilistic

Related to the criticism that EBM insists too much on randomized trials is the concern that EBM either recommends against or fails to recommend treatments, when many people believe they work. Although we sympathize with patients and clinicians who find uncertainty uncomfortable and who appreciate being told what to do, we are distressed by a sense of paternalism and intellectual dishonesty that accompanies recommendations for tests and treatments that go far beyond available data, often making assumptions about patients' values that may be unwarranted. This is particularly problematic when those making the recommendations have a conflict of interest (Hayward 2008), as described in Chapter 6 ("Screening Tests").

A particularly contentious area for EBM is cancer screening. Results of randomized controlled trials suggest that mammographic screening for asymptomatic breast cancer in women aged 40 to 49 has only a small effect on breast cancer mortality (RRR ~15%; estimated NNT to prevent 1 death over 14 years is 1792; Humphrey et al. 2002), with a significant risk (20% to 56% for 10 mammograms) of false-positive results (Armstrong et al. 2007). The low prevalence of breast cancer in this age group, combined with the inaccuracy of the test, means that false positives and the consequent costly and uncomfortable biopsies will occur much more often than true positives. There is also the problem of pseudodisease; we know that some biopsy-proven breast "cancers" never progress to overt disease, but will nonetheless be treated as cancer. Reviewing the data in 1997, an expert panel convened by the National Institutes of Health recommended neither for nor against screening mammography in women aged 40 to 49. Instead, the panel recommended that a woman in this age group be counseled about potential benefits and harms before making her own decision about mammography (NIH 1997). Specialty groups, such as the American College of Radiology and the American College of Obstetricians, and disease-specific advocacy groups, such as the American Cancer Society, disagreed and recommended screening mammography in women aged 40 to 49. In 2006, former director of the National Institutes of Health Bernadine Healy summarized this controversy as part of a *U.S. News and World Report* critique of EBM (Healy 2006):

Remember the mammogram wars over whether women should get them during their 40s? The protagonists were the EBM-ers who said no and the radiologists and oncologists who said yes.

For the naysayers, randomized clinical trials were inadequate to show that the test saved lives, even though it did detect cancers sooner. Such a mammogram program would be costly, and unnecessary biopsies for false positive readings even costlier. But based on their interpretation of clinical evidence, cancer experts maintained that the test saved lives. What's more, they factored in the nature of the disease: more aggressive in younger women and best cured if picked up early. But in 1997 the Department of Health and Human Services gave a thumbs down to recommending that women start having mammograms in their 40s. Women promptly exercised their political clout, which led to an HHS reversal. (In fact, the trend has been for more screening in this age group, not less.)

It is instructive to note that Dr. Healy characterizes as a "thumbs down" the 1997 panel's recommendation that the screening decision be individualized. To some, particularly those concerned about reimbursement by third-party payers (see Criticism #3 below), recommending that a treatment decision be individualized appears to be the same as recommending against it. Dr. Healy failed to make this distinction when discussing prostate cancer screening as well (Box 12.1).

EBM provides an approach to validating research studies and quantitative methods for summarizing their results. Using this approach and these methods, different groups can arrive at different answers about the utility of a treatment or screening program, depending on their prior probabilities and values. (There is no right answer to the question of how many additional false-positive mammograms it is worth to get one more true-positive.) When a group that identifies itself as using the methods of EBM comes to a conclusion with which we disagree, we should review the evidence and how EBM was applied, not blame EBM for the conclusion we do not like.

### 3. EBM has been or might be used by payers as an excuse to deny payment and limit clinician autonomy

A 2007 *Time Magazine* article on EBM says that "insurance companies have been very aggressive in using evidence-based arguments to deny payment for untested treatments" (Gorman 2007). The plaintiff's lawyer in the Merenstein case (Box 12.1) defined EBM as purely a cost-saving method.

We share the concern that the language and methods of EBM may be misappropriated by organizations for which maximizing profit, rather than health, is the goal. A problem arises when the standards of evidence devised to determine whether to recommend population-wide preventive health interventions (which, for reasons described in Chapter 6, should be conservative) are applied to decisions about whether third-party payers will pay for particular tests and treatments (Woolf and George 2000). In this case, judgments and recommendations aimed at preserving physician and patient autonomy can end up preserving neither, if reimbursement for the desired care is denied. On the other hand, the perceived need to force third-party payers to provide coverage may lead to guidelines that are overly aggressive, leading to excess treatment, loss of patient and clinician autonomy, and creation of liability where none should exist (Newman and Maisels 2000).

It will always be necessary to set priorities for the allocation of limited health care resources. Efforts to control health care costs pre-dated EBM and would continue regardless of whether EBM existed. If payers did not use (or claim to use) the

### Box 12.1: EBM as malpractice

We recommend the *JAMA* essay "Winners and Losers" by Dr. Daniel Merenstein (2004), in which he describes his experience of being sued for not obtaining a prostate-specific antigen (PSA) test on a 53-year-old man in 1999. The plaintiff he had not screened was diagnosed in 2002 with incurable prostate cancer. The balance of benefits and risks for PSA testing for prostate cancer in 1999 was at least as questionable as for mammography in women aged 40 to 49 (US Preventive Services Task Force 2002). False positives lead to unnecessary biopsies, and treatments for indolent cancers (pseudodisease) carry the risk of death, incontinence, and impotence. If the patient is unfortunate enough, as in this case, to have an aggressive cancer, it is unclear whether early diagnosis prolongs life, although for the reasons described in Chapter 6, it will appear to do so. As with the NIH panel's recommendation about mammography, the evidence-based recommendation for PSA screening was, in Merenstein's words, "discussing with the patient the risks and benefits, providing thorough informed consent, and coming to a shared decision." Merenstein had documented this discussion and the shared decision not to obtain the PSA test. The plaintiff's lawyer showed that most doctors in the state would have obtained the PSA test without discussing the risks and benefits with the patient. In his closing arguments, the plaintiff's lawyer also put EBM on trial:

> He threw EBM around like a dirty word and named the residency and me as believers in EBM, and our experts as founders of EBM.... He urged the jury to return a verdict to teach residencies not to send any more residents on the street believing in EBM (Merenstein 2004).

The jury found that Merenstein was not liable, but the residency program that trained him in evidence-based practice was – for $1 million – despite the lack of evidence that an earlier diagnosis would have made any difference to the patient.

In her *U.S. News and World Report* essay critical of EBM, here is how Bernadine Healy summarized the case:

> EBM also questions the prostate-specific antigen test, or PSA, for prostate cancer. The evidence-based method concludes that the test brings more harm than benefit, as it leads to unneeded biopsies and surgeries on often slow-growing cancers. This is at odds with the American Cancer Society, which says that men should have annual PSAs starting at age 50, and African-Americans, who have a higher prostate cancer rate, at age 45. This does not help that young primary-care doctor who published a mournful essay in the *Journal of the American Medical Association* in 2004. He did not get a PSA on his 53-year-old patient, based on his dutiful practice of evidence-based medicine. When found to have advanced prostate cancer, the patient sued and won. The jury put its faith in the medical experts who testified that PSAs are the best way to pick up tumors when they are most treatable.

We disagree with Dr. Healy's framing of the issue. The question is not whether the PSA test is the best way to identify prostate tumors when they are most treatable. The questions are whether the expected benefit of the PSA test outweighs the risks of testing and overtreatment and whether patients should have any say in the decision to assume these risks.

methods of EBM to justify denying payment, they would rely on expert panels, common practice, and even more arbitrary justifications. The solution is not to attack EBM, but rather to attack third-party payers who use it inappropriately to limit reasonable care.

## Barriers to the idealized process of evidence-based diagnosis

In Chapters 3 and 4, we learned how to use Bayes's Rule to calculate the post-test probability of disease based on pre-test probability and the LR associated with the test's result. This is an oversimplification of the diagnostic process. How should we estimate the pre-test probability? If we are considering classic diagnostic tests, such as x-rays or laboratories, then the pre-test probability is the probability of disease based on the population prevalence, the patient's history, and the physical exam. But if the test is a physical exam finding, then the pre-test probability is based on whatever information is available prior to examining for that finding. The post-test probability after one test can become the pre-test probability for the next test, but as we discussed in Chapter 8, unless the two tests are independent, the LRs of the results on each sequential test depend on the results of previous tests. Also, clinicians do not do all tests in series, they do many tests in parallel – that is, simultaneously. Finally, as we have pointed out before, the question is not, "Does this patient have disease X?" but "What disease is causing this patient's illness?" Tests help clinicians choose between multiple possible diagnoses.

We will discuss three barriers to the Bayesian process of diagnosis: 1) clinicians do not estimate or even understand probabilities very well; 2) oversimplification of diagnostic problems to fit the evidence-based model can lead to questionable conclusions; and 3) the process is impractical to apply on a patient-by-patient basis.

### Clinicians, probability, and cognitive errors

A barrier for evidence-based diagnosis is that clinicians, like most people, do not estimate or even understand probabilities very well. They show wide variability, inconsistency, and irrationality in their estimates of probabilities. Even when given the pre-test probability, they do not properly use the test result and its LR to calculate post-test probabilities. Interestingly, however, asking clinicians, not for a probability, but for a *clinical decision*, reduces variability, inconsistency, and irrationality.

#### Errors in pre-test probability estimates

Several surveys have shown that different physicians given the same clinical vignette will provide widely different estimates for the probability of disease (Phelps and Levitt 2004; Dolan et al. 1986; Cahan et al. 2003, 2005). In one such survey, Cahan et al. (2003) gave clinicians the history, physical exam, and ECG description of a 58-year-old woman with chest pain. They asked for the probability of multiple different possible diagnoses, including active coronary artery disease, thoracic aortic dissection, esophageal reflux, and biliary colic. The probability estimates for any given diagnosis in the differential varied widely between clinicians. The estimated

> **Box 12.2: Bias**
>
> We have used the term "bias" many times in this book. The dictionary definition of "bias" is: "deviation of the expected value of an estimate from the quantity it estimates." In discussing a bias, we should be clear about what quantity is being systematically under- or overestimated. We have previously discussed multiple biases in clinical research that distort estimates of test accuracy or treatment efficacy. Now, we are discussing biases in clinicians' subjective estimates of disease probability – biases that arise from the use of heuristics. In the literature, the bias is named according to the heuristic from which it results: Representativeness Bias, Availability Bias, and Anchoring Bias.

probability of active coronary artery disease ranged from 1% to 99% with a median of 65% and an interquartile range of 30%. Moreover, the probabilities assigned by an individual physician to each diagnosis in the differential usually summed to much greater than 100%, even though the diagnoses were supposed to be mutually exclusive.

In a classic paper, Tversky and Kahneman (1974) pointed out that we all have difficulty dealing with probabilities and simplify the complex task of assessing probabilities by using heuristics that can lead to severe and systematic errors (i.e., bias; see Box 12.2). A "heuristic" is a rule of thumb used to simplify a problem, such as estimation of a quantity or probability, sometimes at the expense of precision and accuracy. Tversky and Kahneman's example of a heuristic is the subjective estimate of an object's distance from the viewer based on its visual clarity. This leads to overestimates of distance on foggy days and underestimates on clear days. Tversky and Kahneman described three heuristics commonly used to estimate probabilities: representativeness, availability, and adjustment from an anchor. Use of these heuristics can result in biased estimates of disease probability.

*Representativeness.* One of the heuristics used in estimating probability is representativeness, in which likelihood is confused with similarity. In medicine, if a clinical presentation is similar to the typical presentation of a rare disease, the clinician will assign that rare disease a high probability, without taking into account its very low prior probability. For example, among patients who present with chest pain, acute cardiac ischemia is thought to be between 50 and 500 times more likely than thoracic aortic dissection (Burt 1999; Kohn et al. 2005). Because of this, even if the chest pain has a characteristic typical of aortic dissection, such as radiation to the back, the probability of cardiac ischemia may still be at least as high as the probability of aortic dissection. However, many physicians will assign a much higher likelihood to dissection than to ischemia.

*Availability.* Availability is another heuristic used to estimate probabilities. Availability refers to the ease with which instances or occurrences of an event can be brought to mind. Of course, representativeness may be one contributor to availability: the presence of classic symptoms of a rare disease may make it available in memory.

However, other factors affect availability as well. For example, recent events are likely to be more available than earlier events. The Tversky and Kahneman (1974) article points out that "the subjective probability of traffic accidents rises temporarily when one sees a car overturned by the side of the road." An emergency physician is more likely to assign a high probability to aortic dissection if a case was discussed at the last department conference.

One's own experience is obviously more available than the experience of others. For example, surgeons at a hospital were asked to estimate overall (hospital-wide) surgical mortality. The estimates of surgeons from high-mortality specialties (e.g., neurosurgeons) were at least double the estimates of surgeons from low-mortality specialties (e.g., plastic surgeons). Thus, the mortality rate from personally performed operations exerted a disproportionate influence on judgment about the whole hospital's surgical mortality rate (Detmer et al. 1978).

Clinicians often overestimate the probability of a diagnosis with severe consequences because of the anticipated regret if the diagnosis were missed (Bornstein and Emler 2001). This could also be classified as "regret bias." Kahneman and Tversky did not use the term "regret bias," but it is related to use of the availability heuristic, because diagnoses with severe consequences are often more easily brought to mind. We mentioned the Cahan study in which clinicians were surveyed about likely diagnoses in a 58-year-old woman with 2 days of "episodic pressing/burning chest pain." The clinicians assigned aortic dissection a mean probability of 16%, whereas more common (and more likely) problems such as reflux and anxiety were assigned lower probabilities. Perhaps this was because failing to diagnose reflux or anxiety has minor consequences compared with failing to diagnose aortic dissection. When asked for the probability of a particular diagnosis, clinicians usually respond with their level of concern – not the actual likelihood.

Similarly, in Chapter 2 on reliability, we suggested that the same radiologist interpreting the same set of x-rays might be systematically more likely to rate them as abnormal after being sued for missing an abnormality. This is because the lawsuit makes the abnormality more *available* to the radiologist either by increasing its subjective probability or because the level of concern has increased.

*Adjustment from an anchor.* A third heuristic discussed by Tversky and Kahneman is to estimate a probability by starting from an initial value, called the "anchor," and adjusting to reach a final answer. As we shall see, even when the initial value is meaningful, adjustment can be inadequate. But this heuristic is especially problematic when the initial anchor is irrelevant.

For example, Brewer et al. (2007) presented to family physicians (via a mailed survey) a clinical vignette about a 32-year-old woman with cough, pleuritic chest pain, and low-grade fever. First, they established an irrelevant anchor. Half the participants were asked whether the chance of pulmonary embolism was greater or less than 1%; the other half were asked whether the chance was greater or less than 90%. Then, all the participants were asked to give a point estimate of the probability of pulmonary embolism. Physicians in the low anchor group estimated the likelihood of pulmonary embolism at 23% on average, whereas physicians in the high anchor group estimated the likelihood at 53%.

Even when the anchor has some relevance, we can underadjust our probability estimates. In any emergency department, there are critical care rooms for the sickest patients and areas (often multipatient rooms or wards) for the lowest acuity patients. A triage nurse places the patient in an area prior to the emergency physician's initial evaluation. In general, as the emergency physician approaches a patient in the low-acuity area, the chance of a serious condition requiring hospitalization is very low. But, one of the more common errors in emergency medicine is to send a patient home from the multipatient ward who would have been admitted from a critical care room. This is probably anchoring bias; the patient in the ward starts out with a low probability of serious illness that the emergency physician insufficiently adjusts upward. This phenomenon has also been called "triage cueing bias"(Croskerry and Wears 2003).

### Errors in post-test probability estimates

The discussion of adjusting from an anchor and its possible effect on pre-test probability estimates naturally leads to a discussion of cognitive bias in test interpretation. As mentioned in the introduction to this section, the pre-test probability for one test can be the post-test probability from a prior test, and many tests are done in parallel rather than in series. Because of this, the distinction between cognitive bias in test interpretation and cognitive bias in estimating pre-test probabilities is somewhat arbitrary. Attempts have been made to name the cognitive biases that contribute to our misinterpretation of test results (Dawson and Arkes 1987). For example, "confirmation bias" consists of cognitive "cherry-picking"; unconsciously, we both pay more attention to test results that support our initial impression and misinterpret nonspecific findings as confirmatory. "Premature closure" is choosing (and often labeling a patient with) a specific diagnosis that is not sufficiently supported by the test results. This can occur because of the patient's or our own discomfort with uncertainty. Confirmation bias and premature closure can be especially problematic if we stake ego on our initial impression by mentioning it to the patient or a member of the house staff, or if we are fatigued or under time pressure. Unlike representativeness and availability bias, cognitive errors in test interpretation, such as confirmation bias and premature closure, do not arise from commonly used heuristics for estimating probabilities.

*Intuition versus math.* Anchoring bias occurs when we are influenced by an irrelevant anchor or underuse new information to adjust from a relevant anchor. On the other hand, we often tend to overadjust probabilities of disease based on positive test results. Recall the example in Chapter 3 of a positive screening mammogram in a 45-year-old woman. The prevalence of breast cancer was 2.8/1,000. Before we teach probability updating in our class, we ask our students to estimate the probability of cancer given the prevalence, test characteristics, and the positive mammogram. The answers tend to exceed 50%. We saw in Chapter 3 that, assuming a sensitivity of 75% and a specificity of 93%, the actual answer is about 3%. This systematic bias is obviously not due to underadjustment from the anchor of 2.8/1,000. Rather, it represents failure to consider the very low pre-test probability. Using a mammography example similar to this one, Eddy (1982) concluded that physicians grossly overestimate probability of disease in patients with positive screening tests for rare diseases.

We spent Chapters 3 and 4 teaching you the mathematics of adjusting an initial pre-test probability to get a post-test probability, but as shown in Box 12.3, if you rely on your intuition instead of the math, you may get it wrong.

---

**Box 12.3**

Without doing any mental arithmetic, try answering the following problem adapted from Raiffa (1968):

There are two large, outwardly identical bags filled with red and white marbles. In Bag R3W1, 3/4 of the marbles are red and 1/4 are white. In Bag W3R1, 3/4 are white and 1/4 are red. You have been given one of the 2 bags, and are trying to figure out which one you got. You draw 12 marbles and find that 4 are white and 8 are red. (To simplify the math, we'll assume you drew them in that order, although it doesn't actually matter.) The bags hold thousands of marbles, so you don't have to worry about sampling without replacement versus with replacement. Keep in mind that the sample held predominantly *red* marbles. This obviously *lowers* likelihood that you started out with Bag W3R1, which has 3/4 white marbles. What is the probability that you got Bag W3R1, with its 3/4 white marbles and only 1/4 red marbles?

a)      >50%
b)      35–50%
c)      20–34%
d)      5–19%
e)      <5%

Circle your answer before reading on.

The pre-test odds = 1:1.

The probability of the sample[1] given Bag W3R1, with its 3/4 white balls is

$$P(4 \text{ white, 8 red} \mid \text{W3R1}) = 3/4 \times 3/4 \times 3/4 \times 3/4 \times 1/4 \times 1/4 \times 1/4 \times 1/4 \times 1/4$$
$$\times 1/4 \times 1/4 \times 1/4.$$

$$P(4 \text{ white, 8 red} \mid \text{R3W1}) = (3/4)^4 \times (1/4)^8$$

The probability of the sample given Bag R3W1, which contains only 1/4 white balls is

$$P(4 \text{ white, 8 red} \mid \text{W3R1}) = 1/4 \times 1/4 \times 1/4 \times 1/4 \times 3/4 \times 3/4 \times 3/4 \times 3/4 \times 3/4$$
$$\times 3/4 \times 3/4 \times 3/4.$$

$$P(4 \text{ white, 8 red} \mid \text{R3W1}) = (1/4)^4 \times (3/4)^8$$

---

[1] This is a sample with one specific sequence of 4 white and 8 red marbles. If we wanted the probability of *any* combination of 8 red and 4 white marbles, we would have to multiply by a factor of $(12 \times 11 \times 10 \times 9)/(4 \times 3 \times 2 \times 1)$, but this would be in both the numerator and denominator of the LR, and hence would cancel out anyway.

The LR is

$$LR = \frac{P(4 \text{ white, } 8 \text{ red} \mid W3R1)}{P(4 \text{ white, } 8 \text{ red} \mid R3W1)}$$

$$LR = \frac{(3/4)^4 \times (1/4)^8}{(3/4)^8 \times (1/4)^4} = \frac{(1/4)^4}{(3/4)^4}$$

$$= \frac{1}{3^4}$$

$$= 1/81$$

Post-test odds is pre-test odds times the LR
Post-test odds = $1 \times 1/81 = 0.012 \approx$ post-test probability.
So, the correct answer is (e).
How did you do? Most people exhibit insufficient adjustment from the pre-test probability of 50% and answer (b) or (c).

This is illustrated by a study by Sox et al. (2006), who asked pediatricians for the post-test probability of pertussis given a pre-test probability of 30% and a negative pertussis direct fluorescent antibody (DFA) test. One-third of the physicians were given the sensitivity (50%) and specificity (95%) of the DFA; one-third were given the test characteristics explained in nontechnical terms; and one-third received no information about test characteristics.

The correct post-test probability is 18%.[2] Two-thirds of the respondents estimated a post-test probability *higher than* the pre-test probability of 30%, despite the negative DFA result. This was *worse* in the two groups that were given the test's characteristics. We hope readers of this book would do better!

### Probability estimates versus decision making

When clinicians estimate disease probabilities, we use heuristics that can result in significant biases. Also, despite the medical school and CME courses on clinical epidemiology and EBM, and despite the nomograms, slide-rules, and on-line calculators designed to make the process easier, many clinicians still cannot properly update pre-test probabilities based on the results of a diagnostic test. On the other hand, clinicians are probably more consistent and rational in their clinical decision making than they are in their probability estimates. In the literature on cognitive biases, this is the distinction between judgment (probability estimates) and choice (decision making) (Kahneman et al. 1982; Brewer et al. 2007).

Although experienced clinicians do not estimate or update probabilities well, they often make good decisions that take into account varying presentations and consequences of error. In the study of Brewer et al. (2007), physician estimates for the probability of pulmonary embolism were influenced by the irrelevant anchors of 1% and 90%. However, the authors went on to ask the physicians for a decision

---

[2] You can just about do this in your head. Convert 30% probability to pre-test odds of 3/7. Caculate LR(−) = 50%/95% ≈ 1/2. Post-test odds = 3/7 × 1/2 = 3/14. Convert to post-test probability = 3/17 ≈ 0.18.

about next steps.[3] Although the initial anchor affected probability estimates, it did not appear to affect the treatment decisions. In fact, the physicians in the low anchor group were slightly more aggressive about testing and treating for pulmonary embolism. Similarly, although doctors may not be very good at estimating the probability of serious illness, they may do at least as well as decision rules at deciding whom to admit and treat (Pantell et al. 2004; Tierney et al. 1985; Davison et al. 1990).

This is not to say that cognitive errors do not affect patient outcomes. In *How Doctors Think*," Groopman (2007) gives multiple examples of cognitive errors in diagnosis resulting from the biases mentioned above and contributed to by time pressure, fatigue, and cultural barriers. Groopman's choice for a book title is itself an indication of the importance of cognitive error in medicine. Of course, we all focus on the cognitive errors leading to "misses," failures to identify a serious diagnosis, which lead to the most dramatic stories. But more commonly, flawed thinking leads to overtesting, which is much more mundane. For example, unnecessary tests, like an obligatory throat culture after a negative rapid strep test (Problem 3.5), are often recommended because clinicians misunderstand and miscalculate the implications of imperfect sensitivity (a small but non-zero false-negative rate).

## Oversimplification of the diagnostic problem

Another problem with evidence-based diagnosis is that its application sometimes entails oversimplification that leads to highly questionable conclusions.

Cardall et al (2004) recommend against obtaining a WBC count to determine whether a patient with abdominal pain has appendicitis, because it is "not clinically useful" for distinguishing between patients with and without appendicitis. But their study showed that a WBC $\geq 15,000/\mu L$ has an LR of 3.2 for appendicitis. Moreover, the study failed to adequately consider that the WBC count is a continuous test; a WBC count of $28,000/\mu L$ or $500/\mu L$ would appropriately affect a clinician's management decisions. Also, when confronted by a patient with abdominal pain, the question is not whether the patient has appendicitis; the questions are what the patient does have and whether additional testing (e.g., a CT scan) can help identify the problem. A markedly elevated WBC count is associated with other conditions, such as diverticulitis and small bowel obstruction, which are identifiable on CT. Finally, the study did not consider something that clinicians do consider – the WBC count is always part of a complete blood count, which provides a hematocrit and a platelet count as well, both of which may help with diagnosis and treatment decisions.

Experienced clinicians are also justifiably concerned about evidence-based diagnosis when a book on the subject pronounces the electrocardiogram as "useless testing" in identifying which patients with acute chest pain to admit to the hospital (Knottnerus and Van Weel 2002).

---

[3] The choices were: normal care; lung scan; pulmonary angiogram; hospitalize; and treat with anticoagulant.

Making a multilevel test dichotomous or failure to adequately consider the full range of possible test results are oversimplifications addressed in Chapter 4. The multiplicity of possible diagnoses to explain a patient's illness is more difficult to accommodate.

### Is evidence-based diagnosis practical?

The main problem with the step-by-step Bayesian process of evidence-based diagnosis is that it is impractical for clinicians to apply on a patient-by-patient basis. According to Croskerry (2002), in their "flesh-and-blood decision making," emergency physicians are not and cannot be formal Bayesians. Instead, they have developed several decision-making strategies that reduce decision complexity and build economy and redundancy into the process. The primary strategy is to make a treatment/disposition decision fairly soon after the presentation of a patient at the emergency department, or to commit to a formal work-up involving an array of tests, imaging techniques, and consultations.

MAK is an emergency physician in a nonteaching, community hospital who sees, without the interposition of medical students or residents, approximately 1,500 patients per year. Many of these patients, such as those with chest or abdominal pain, fever, shortness of breath, or altered mental status, present significant diagnostic problems. TBN is a pediatrician at a teaching hospital who attends in an urgent care clinic and a newborn nursery, where the prevalence of serious illness is lower, but diagnostic barriers still exist. If anyone were going to apply the step-by-step Bayesian approach to diagnosis, the co-authors of a book on evidence-based diagnosis would. But we almost never, on a patient-by-patient basis, estimate pre-test probabilities and then update them using the results of the tests that we order. We do use the basic logic of evidence-based diagnosis with many of the patients we see. For example, material covered in this text has helped us:

- decide not to order tests (e.g., a head CT on a child with a minor head injury) when the disease is so unlikely that the pain, risk, and cost (e.g., radiation exposure) of testing are not worth the negligible chance of a positive result.
- avoid ordering nonspecific tests (e.g., myeloperoxidase and C-reactive protein).
- accept some negative initial tests (e.g., rapid strep test or urinalysis) without ordering confirmatory tests (e.g., throat or urine cultures).
- interpret tests (e.g, BNP) along a whole range of possible values, rather than dichotomizing them as either positive or negative.
- act on mildly abnormal test results (e.g., a slightly elevated D-dimer or WBC count) when our level of concern is high but wait when we get the same results on patients about whom we are less concerned.
- become more aware of how our own biases and cognitive limitations affect our ability to diagnose and treat disease.

One way to address the practical barriers to the step-by-step Bayesian approach is to minimize the need for front-line clinicians to estimate or deal with probabilities by providing them with clinical decision rules and guidelines, to be discussed in the next section.

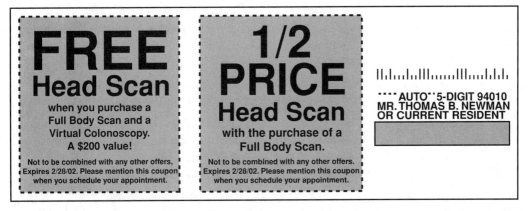

Figure 12.1 Example of direct-to-consumer advertising from an imaging center, sent via direct mail to TBN.

## The future of evidence-based diagnosis

As we come to the end of this book, we cannot resist the temptation to speculate about the direction in which medical tests are moving, and how the material in this book might help readers keep up.

One direction seems clear: more and more new tests will be offered, and they will need to be critically evaluated. These tests will take advantage of advances in technology, particularly in genetics, molecular biology, and imaging. Increasingly, we fear, they may be promoted directly to consumers (Fig. 12.1), who are ill-equipped to critically evaluate the claims of the promoters.

Clinicians, already drowning in a sea of data, will increasingly rely on decision rules and guidelines, sometimes implemented as computer-based decision aids, to assist with deciding which tests to order and how to interpret the results. This will help to overcome both knowledge gaps about pre-test probabilities and LRs, as well as cognitive errors in probability estimation and updating. The authors of the decision rules and guidelines evaluate treatment effectiveness, determine test characteristics, estimate pretest probabilities, do the Bayesian updating for a range of clinical scenarios, and then provide their recommendations to clinicians. However, clinicians will need to be skeptical consumers of these decision rules and guidelines, just as they are of individual tests. As shown in this book, decisions about which tests to order depend not only on the costs and accuracy of tests, but on the efficacy and risks of different treatment options, and assessment of these may depend on the patient's values. For all of the reasons discussed in Chapter 6, it will be important to discern whose values and whose perspective are reflected in any such decision aids. The material in this text should help us select and interpret diagnostic and screening tests so as to maximize the benefit to our patients' health.

## Summary

1. Evidence-based medicine has been criticized for being overly reliant on evidence from randomized controlled trials, overly skeptical about the efficacy of many

treatments, and an excuse for insurance companies to deny coverage for treatments. These valid concerns should give rise to caution about the application of EBM, not to its abandonment.

2. Evidence-based diagnosis as a step-by-step Bayesian process faces the challenge that clinicians often do not deal well with probabilities, either estimating pre-test probabilities or interpreting tests and calculating post-test probabilities. Despite this, experienced clinicians often make good clinical decisions.

3. However, with knowledge of evidence-based diagnosis and understanding of our cognitive biases and limitations, we can do even better.

4. Clinicians, as skeptical consumers, can use the methods of evidence-based diagnosis to evaluate and use the increasing number of individual tests, clinical decision rules, and practice guidelines that appear in the literature and the marketplace.

# References

Armstrong, K., E. Moye, et al. (2007). "Screening mammography in women 40 to 49 years of age: a systematic review for the American College of Physicians." *Ann Intern Med* **146**(7): 516–26.

Bornstein, B. H., and A. C. Emler (2001). "Rationality in medical decision making: a review of the literature on doctors' decision-making biases." *J Eval Clin Pract* **7**(2): 97–107.

Brewer, N. T., G. B. Chapman, et al. (2007). "The influence of irrelevant anchors on the judgments and choices of doctors and patients." *Med Decis Making* **27**(2): 203–11.

Burt, C. W. (1999). "Summary statistics for acute cardiac ischemia and chest pain visits to United States EDs, 1995–1996." *Am J Emerg Med* **17**(6): 552–9.

Cahan, A., D. Gilon, et al. (2003). "Probabilistic reasoning and clinical decision-making: do doctors overestimate diagnostic probabilities?" *QJM* **96**(10): 763–9.

Cahan, A., D. Gilon, et al. (2005). "Clinical experience did not reduce the variance in physicians' estimates of pretest probability in a cross-sectional survey." *J Clin Epidemiol* **58**(11): 1211–6.

Cardall, T., J. Glasser, et al. (2004). "Clinical value of the total white blood cell count and temperature in the evaluation of patients with suspected appendicitis." *Acad Emerg Med* **11**(10): 1021–7.

Croskerry, P. (2002). "Achieving quality in clinical decision making: cognitive strategies and detection of bias." *Acad Emerg Med* **9**(11): 1184–204.

Croskerry, P., and R. Wears (2003). Safety errors in emergency medicine. In: *Emergency Medicine Secrets*. Markovchik. VJ and Pons. PT. Philadelphia, PA, Hanley and Belfus.

Davison, G., A. L. Suchman, et al. (1990). "Reducing unnecessary coronary care unit admissions: a comparison of three decision aids [see comments]." *J Gen Intern Med* **5**(6): 474–9.

Dawson, N. V., and H. R. Arkes (1987). "Systematic errors in medical decision making: judgment limitations." *J Gen Intern Med* **2**(3): 183–7.

Detmer, D. E., D. G. Fryback, et al. (1978). "Heuristics and biases in medical decision-making." *J Med Educ* **53**(8): 682–3.

Dolan, J. G., D. R. Bordley, et al. (1986). "An evaluation of clinicians' subjective prior probability estimates." *Med Decis Making* **6**(4): 216–23.

Eddy, D. M. (1982). Probabilistic reasoning in clinical medicine: problems and opportunities. In: *Judgment Under Uncertainty: Heuristics and Biases*. D. Kahneman, P. Slovic, and A. Tversky, editors. Cambridge, Cambridge University Press, pp. 249–267.

Gorman, C. (2007). "Are Doctors Just Playing Hunches?" *Time Magazine*. February 15, 2007.

Groopman, J. (2007). How Doctors Think. New York: Houghton Mifflin.

Grahame-Smith, D. (1995). "Evidence based medicine: Socratic dissent [see comments]." *Br Med J* **310**(6987): 1126–7.

Hayward, R. (2008). "Access to clinically-detailed patient information." *Med Care* **46**(3): 229.

Healy, B. (2006). "Who Says What's Best?" *U.S. News and World Report.*

Humphrey, L. L., M. Helfand, et al. (2002). "Breast cancer screening: a summary of the evidence for the U.S. Preventive Services Task Force." *Ann Intern Med* **137**(5 Part 1): 347–60.

Kahneman, D., P. Slovic, et al. (1982). *Judgment Under Uncertainty: Heuristics and Biases.* Cambridge, Cambridge University Press.

Knottnerus, J. A., and C. Van Weel (2002). General Introduction: evaluation of diagnostic procedures. In: *The Evidence Base of Clinical Diagnosis.* J. A. Knottnerus, editor. London, BMJ Books, pp. 1–18.

Kohn, M. A., E. Kwan, et al. (2005). "Prevalence of acute myocardial infarction and other serious diagnoses in patients presenting to an urban emergency department with chest pain." *J Emerg Med* **29**(4): 383–90.

Lancet (1995). "Evidence-based medicine, in its place." *Lancet* **346**(8978): 785.

Merenstein, D. (2004). "A piece of my mind. Winners and losers." *JAMA* **291**(1): 15–6.

Newman, T. B., and M. J. Maisels (2000). "Less aggressive treatment of neonatal jaundice and reports of kernicterus: lessons about practice guidelines." *Pediatrics* **105**(1 Pt 3): 242–5.

NIH (1997). "NIH Consensus Statement. Breast cancer screening for women ages 40–49." *NIH Consens Statement* **15**(1): 1–35.

Pantell, R. H., T. B. Newman, et al. (2004). "Management and outcomes of care of fever in early infancy." *JAMA* **291**(10): 1203–12.

Phelps, M. A., and M. A. Levitt (2004). "Pretest probability estimates: a pitfall to the clinical utility of evidence-based medicine?" *Acad Emerg Med* **11**(6): 692–4.

Raiffa, H. (1968). *Decision Analysis: Introductory Lectures on Choices Under Uncertainty.* Reading, MA, Addison–Wesley.

Smith, G. C., and J. P. Pell (2003). "Parachute use to prevent death and major trauma related to gravitational challenge: systematic review of randomised controlled trials." *Br Med J* **327**(7429): 1459–61.

Sox, C. M., T. D. Koepsell, et al. (2006). "Pediatricians' clinical decision making: results of 2 randomized controlled trials of test performance characteristics." *Arch Pediatr Adolesc Med* **160**(5): 487–92.

Tierney, W. M., B. J. Roth, et al. (1985). "Predictors of myocardial infarction in emergency room patients." *Crit Care Med* **13**(7): 526–31.

Tversky, A., and D. Kahneman (1974). "Judgment under uncertainty: heuristics and biases." *Science* **185**: 1124–31.

US Preventive Services Task Force (2002). "Screening for prostate cancer: recommendation and rationale." *Ann Intern Med* **137**(11): 915–6.

Woolf, S. H., and J. N. George (2000). "Evidence-based medicine. Interpreting studies and setting policy." *Hematol Oncol Clin North Am* **14**(4): 761–84.

# Answers to problems

## Chapter 1 Problem answers: understanding diagnosis

1. A diagnosis of rotavirus would not often affect treatment decisions, as treatment will generally just be hydration. It might affect decisions about other tests to determine the cause of the diarrhea, although we suspect this is an uncommon justification because when people send stool samples to try to identify an organism it is typically all at once, before the result of the rotavirus test would be available. It might affect decisions about isolation, except that we think one should assume that all childhood diarrhea is quite infectious. The main use would be in tracking an epidemic – for example, of diarrhea on an inpatient ward – or for estimating the impact of a vaccine. Sporadic testing by individual clinicians is unlikely to be very helpful for the latter purpose.

2. Although this infant does not meet the strict definition of colic used in the randomized trials, he has an entity we might call "crying distressing enough to try a formula change." In this case, the treatment is benign, and the symptom is highly distressing. There is no biological reason to think that benefits of a formula change will exceed the risks and costs only if the crying is at least 3 hours a day, three times a week.

3. Whether metastatic undifferentiated carcinoma is a sufficient diagnosis depends on what decisions are to be made and how difficult it will be to make a more specific diagnosis. Although we suspect the prognosis is grim no matter what the primary is, it is possible that there are some diagnoses for which he would choose chemotherapy. On the other hand, we did not tell you much about the patient – some 86-year-olds are much better candidates for chemotherapy than others, either because of underlying comorbidities or patient preferences.

   If this were our family member, and the additional workup was going to be risky or invasive, we would want an estimate of the likelihood that a more strenuous search would identify something for which treatment would be a reasonable option and how much he might gain from such treatment. The most important thing is to realize that the decision to pursue a more specific diagnosis should be just that – a decision. It should not be automatic.

4. Once again, it comes down to thinking about "what decision is this test going to help me make?" If the goal of the VCUG is to diagnose reflux so you can treat with antibiotics, it is helping you to avoid two kinds of mistakes:

   a) Failing to treat a patient who does have vesicoureteral reflux with prophylactic antibiotics; and

   b) Prescribing prophylactic antibiotics to a patient with a history of UTI but without vesicoureteral reflux.

It is not clear whether either of these two "mistakes" is actually bad, because there is no evidence that the antibiotics work in either setting. Therefore, it is hard to justify putting a child through the trauma of a VCUG to avoid making these mistakes.

## Chapter 2 Problem answers: reliability and measurement error

1a. $(16 + 14)/60 = 30/60 = 0.5 = 50\%$

1b. $(16 + 3)/60 = 19/60 = 0.317 = 31.7\%$

1c. $(16 + 27)/60 = 43/60 = 0.7167 = 71.7\%$

1d. Expected numbers in cells:

|  | Angina | Atypical CP |
|---|---|---|
| **Angina** | $(19 \times 30)/60 = 9.5$ | |
| **Atypical CP** | | $(41 \times 30)/60 = 20.5$ |

so, the expected agreement is: $(9.5 + 20.5)/60 = 0.5 = 50\%$.

1e. kappa = (observed − expected)/(100% − expected)

$$= (71.7\% - 50\%)/(100\% - 50\%)$$

$$= 21.7\%/50\%$$

$$= 0.43$$

1f. The disagreements are unbalanced: the diagnosis based on ICD-9 codes appears to have been looser than the consensus. Although one can see this by looking at the marginals, it is more dramatic looking for asymmetry along the diagonal, where there were only 3 cases where the consensus was angina and the ICD-9 code was not, whereas there were 14 where the ICD-9 code was for angina and the consensus was not.

This suggests that the prevalence of unstable angina could be falsely high in a study by these investigators in which the diagnosis was based on ICD-9 codes.

2a. Observed Agreement $= (3 + 3)/10 = 6/10 = 60\%$

Expected Agreement $= (0.5 \times 5 + 0.5 \times 5)/10 = (2.5 + 2.5)/10 = 5/10 = 50\%$

Kappa $= (60\% - 50\%)/(100\% - 50\%) = 10\%/50\% = 0.20$

2b. Observed Agreement $= (5 + 1)/10 = 60\%$

Expected Agreement $= (0.7 \times 7 + 0.3 \times 3)/10 = (4.9 + 0.9)/10 = 5.8/10 = 58\%$

Kappa $= (60\% - 58\%)/(100\% - 58\%) = 2\%/42\% = 0.048$

2c. You can think of the second kappa calculation as assuming that the two physicians knew ahead of time that the right lower quadrant would be tender in 7 out of the 10 patients. The kappa of 0.048 says that they really didn't do much better than if they each had just skipped the exam and randomly selected the 7 patients to classify as tender. If the two observers agree that the prevalence of the finding is very high or very low, it is hard for them to have a high kappa.

2d. Observed Agreement $= (3 + 3)/10 = 60\%$

Expected Agreement $= (0.7 \times 3 + 0.3 \times 7)/10 = (2.1 + 2.1)/10 = 4.2/10 = 42\%$.

Kappa $= (60\% - 42\%)/(100\% - 42\%) = 18\%/58\% = 0.31$

2e. The disagreements were unbalanced; the surgeon systematically said "not tender" when the emergency physician said "tender." As a result, the prevalence estimates are different; the surgeon felt that only 3 out of 10 patients had tenderness, whereas the emergency physician felt that 7 out of 10 had tenderness. Just as kappa gave them no credit for agreeing on the prevalence in part (c), it takes away nothing for disagreeing on the prevalence in part (d), so the kappa of 0.31 indicates fair agreement. (Note, however, that with this level of unbalanced disagreement, the kappa observed in part (d) is as high as it can be; there is no way to keep these marginals and place numbers inside the table that will give a higher kappa.)

3. If observed agreement is greater than expected agreement, kappa will be greater than 0. To get the kappa above 0 with observed agreement less than 50%, you need an expected agreement much less than 50%. One can construct such a 2 × 2 table by making the marginals disparate. This decreases the expected agreement and leads to a higher kappa.

Here's a simple example:

| | **Obs #1** | | |
|---|---|---|---|
| **Obs #2** | **Abnormal** | **Normal** | **Total** |
| **Abnormal** | 1 | 0 | 1 |
| **Normal** | 3 | 1 | 4 |
| **Total** | 4 | 1 | 5 |

Observed agreement $= (1 + 1)/5 = 40\%$

Expected agreement $= (1/5 \times 4 + 4/5 \times 1)/5 = (0.8 + 0.8)/5 = 1.6/5 = 32\%$

Kappa $= (40\% - 32\%)/(100\% - 32\%) = 0.118$

4a.

|   | 1 | 2 | 3 | 4 | 5 |
|---|---|---|---|---|---|
| 1 | 1 | 0.9375 | 0.75 | 0.4375 | 0 |
| 2 | 0.9375 | 1 | 0.9375 | 0.75 | 0.4375 |
| 3 | 0.75 | 0.9375 | 1 | 0.9375 | 0.75 |
| 4 | 0.4375 | 0.75 | 0.9375 | 1 | 0.9375 |
| 5 | 0 | 0.4375 | 0.75 | 0.9375 | 1 |

The quadratic weights are shown above. The weighted kappa is higher than unweighted kappa because there is much more partial agreement than would be expected based on the marginals alone. As shown above, quadratic weighted kappa is very generous with "partial credit." In fact, it gives 44% credit for disagreements that are 3 categories apart. This means that the observers would get 44% "credit" if one said that the findings were nonspecific and the other said that the findings showed clear evidence of penetration.

4b.

i) The exclusion would probably increase kappa by limiting the comparison only to photos that all raters agreed were "interpretable."

ii) They could have included a 6th category in the grid, for "unable to interpret," to see if the raters agreed on that rating. This would have precluded use of weighted kappa, however, unless they could place "unable to interpret" on the ordinal scale of the findings. Alternatively, they could have combined "unable to interpret" with "nonspecific findings" – in both cases the rater is making no judgment about sexual abuse – which would preserve the ability to calculate weighted kappa.

4c. The estimates of kappa from this study are probably higher than would be obtained with less experienced examiners. If the conclusion of the study is that inter-rater reliability is not very good, this would only be strengthened by the high level of experience of the examiners. On the other hand, although it seems unlikely in this setting, it is worth at least considering the possibility that they see a referral population in whom findings are especially difficult to interpret.

4d. This is a fascinating and counter-intuitive finding. One would expect kappa to increase with provision of more information. The drop in kappa is probably due to some combination of:

1. Interobserver agreement on interpretation of the history is worse than agreement on physical findings. The lower kappa when history is provided suggests a) that they are using the history to interpret the physical examination, and b) they disagree about how to do this.

2. The sample size was higher when the history was provided, because fewer photographs were regarded as uninterpretable. It looks like perhaps the agreement on these photos was very poor.

3. The difference could be due to chance. Confidence intervals are not provided, but given the sample size and the consistency and magnitude of the difference, it seems chance is probably not the whole explanation.

**Note:** If the history increased the agreement on the marginals, this could lead to a decrease in kappa. However, we can't think of any mechanism by which telling clinicians the history would lead to greater agreement on the marginals without correspondingly greater agreement within the table.

5a. Observed Agreement $= (30 + 4 + 1 + 28 + 1)/116 = 64/116 = 55.2\%$

Expected Agreement:

|  |  | Second | | | | | |
|---|---|---|---|---|---|---|---|
|  |  | 1 | 2 | 3 | 4 | 5 | Total |
|  | 1 | 12.4 |  |  |  |  | 41 |
| First | 2 |  | 1.8 |  |  |  | 14 |
|  | 3 |  |  | 0.2 |  |  | 2 |
|  | 4 |  |  |  | 18.6 |  | 44 |
|  | 5 |  |  |  |  | 0.6 | 15 |
|  | Total | 35 | 15 | 12 | 49 | 5 | 116 |

Expected Agreement: We won't show all the calculations; the expected agreement in the upper left cell is $(41/116) \times 35 = 12.4$, and other cells are calculated similarly.

$(12.4 + 1.8 + 0.2 + 18.6 + 0.6)/116 = 33.6/116 = 29.0\%$.

So kappa: $(55.2\% - 29.0\%)/(100\% - 29.0\%) = 0.37$, as reported by the authors.

5b.

| Verbal GCS subscore |  | Second measure (within 5 minutes) | | | | | |
|---|---|---|---|---|---|---|---|
|  |  | 1 | 2 | 3 | 4 | 5 | Total |
|  | 1 | 12 | 5 | 2 | 4 | 0 | 23 |
| First | 2 | 2 | 4 | 3 | 4 | 1 | 14 |
| Measure | 3 | 0 | 0 | 1 | 1 | 0 | 2 |
|  | 4 | 2 | 5 | 6 | 28 | 3 | 44 |
|  | 5 | 1 | 1 | 0 | 12 | 1 | 15 |
|  | Total | 17 | 15 | 12 | 49 | 5 | 98 |

The only difference is the cell (1,1) contains $30 - 18 = 12$, and the marginal totals have been changed accordingly.

Calculation of kappa:

Observed Agreement $= (12 + 4 + 1 + 28 + 1)/98 = 46/98 = 46.9\%$

Expected Agreement:

| Verbal GCS subscore | | Second measure (within 5 minutes) | | | | | |
|---|---|---|---|---|---|---|---|
| | | 1 | 2 | 3 | 4 | 5 | Total |
| | 1 | 4.0 | | | | | 23 |
| First | 2 | | 2.1 | | | | 14 |
| Measure | 3 | | | 0.2 | | | 2 |
| | 4 | | | | 22.0 | | 44 |
| | 5 | | | | | 0.8 | 15 |
| | Total | 17 | 15 | 12 | 49 | 5 | 98 |

Expected Agreement $= (4.0 + 2.1 + 0.2 + 22.0 + 0.8)/98 = 29.1/98 = 29.7\%$
Kappa $= (46.9\% - 29.7\%)/(100\% - 29.7\%) = 0.24$. This is what the authors reported.

5c. Kappa should be (and is) lower for the subset excluding the 18 intubated patients because they were exact agreements (1 for both observers). Eliminating agreements reduces kappa.

5d.

| | | Second | | | | |
|---|---|---|---|---|---|---|
| | | 1 | 2 | 3 | 4 | 5 |
| | 1 | 1 | 0.5 | 0 | 0 | 0 |
| First | 2 | 0.5 | 1 | 0.5 | 0 | 0 |
| | 3 | 0 | 0.5 | 1 | 0.5 | 0 |
| | 4 | 0 | 0 | 0.5 | 1 | 0.5 |
| | 5 | 0 | 0 | 0 | 0.5 | 1 |

Of course, this is a 5 × 5 version of Table 2.12.

    Weighted Kappa calculation:

Observed Weighted Agreement =
$64 + 0.5(5 + 3 + 1 + 3 + 2 + 0 + 6 + 12) = 64 + 0.5(32) = 80$
Observed % Agreement $= 80/116 = 69.0\%$

Expected Agreement:

| | | Second | | | | |
|---|---|---|---|---|---|---|
| | | 1 | 2 | 3 | 4 | 5 |
| | 1 | 12.4 | 5.3 | 4.2 | 17.3 | 1.8 |
| First | 2 | 4.2 | 1.8 | 1.4 | 5.9 | 0.6 |
| | 3 | 0.6 | 0.3 | 0.2 | 0.8 | 0.1 |
| | 4 | 13.3 | 5.7 | 4.6 | 18.6 | 1.9 |
| | 5 | 4.5 | 1.9 | 1.6 | 6.3 | 0.6 |

Expected Weighted Agreement =
$33.6 + 0.5(4.2 + 0.3 + 4.6 + 6.3 + 5.3 + 1.4 + 0.8 + 1.9) =$
$33.6 + 0.5(24.8) = 33.6 + 12.4 = 46$

Expected Weighted % Agreement =
46/116 = 39.7%
Kappa: (69.0% − 39.7%)/(100% − 39.7%) = 0.48

5e. The investigators could estimate the importance of the effect by having the same examiner score the patient twice, 5 minutes apart. If one can assume intra-rater reliability is high, then any changes in the score would presumably represent true changes in the patient's mental status.

Alternatively the study could have two raters measure the GCS simultaneously. For example, both raters could observe a third person (e.g., the Emergency Department resident) examining the patient for mental status. They could then independently record their scores based on responses elicited by the neutral examiner. Similarly, investigators could videotape a third person's exam and then have the observers separately watch the videotape. However, both of these strategies may overestimate real-world reproducibility by eliminating sources of variation in how the score is elicited.

6a. It is hard to tell, because the line in the graph is the regression line, not the line of identity. If you draw the line of identity (easiest if you draw the line from (0,0) to (90,90), you will see that most of the points are below the line, meaning that CT gives the higher measurement:

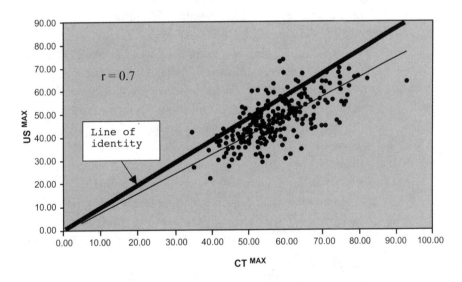

6b. The correlation coefficient is not of much help unless it is low, in which case you know the test is pretty useless. This coefficient 0.7 really is not very good. But even if it were 0.99, the $CT^{max}$ could still be consistently 20 mm or 50% higher than $US^{max}$.

6c. A Bland–Altman plot.

6d. Now it should be clear that CT gives higher diameter measurements. On average, the diameter according to CT was 9.4 mm (almost 1 cm) greater than by US.

6e. The authors concluded no, and we agree.

## Chapter 3 Problem answers: dichotomous tests

1. You would want to know the positive predictive value, because what you really want to know is "What is the probability that I actually have Grunderschnauzer disease given that I have a positive test?" (Of course you also want to know what Grunderschnauzer disease is, but that is not the question. For the record, it does not exist.)

2a.

|          | Cat scratch | Control | Total |
|----------|-------------|---------|-------|
| Test+    | 38          | 4       | 42    |
| Test−    | 7           | 108     | 115   |
| Total    | 45          | 112     | 157   |

2b. The calculation is not correct, because the study design does not permit calculation of predictive value. The authors apparently calculated $38/42 = 91\%$ as the positive predictive value. This would be correct if they had employed cross-sectional sampling, and $45/157$ was the prevalence or prior probability of Cat Scratch Disease. But in this study the cases of Cat Scratch Disease and the controls were sampled separately, so the ratio of cases to controls was determined by the investigators, rather than reflecting a prior probability, and predictive value cannot be determined.

3. We disagree. The decision to culture should be based on the (posterior) probability of Group A Streptococcal infection after a negative OIA (i.e.,$1 -$ Negative Predictive Value), not on the "false-negative rate" (i.e., $1 -$ Sensitivity) as given here. Presumably there is some prior (before culture) probability of strep so low that the culture is not worth doing. Let's say it is 10%. That is, if the prior probability of strep is less than 10%, it means that we would need to do more than 10 throat cultures on such patients for each one that is positive, and it is not worth that much effort to diagnose strep throat.

   If that's the case, then if, for example, the prior probability of strep (before OIA) were about 20% and the OIA were negative, then the estimated probability of strep before culture would decline to only about 2.5%; a throat culture would not need to be processed after a negative OIA.

   Of course, if the prior probability is high (more than 54%), then even if the OIG is negative, the posterior probability will be more than 10%, and a culture will be indicated. But if the prior probability were very high, it might make sense just to treat the patient and skip all of the tests!

   We think one reason why it is so common to see recommendations based on sensitivity and specificity, as this one was, rather than predictive value, is that most of us hate to admit to uncertainty, and therefore we like rules that just tell us what to do, rather than asking us to do hard things like estimate prior probabilities. (See Chapter 12 on "Challenges for Evidence-Based Diagnosis.")

4a. Recall a way to remember the definition of LR was WOWO ("with over without") – the probability of the finding in those With the disease Over the probability of the finding in those WithOut the disease. Because the "disease" in this case is a positive CT scan, the LR is about $61\%/33\% = 1.85$; the LR of 11 in the table is a mistake.

4b. Of 180 subjects with drug or alcohol intoxication, 22 had a positive CT scan. So the numerator of the prevalence ratio is $22/180$. Of $520 - 180 = 340$ subjects who did not have drug or alcohol intoxication, $36 - 22 = 14$ had a positive CT scan. So the denominator is $14/340$. So the prevalence ratio is $22/180/(13/340) = 2.97$. It still is not clear where the number 11 in the table came from.

4c. Because prior probability is 10%, prior odds $= 1{:}9$. Given the LR of 1.85, the posterior odds are $1{:}9 \times 1.85 = 1.85{:}9$, so posterior probability $= 1.85/10.85 = 17\%$.

5a. Positive predictive value

5b.
- i) $106/146 = 72.6\%$
- ii) $75/112 = 67\%$
- iii) $(1 - \text{Negative Predictive Value})$ or the posterior probability of immune failure after a negative test
- iv) $31/106 = 29.2\%$
- v) $37/40 = 92.5\%$

5c. It's an example of a test that is more helpful when positive $[\text{LR}(+) = 3.9]$ than negative $[\text{LR}(-) = 0.76]$, but even the positive LR is not very high. On the other hand, the price is right. Our guess is that, if the diagnosis of immune failure were an important one to make, you would want a more definitive test.

6a. The graph looks just like Figure 3.2 except that $C = \$40$ and $B = \$60$ and the x-axis is the probability of strep throat.

6b. $C/(C + B) = \$40/(\$40 + \$60) = 0.4$. It's where the lines cross on the graph.

6c. $\text{LR}+ = 90/9 = 10$. Since the treatment threshold is $P = 40\%$, the treatment threshold odds $= 2{:}3 = $ post test odds. So we divide these post-test odds by the $\text{LR}+$ to get the No Treat-Test threshold Odds:

$$(2/3)/10 = 2/30 \rightarrow P = 2/32 = 1/16 = .0625$$

$\text{LR}- = 10/91 = 0.1099$. So we divide the post-test odds of $2{:}3$ by $\text{LR}-$ to get Test-Treat threshold Odds:

$$(2/3)/0.1099 = 6.07 \rightarrow P = 6.07/7.07 = .87.$$

6d. The most that a perfect test can save you in misclassification costs is $0.4(\$60) = 0.6(\$40) = \$24$, so it is *never* worth doing the \$30 test. The test line is higher than the intersection of the No Treat and Treat lines, so not treating or treating empirically will always be a lower cost option than testing.

6e. Testing is the lowest cost strategy between $P = 30/160 = .1875$ and $P = 1 - 30/40 = 0.25$. The key concept here is that when the sore throat is more severe, the benefit of treating it (or the cost of not treating it) is greater. Therefore it is worth more to make the diagnosis. But because T is almost as high as C, there is only a narrow range where testing is better than treating without testing.

## Chapter 4 Problem answers: multilevel and continuous tests

1a. (Note that you should plot this using descending ranks, because higher test results indicate pregnancy.)

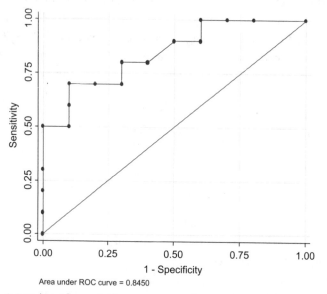

Area under ROC curve = 0.8450

1b. 0.845 (84.5 boxes). Shortcut: count boxes above the curve and subtract from 100!

1c. It is easiest to do the ranks in two columns, as shown below:

| Pregnant | | Not Pregnant | |
|---|---|---|---|
| Result | Rank | Result | Rank |
| 32 | 1 | | |
| 30 | 2 | | |
| 26 | 3 | | |
| 23 | 4.5 | | |
| 23 | 4.5 | | |
| | | 21 | 6 |
| 20 | 7 | | |
| 18 | 8 | | |
| | | 17 | 9 |
| | | 16 | 10 |
| 15 | 11 | | |
| | | 13 | 12 |
| 7 | 13.5 | 7 | 13.5 |
| | | 5 | 15 |
| 4 | 16 | | |
| | | 3 | 17 |
| | | 2 | 18 |
| | | 1 | 19.5 |
| | | 1 | 19.5 |
| Total | 70.5 | | |

1d. $S = 70.5$ (sum of ranks in pregnant group)

$S_{min} = d(d + 1)/2 = (10)(11)/2 = 55$

$S_{max} = dn + S_{min} = (10)(10) + 55 = 155$

1e. $c = (S_{max} - S)/(S_{max} - S_{min}) = (155 - 70.5)/(155 - 55) = 0.845$

1f. If you create a table by counting up the number of people who were pregnant vs. not with test results of $<10$, $10-20$, and $>20$, you can easily calculate the LR (see table below). Recall that $LR = P(\text{result}|\text{pregnant})/P(\text{result}|\text{not pregnant})$

|        | Pregnant | Not pregnant | LR |
|--------|----------|--------------|----|
| **>20**   | 5 | 1 | $(5/10)/(1/10) = 5$ |
| **10–20** | 3 | 3 | $(3/10)/(3/10) = 1$ |
| **<10**   | 2 | 6 | $(2/10)/(6/10) = 1/3$ |
| **Total** | 10 | 10 | |

1g. Posterior odds $= (1)(1/3) = 1/3$

Posterior probability $= \dfrac{1/3}{(1 + 1/3)} = 1/4\ (25\%)$

1h. With a sample size of only 10 subjects per group, it is hard to say anything for sure – the 95% CI for the AUROC curve goes up almost to 1. But it certainly does not look promising. If the LRs above are correct, the test is not powerful enough to affect clinical decisions and much better tests are readily available. Thinking about it more intuitively: Who wants to know that there is a 25% chance *after* a pregnancy test that she's pregnant? Even for a high test value, with the LR of 5 (with the same 50% pretest probability), we'd only be able to say that there's an 83% chance she's pregnant. This is not good enough!

2a. It's pretty useless. The distribution of CRPs in those with major coronary events must have been about the same as those without major coronary events, because the ROC curve has a slope of about 1.

2b. The disease in this figure is "major adverse coronary events within 30 days." MI is a major adverse coronary event, and it was defined by Troponin T of at least 0.1 ng/mL. Therefore, it is impossible to have a false positive result – everyone whose Troponin T was at least 0.1 ng/mL is a true positive by definition.

  About 58% of the D+ patients had an MI as their major adverse event. So the point on the Troponin T ROC curve at Sensitivity $= 58\%$, Specificity $= 100\%$ corresponds to a Troponin T cut-point of 0.1 ng/mL. The points higher on that ROC curve correspond to Troponin T's of $<0.1$ ng/mL. Using the index test in the definition of the D+ group is called "Incorporation Bias." We will return to this in Chapter 5.

2c.

  i) $LR(\text{High}) = 2$   $LR(\text{Med}) = 1$   $LR(\text{Low}) = 0.5$

  ii) The threshold probability $= 1/5$, so threshold odds $= 1:4$.

   Divide by $LR(\text{High})$ to get $1:8$, then convert back to probability to get $1/9$.

   Divide by $LR(\text{Low})$ to get $1:2$, then convert back to probability to get $1/3$.

   So the range of prior probabilities where the test might help is from $1/9$ to $1/3$ (11% to 33%).

2d. You just need to picture the little man walking. At the lower left part of the ROC curve, he is going up pretty steeply; this means that more people *with* than *without* major adverse coronary events have these (high) CK-MB levels. Then he levels off, suggesting we've moved into a normal, reassuring range – that is, that CK-MB levels in this range are more common in folks without an adverse coronary event. Then he goes up approximately diagonally, suggesting that similar numbers of those with and without the outcome have low CK-MB levels.

Your first instinct is probably to say the distribution of CK-MB levels in those with disease must be bimodal. But, in fact, the distributions of CK-MB levels in both those with and those without disease could be unimodal but with different variances. As shown in the figure below, if the variance for CK-MB is greater in those with major coronary events, an ROC curve similar to that in (C) of the figure could be obtained. In the figure below, sections C, B, and A in the graph correspond to the labeled sections of the ROC curve below:

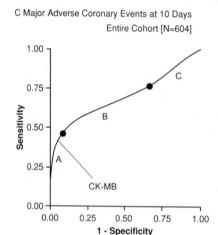

C Major Adverse Coronary Events at 10 Days
Entire Cohort [N=604]

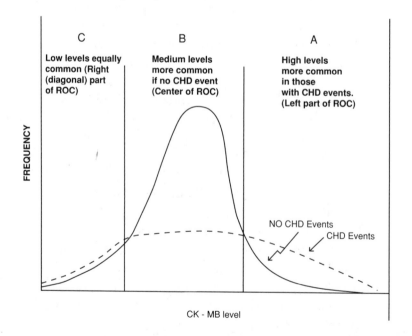

3a. Accuracy is (True Positives + True Negatives)/Total Sample Size. This is equivalent to the weighted average of sensitivity and specificity, weighted by the prevalence of disease (p):

Accuracy = p × (Sensitivity) + (1 − p) × (Specificity)

You may have reasonably concluded that they calculated accuracy as

(Sensitivity + Specificity)/2,

but that is only because (after some inappropriate exclusions from the no CHF group) the prevalence of CHF in this study was very close to 50%.

3b. This study provides a nice example of how understanding ROC curves and LRs can help you compensate for suboptimal reporting of results of a study of a diagnostic test.

What you should notice about the ROC curve is that the slope in the area between values of about 80 and 150 is roughly constant and close to 1. (Actually, it's too bad they did not label the point where the slope changes, a bit to the left of the 150 pg/mL value. This would be a higher value, like 300.) Thus, when the result is in the range 80–150, the test provides very little information, and the posterior probability will be almost the same as the prior probability. From the table under the graph, you can calculate the LR. You can see from the "Sensitivity" column that 93% of CHF patients had a BNP >80, whereas 85% had BNP >150. Therefore, there must have been 8% with levels between 80 and 150.

BNP results above 150 have an LR of about 5: P(BNP > 150|CHF) = 85%; P(BNP > 150|no CHF) = 1− 83% = 17%; LR = 85%/17% = 5. Values below 50 have an LR of about 0.05: P(BNP < 50|CHF) = 100% − 97% = 3%; P(BNP < 50|no CHF) = 62%; LR = 3%/62% = 0.05. To get the LR for values between 50 and 80, we need to subtract sensitivities and specificities: P(BNP 50–80|CHF) = 97% − 93% = 4%; P(BNP 50–80|no CHF = 74% − 62% = 12%; LR = 4%/12% = 0.33.

Note that you could also just look at the slope of the ROC curve in the little segment between BNP = 125 and BNP = 150 to get the LR for your patient from the night before. If you do this, you get an LR of 0.5 (2%/4%). But biologically it is not very plausible that the slope of the ROC curve would decline non-monotonically. (The LR for a result between 80 and 100 is 3%/2% = 1.5, whereas it should be a little lower, not higher than that for 125–150.) So this approach is less satisfactory.

It's also worth noting the contrast between our estimated LR of 1 and just using the positive predictive value for BNP >125 (80%). Also, consider this: the patient last night had a value >125, which should give him a PPV of 80% – that is, an 80% chance of having CHF. But he also had a value of <150, which has a negative predictive value of 85% – that is, an 85% chance that he does not have CHF! This shows the problem with dichotomizing results of continuous tests.

Physicians experienced with BNP levels use them when a patient has more than one potential underlying cause for shortness of breath, like emphysema versus CHF. BNP levels are mainly helpful when they are <100 or >500.

4a. Specificity.

4b. You would favor the initiative because presumably there are some guilty defendants that 10 or 11 but not 12 jurors would vote to convict.

4c. Both ROC curves should plot sensitivity (y-axis) versus 1 − Specificity (x-axis) and have the 12-juror point closer to the origin than the 10-juror point.

The "Support" curve should rise steeply between the 12 and 10 points – that is, sensitivity increases with little or no decrease in specificity. This means that many more guilty criminals would be convicted with little or no increase in conviction of innocent defendants.

The "Oppose" curve should move horizontally a lot, and not very far vertically, between 12 and 10. This would mean that requiring only 10 jurors to convict would lead to many more innocent people being convicted and not very many more guilty people.

4d. The most obvious reason is that they have different values – that is, that they have different answers to the question, "How many guilty defendants are you willing to acquit to avoid convicting one innocent one?"

A more subtle reason is that they might also differ on their estimates of the prevalence/prior probability of guilt among persons brought to trial. Remember that the frequency of false-positive and false-negative errors depends on prior probability. For example, if your prior probability is very high, most positive results will be true positives and most negative results will be false negatives. If the prior probability is low (as was the case in the mammography example in Chapter 3), most of the positive results will be false positives and most negative results will be true negatives. Thus, even with the same values, someone who thought that the overwhelming majority of people put on trial are guilty would be more likely to support the initiative than someone who thought a lot of innocent people are tried.

5a.

| | Bacterial Meningitis or Bacteremia | | | | |
|---|---|---|---|---|---|
| | Yes | | No | | |
| WBC count (/μL) | Number | % | Number | % | LR |
| 0–4999 | 5 | 7.94 | 96 | 4.41 | **1.8** |
| 5000–11999 | 21 | 33.33 | 1240 | 56.91 | **0.59** |
| 12000–19999 | 22 | 34.92 | 691 | 31.71 | **1.1** |
| >19999 | 15 | 23.81 | 152 | 6.98 | **3.4** |
| **Total** | **63** | **100.00** | **2179** | **100.00** | |

5b. Post-test odds = pre-test odds × LR (15,000)

LR (15,000) = 1.1.

Pre-test probability = 0.04, so pretest odds = 4/96 = 0.042.

Therefore, post-test odds = 0.042 × 1.10 = 0.046.

And post-test probability = 0.046/(1 + 0.046) = 0.044 = 4.4%.

Or you could have recognized that the LR is only a little above 1, and concluded that the post-test probability would be only a little above the pre-test probability of 4%.

5c.

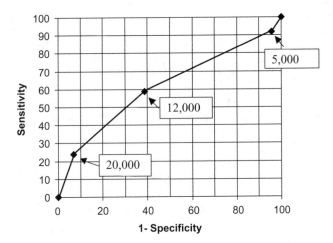

5d. The AUROC curve might not be a good measure of the discrimination of the test because the ROC curve slope does not decrease consistently (i.e., the ROC curve is not concave). The D+ (bacteremic) infants have a higher probability of both very low and very high WBC counts than the D− infants.

5e. The WBC interval with the lowest (most reassuring) LR is 5,000–11,999 with an LR of 0.59.

5f. The lowest pre-test probability at which we should admit regardless of the WBC count is a pre-test probability that is still high enough to exceed the admission threshold of 1%, even if the WBC count is maximally reassuring. From part (e), the most reassuring result is a WBC count of 5,000–11,999, with an LR of 0.59. Therefore, we should admit at the lowest pre-test odds such that pre-test odds × 0.59 > 0.01 (No need to convert 0.01 to odds.)

Lowest pre-test odds = 0.01/0.59 = 0.017 (again, no need to convert back to probability).

So, if the pre-test probability of bacteremia/meningitis is 0.017 or greater, you will admit regardless of the WBC count.

6a. Picture an X-shaped graph like those we introduced in Chapter 3. What we are saying is that missing trisomy 21 is 30 times worse than doing a chorionic villus sample on a normal fetus. So B must be 30 times C, so our threshold odds are C/B = 1/30 and threshold probability must be 1/31 = 3.2%.

6b. If the pre-test probability is 1%, the question is: what value of the NT will lead to a posterior probability of 3.2% or more. Again, because all probabilities for this problem are less than 3.2%, we can skip the odds step and just look for an LR more than 3.2, which will be needed to get the prior probability from 1% to 3.2%. Looking at the table, we can see that a NT of ≥3.5 mm will have an LR of at least 3.6 so that would be the NT measurement that should prompt CVS.

6c. We can just add up the percentages with trisomy 21 who would test positive to get Sensitivity = 31.2% + 12.3% + 20.1% = 63.6%. (If we add up the numbers themselves, rather than the percentages, then divide by the number with trisomy 21, we get 63.7%; using the percentages is a little easier but introduces a tiny rounding error.)

For Specificity, we add up those who would test negative: $28.7\% + 62.1\% = 90.8\%$.

## Chapter 5 Problem answers: studies of diagnostic tests

1a. vWF activity, vWF antigen, and factor VIIIc

1b. Presence of a personal and family history of bleeding symptoms and a documented abnormality of vWF activity or vWF antigen.

1c. Sensitivities

1d. The "gold standard" for diagnosis included two of the tests they were evaluating! This is incorporation bias and would bias sensitivity up and specificity up. (The abstract did not report specificities.). A fine point – there may also be some spectrum bias in the no disease (D−) group because they appear to have been well children, not children with symptoms suggestive of Von Willebrand's disease. That could also bias the specificity up.

2a. Study 1 (Morrison et al.):

|  | Microscopy | | | |
|---|---|---|---|---|
|  | Abnormal (+) | Normal (−) | Total | |
| Chemstrip-9 (+) | 470 | 248 | 718 | Positive Predictive Value = 470/718 = 65% |
| Chemstrip-9 (−) | 103 | 179 | 282 | Negative Predictive Value = 179/282 = 63% |
| Total | 573 | 427 | 1000 | |
|  | Sensitivity = 470/573 = 82% | Specificity = 179/427 = 42% | | |

Study 2 (Hamoudi et al.):

|  | Microscopy | | | |
|---|---|---|---|---|
|  | Abnormal (+) | Normal (−) | Total | |
| Chemstrip-9 (+) | 310 | 11 | 321 | Positive Predictive Value = 310/321 = 96.6% |
| Chemstrip-9 (−) | 27 | 668 | 695 | Negative Predictive Value = 668/695 = 96.1% |
| Total | 337 | 679 | 1016 | |
|  | Sensitivity = 310/337 = 92% | Specificity = 668/679 = 98% | | |

2b. The 36% they report is (1 − Negative Predictive Value). (The numbers above give 35%, presumably because of rounding error.) The standard definition is 1 − Sensitivity, which would be 1 − 82% = 18% in this case.

2c. Both studies address the same research question, and their basic designs (cross-sectional studies) are also the same. Possible differences are:

    i) The subjects differ between the studies. The "disease" in this case is not really a disease; it is the result of urine microscopy. Still, urine microscopy is not naturally dichotomous, so there could be a spectrum of abnormalities that might differ between the two studies. For example, if in the Morrison study, many of those with abnormal microscopy were just barely abnormal, whereas in the Hamoudi study the abnormalities were more severe, this would explain the differing sensitivities.

    ii) The predictor variable (in this case the dipstick) might have been measured differently. The urine dipstick is actually a combination of multiple tests, and the abstract of the Morrison study does not indicate which tests were used to arrive at an overall positive or negative result. Also, perhaps the skill or training at reading the dipsticks was less in the first study. Note that the discrepant results are probably not simply because the threshold for calling the dipstick abnormal varied between the studies. If that were the case, you would expect a trade-off between sensitivity and specificity, rather than both being higher in one study, as was observed.

    iii) The outcome variable, in this case, the urine microscopy, might have been measured differently in the two studies. If microscopy were done less skillfully in the first study, this would make it appear that the dipstick performed less well, when in fact, it was due to the gold standard being more often incorrect. Alternatively, perhaps there was a difference in blinding. If those doing microscopy in the second study were aware of the dipstick result, they might have been more likely to have concordant results of microscopy.

3a. There is a problem with the spectrum of the "nondisease" group. It doesn't include the women who had an abnormal intrauterine pregnancy and went on to abort, only women who turned out to have a normal pregnancy. Those who did abort probably had lower HCG levels.

3b. The sensitivity estimate is probably about right. The sensitivity of a test is affected by the spectrum of disease in your sample. In this study, there is no reason to suspect an unrepresentative range of severity of ectopic pregnancies, so the sensitivity of the HCG for detecting an ectopic should be fine.

3c. Too high: The specificity of tests can be affected by the spectrum of "nondisease." In this case, the "nondisease" group is missing women with an abnormal intrauterine pregnancy – that is, the women who went on to have a spontaneous abortion. These women may have had lower HCG levels than the women who did not abort. Therefore, excluding them will make the specificity look falsely high: it is easier for the test to discriminate between ectopic pregnancies and normal intrauterine pregnancies than between ectopic pregnancies and abnormal intrauterine pregnancies.

4a.

|        | Intussusception | No intussusception | Total |
|--------|-----------------|--------------------|-------|
| US+    | 37              | 7                  | 44    |
| US−    | 3               | $18 + 86 = 104$    | 107   |
| Total  | 40              | 111                | 151   |

4b. Sensitivity $= 37/40 = 93\%$ (not $37/44 = 84\%$, which is the positive predictive value). Specificity $= 104/111 = 94\%$ (not $104/107 = 97\%$, which is the negative predictive value). Accuracy $= (37 + 104)/151 = 93\%$. (Correct)

4c. Yes, it's a "cross-sectional" sampling scheme – that is, they did not sample children with and without intussusception separately. PPV $= 84\%$, NPV $= 97\%$.

4d. Double gold standard bias.

4e. None. Those 86 patients with negative ultrasounds who had negative observation periods would also have had negative contrast enemas if they had received that "gold standard."

4f. Both sensitivity and specificity would be falsely increased. For spontaneously resolving cases for which the contrast enema is done only if the ultrasound is positive, the ultrasound can never give a wrong answer.

4g. Just as the ultrasound can never give a wrong answer in the case of self-resolving intussusception, it can never give a right answer for cases of intussusception not present at the time of the air enema, that develop during the follow-up period.

Thus, both sensitivity and specificity would be falsely decreased.

5a. Sensitivity is not affected by the types of conditions in the nondiseased or D− group. If the spectrum of severity in the patients with CHF was appropriate, not tilted toward especially severe or especially mild CHF, then the BNP's sensitivity should not be biased. (Although it has been argued that some of the patients with CHF in this study had such obvious CHF that no BNP test was required.)

It seems that the patients with an obvious non-CHF diagnosis would have lower BNPs than non-CHF patients with pulmonary embolism, COPD exacerbations, and other things that might be confused with CHF. Certainly, the 72 patients with a history of left ventricular dysfunction had higher BNPs, and they were excluded from the D− group. Therefore, the spectrum of nondisease was too "easy" and the specificity was biased up.

If the sensitivity is about right and the specificity is biased up, the LR(+) will also be biased up.

5b. Because the chest x-ray was used by the cardiologist to determine whether a patient had CHF, the high sensitivity and specificity could mean only that the heart size was one of the main things that the cardiologists were looking at. Both sensitivity and specificity are likely to be biased up relative to what they would be if the cardiologists were blinded to the chest x-ray. This is incorporation bias.

6a. False. Verification bias tends to increase sensitivity and decrease specificity. If a few of those "children who could hop around without pain" actually had appendicitis and were excluded from the study, this would falsely *decrease* false negatives and falsely *increase* the sensitivity of the finding for appendicitis.

6b. False. When there is spontaneous resolution of disease, double gold standard bias makes both sensitivity and specificity falsely high. In this case, children able to jump whose appendicitis is allowed to resolve would get counted as true-negatives, rather than false-negatives, thus *increasing* rather than decreasing the apparent sensitivity of the finding.

## Chapter 6 Problem answers: screening tests

1a. Lead time bias. Because time to renal failure was measured beginning with the time of the biopsy, earlier biopsy will mean greater time to renal failure.

(Length time bias is possible if biopsy was deferred in sicker patients, but it seems more likely that length time bias would go the other way: people biopsied early are more likely to be having a rapidly progressive course.)

1b. This is probably volunteer bias: people who turn in more Hemoccult cards are probably more health-conscious and less likely to smoke.

1c. This could be stage migration bias. The overall death rate might be the same. There may only have been a shift of patients from the ward to the ICU. These former ward patients are not as sick as other ICU patients, but are sicker than average ward patients. So the average level of illness of both ICU and ward patients has declined, but more patients are going into the ICU.

Another reason why death rates on the ward could decline is that patients who previously might have been sent home from the emergency department are now admitted (perhaps because they have a $pCO_2$ of 41–44 mm Hg), thus reducing the average severity of illness among the ward patients.

2a. True

2b. False, sticky diagnosis bias would make screening look worse, not better.

2c. True, this is exactly what length-time bias does

2d. False, it is common for pseudodisease to be confirmed pathologically, as it was in the Mayo Lung Study.

2e. False, there are lots of problems with this study, including:

   i) No comparison group, except the inappropriate comparison to historical 5% survival for lung cancer diagnosed at all stages. The comparison group you would want would be similar people who were not screened.

   ii) Lead and length-time bias as mentioned above.

   iii) Pseudodisease.

   These problems are well catalogued in the Letters to the Editor prompted by this paper. See *N Engl J Med* 2007 Feb 15;**356**(7):743–7.

3a. Yes. In fact, the 0.19% AAA-related death rate in the invited group is 42% lower (95% CI 22% to 58%; P = 0.0002) than the risk in the control group. (We will discuss relative risk reductions like this in Chapter 9, and confidence intervals and P-values in Chapter 11.)

3b. Chance is a reasonable explanation: The observed relative reduction in all cause mortality was only 2.4% (95% CI: 6.4% reduction to 1.8% increase; P = 0.27). Alternatively or in addition, it is possible that invitation to screening led to cointerventions (e.g., treatment of hypertension) that reduced non-AAA mortality. Finally, some deaths attributed to other causes (in both groups) may actually have been due to AAA (misclassification of outcome).

3c. The most likely explanation is volunteer or selection bias. Those interested enough in their health to attend screening may have other, better health habits and some of those who did not attend screening may have been too sick to do so.

Remember that lead time and length-time bias do not occur when the whole group receiving an intervention is compared with the whole group not receiving it. They only occur when survival of those with disease is compared. Misclassification of outcome is not plausible, because the outcome is total mortality. Misclassification of exposure (i.e., not being able to tell who got scanned) also seems unlikely. They may have coded it wrong in a few, but this is a huge effect. This seems like much too big a difference to be due to co-interventions, but co-interventions may have contributed a little. Chance is not a viable explanation. These numbers are huge — the P-value is about $10^{-72}$.

3d. The "as treated" comparison appears not to be biased because the AAA death rate in nonscanned patients (0.33%) is the same as the death rate in uninvited patients (0.33%). This suggests that, for this particular cause of death (AAA), the volunteer bias that led to differences in total mortality was not important.

4a. In this example, the entire population was screened, and it is difficult to think about lead-time bias when there is no unscreened group, but bear with us. With lead-time bias, you can assume that the natural history of the disease (recurrent medulloblastoma) is the same for all patients. There is a "latent" or detectable preclinical phase during which the disease can be identified by screening before signs and symptoms develop. The length of that latent phase is the upper limit for lead-time bias, because in order to get that amount of additional survival you would need for each patient to be screened on the first day their disease was detectable by scanning. If this latent phase were longer than the 6-month screening interval, all of the recurrences would have been detected on screening. If the latent period were 3 months long, we would expect about half of the recurrences to be detected by screening, because half would become detectable by scanning (but not yet symptomatic) in the 3 months before a scan and they would get a maximum of 3 months, but an average of more like 1.5 months of additional survival. The other half, whose tumors became detectable in the 3 months after a scan would become symptomatic before their next scan. Since only about one-sixth of the cases were detected on screening, the latent phase is likely to be about 1 month; one-sixth of the patients would enter the latent phase in the month before scanning and have a positive screen, whereas the other five-sixths would enter the latent phase in the 5 months after scanning and become symptomatic before the next screen. The maximum lead-time bias is 1 month, and the average lead-time bias should be about 2 weeks. So, lead-time bias cannot explain the 16-month difference in median survival between the two groups.

4b. This study is definitely subject to length-time bias. The entire study population was being screened; only individuals with the disease were considered; and those with disease diagnosed by screening were compared with those diagnosed from symptoms. The 4 patients whose recurrence was identified on a screening scan prior to developing signs or symptoms may have had more slowly progressive disease and remained in the detectable preclinical phase longer. Their disease still (tragically) progressed to death, but it did so more slowly than for the others, so they had longer median survival.

If there had been some survivors in this group whose recurrence was detected by scanning, it would have been hard to know what to conclude – there would be no way to distinguish between the explanation that the therapy was effective for cancers caught early and length bias (or even pseudodisease). However, because there were no survivors, you can put an upper limit on the number of life years gained, and therefore a lower limit on number of scans per year of life gained. The authors had to do 794 scans to identify 4 patients with recurrences that had not yet become symptomatic. These 4 lived an average of 15 months longer. If you ignore the possible couple of weeks of lead-time bias, even if we completely ignore length bias, we've gained at most $4 \times 15 = 60$ person-months of (probably not very high-quality) life by doing 794 scans. So this is at least 13 scans per month of life gained.

5. The overall survival could be just as high in the South. This is a nice example of possible "stage migration bias." In this case, rather than better diagnostic tests moving patients from lower to higher cancer stages, better diagnosis moves children from the no CHD group into the CHD group. This would lead to better survival in both CHD and non-CHD patients in the region where more CHD was diagnosed, even if there were no actual survival benefit.

## Chapter 7 Problem answers: prognostic tests

1a. Optimistic. The actual disease-free survival in this group was $3/12 = 25\%$.

1b. This is the only group for whom the doctors were a little too pessimistic (the point is above the diagonal line). It looks like 2 of the 48 patients (4.2%) actually survived, disease-free, for 5 years.

2a. These inclusion criteria are heterogeneous. The majority of subjects (172/197) were identified by screening for CMV. But 25 of the 197 subjects (13%) came from a variety of sources, including newborns with symptoms. These 25 subjects would likely have worse CMV with a higher risk of bad outcomes than the 172 subjects identified by screening, making the prognosis for the study as a whole appear worse.

2b. In a best-case scenario, it is possible that all cases of hearing loss came from the 25 subjects referred from outside. In that case, *none* of the 172 subjects identified by screening would develop hearing loss. On the other hand, the risk in the 25 referral patients could be no higher than the risk in those picked up by screening. (It is hard to come up with a mechanism whereby the risk in referral patients would be *lower* than in those identified by screening.) If that is the case, then the upper limit for the risk of hearing loss in an asymptomatic infant would be $24/197 = \sim12\%$.

(Note that, if all 24 of those with hearing loss came from the 172 subjects identified by screening, then the risk of sensorineural hearing loss could be as high as $24/172 = 14\%$, but this seems unlikely, as it would imply selective referral of lower-risk subjects in the outborn group, so we don't think that answer is as good.)

2c. If we assume that all cases of hearing loss were in the group referred from outside, then the upper limit would be $\sim24/25$, or about 96%. The lower limit would 12% if we assume (as above) that the prognosis in referred children is the same as in the infants identified by screening. (Again, an estimate <12% is not plausible for the reason discussed under part b.)

3a. As the authors wrote, their new prediction rule needs to be externally validated (in another population of low back pain patients). If in the validation study its discrimination were still better than the GP's estimates, it would be important to consider how much additional time it takes the patient and physician, and whether it changes management often enough and favorably enough to justify the extra time it takes to do.

3b. The most likely reason there are only 6 points on the graph is that large numbers of the ratings were the same. For example, 30% of the subjects might have been rated as having a 50% probability of bad outcome. If that were the case, then there would be at least 2 deciles for which exactly 50% was the average predicted probability, and these 2 deciles would leave only a single point on the graph.

4a. We don't think the conclusion would be affected. Even if the CACS predicted events as well in this low-risk group (and Pletcher et al. are correct that the data presented provide virtually no evidence to the contrary), the CACS would not be likely to be cost-effective because the prevalence of high CACS scores would be expected to be low and therefore the number of scans needing to be done to find one result that would change management would likely be high. (Pletcher et al. point this out in the next sentence of their letter.)

4b. They could stratify on treatments received and compare the CACS and FRS separately among those who were and were not treated.

5a. It seems likely that deaths could be due to multiple causes unrelated to bone, and hence including them would diminish the apparent strength of the association between Ntx and outcome (as they would be less associated with Ntx levels than skeletal events would be). However, if Ntx were at most weakly associated with skeletal events, but strongly associated with general severity of illness and death, it could also lead to a spuriously strong association between the composite outcome of skeletal events and deaths. If the number of deaths was small, it probably does not make much difference.

5b. No. The risk in the >100 group was $41/56 = 73\%$ and the risk in the <100 group was $8/65 = 12\%$. 73%/12% is about 6, not 19. (They confused the odds ratio with the risk ratio. We'll see more examples of this in Chapter 9.)

5c. We disagree. All of the subjects in the study were taking bisphosphonates, so the results provide no information about who might and might not benefit those medicines. In fact, an interpretation opposite to that of the authors also is plausible – the subjects who had increased bone turnover and increased fractures while on bisphophonates could be those who were *unresponsive* to the medication, and did not benefit from treatment, whereas those with lower Ntx levels had fewer fractures because in them the treatment was more effective!

6a. Unless the other causes of death were at least as strongly associated with disruptive *TP53* mutations as deaths due to head and neck cancer, inclusion of these other deaths in the outcome would attenuate the apparent magnitude of the association.

6b. The authors could have explored the association between *TP53* and death from other and unknown causes separately. If, for example, the association with *TP53* were almost as strong in the group who died from unknown causes, but not other causes, it would suggest that many of those deaths were, in fact, due to head and neck cancer. Although it might be tempting simply to exclude the subjects who died of other or unknown causes, it would be better to consider their time period at risk of death of head and neck cancer and consider them "censored" at the time of death from another cause.

6c. The hazard ratio for the *TP53* mutation is the same in the multivariate model as in the bivariate model. That is, including the nodal stage in the model did not at all attenuate the association with the *TP53* mutation. This suggests that the mutation does, in fact, provide new information.

6d. We would want to know the cost and inconvenience of the test, and if these are significant, what decisions it is supposed to help with and prognosis thresholds for those decisions. We also would need some estimate of the importance of those decisions – that is, the potential harmful consequences of basing them on a less accurate prognosis. Finally, even if the hazard ratios are generalizable, we'd want to know if absolute probabilities of survival are generalizable as well, because treatment decisions would presumably be based on these absolute probabilities. In summary, the key questions to ask are what you would do differently depending on the result of the test and how important those decisions are for optimizing outcomes.

## Chapter 8 Problem answers: multiple tests

1a.

Rearranging the numbers in "Table 4" gives:

|  | Appendicitis+ | Appendicitis− | Total |
|---|---|---|---|
| US+ | 102 | 11 | 113 |
| US− | 33 | 171 | 204 |
| **Total** | 135 | 182 | 317 |

Sensitivity $= 102/135 = 76\%$
Specificity $= 171/182 = 94\%$
LR$(+) = 12.5$
LR$(-) = 0.26$

| | Appendicitis+ | Appendicitis− | Total |
|---|---|---|---|
| **CT+** | 131 | 12 | 133 |
| **CT−** | 4 | 170 | 174 |
| **Total** | 135 | 182 | 317 |

Sensitivity $= 131/135 = 97\%$
Specificity $= 170/182 = 93\%$
LR(+) $= 14.7$
LR(−) $= 0.03$

1b.

Probability $= 10\% \rightarrow$ odds $= 1{:}9 = 1/9$
Posterior odds $= 12.5 \times 14.7 \times 1/9 = 20.4$
Posterior probability $= 95.3\%$

1c.

| | | Appendicitis | | | | |
|---|---|---|---|---|---|---|
| **Ultrasound+** | **CT Scan+** | **Yes** | **%** | **No** | **%** | **LR** |
| Yes | Yes | 100 | 74.1 | 3 | 1.6 | 44.9 |
| Yes | No | 2 | 1.5 | 8 | 4.4 | 0.34 |
| No | Yes | 31 | 23.0 | 9 | 4.9 | 4.6 |
| No | No | 2 | 1.5 | 162 | 89.0 | 0.02 |
| | Total | 135 | 100 | 182 | 100 | |

Posterior odds $= 44.9 \times 1/9 = 5.0$
Posterior probability $= 5/6 = 83\%$

1d. We can tell that the two tests are not independent, because the LR for both tests being positive is different from the product of the LRs for the tests considered separately. This may be because both tests tend to identify the same subset of patients with appendicitis who have appendixes that look abnormal, and/or both may be fooled by the same subset of patients without appendicitis who have appendixes that look abnormal.

2a. It looks like the figure was created from some sort of recursive partitioning analysis (also known as CART = Classification and Regression Trees), but if the authors used CART, they appear to have collapsed the resulting decision tree in some places. (With CART each node contains a single dichotomous question.)

2b. He would be classified as high risk

2c. The decision rule does not help with the decision to give IVIG because the patients used for this decision tree all got it. Although none of the kids in the study with <50% PMNs developed an aneurysm (0/123), you don't know what would have happened if they had not received IVIG.

2d. Yes. The problem is that the investigators tested many different classification schemes on the validation sets, then picked the one to publish that did the best. This is subtly apparent by the plural "instruments" in the "Methods" section. It is okay to test many different combinations of variables on your derivation set until you come up with a combination that looks good. But then, you should take that *one* "best fit" and test it in your validation set to see how it does. If you test many possible decision rules in both your derivation set and validation sets and report the one that did best in both, then essentially all you've done is develop the rule in one big derivation set, and the results are subject to over-fitting.

3a. A 5-month-old boy with a fever of 39.5°C and a WBC count of $20 \times 10^3/\mu L$ would fall below the upper ("treat fewer") line, and hence we would not treat.

3b. If the fever was 41°C, a WBC of 20,000 would put him above the line, and we would treat.

3c. To keep risk constant, the WBC count threshold has to decrease as the temperature increases.

3d. The "treat more" line needs to be lower so that for a given temperature, it does not take as high a WBC to be treated, leading to more infants being treated.

4a. Low risk. Note that "risk factors" are not the standard cardiac risk factors of male sex, smoking, family history, and high cholesterol. This patient has one "risk factor" as defined in this study – pain the same as that associated with a prior MI.

4b. $483/10682 = 4.5\%$

4c. $55/1511 = 3.6\%$

4d.

The prior odds are: $0.036/(1 - 0.036) = 0.037$
The LR for high risk is $(222/483)/(812/10,199) = 5.77$
Multiply by LR: $0.037 \times 5.77 = 0.21$
Convert back to prob: $0.21/1.21 = 0.17$
So our patient's risk will be about 17%.

## Chapter 9 Problem answers: quantifying treatment effects

1a. In general it's best to use *risks* to refer to risks of bad outcomes. In this case, the bad outcome is persistence of the effusion. So the risk of persistent effusion is $(100\% - 30\% =)$ 70% with amoxicillin and $(100\% - 14\% =)$ 86% with placebo. It's also easiest to do the RR before the RRR:

RR $= 0.70/0.86 = 0.81$
RRR $= 1 - 0.81 = 0.19$ (or alternatively, RRR $= (0.86 - 0.70)/0.86 = 0.19$)
Those treated with amoxicillin had a 19% lower risk of persistent effusion.
ARR $= 0.86 - 0.70 = 0.16$ (note you can also get this the other way, i.e., $30\% - 14\%$.)
NNT $= 1/0.16 = 6.25$

1b. The RRR and ARR are similar in this study because the risk of persistent effusion in the control group is so high, 86%. ARR = Risk(Placebo) × RRR. If Risk(Placebo) ≈ 1, then ARR ≈ RRR.

1c. We don't agree with the decision to exclude children who developed acute OM. These children were probably more likely to have persistent OME, because OME is a risk factor for acute OM. Because acute OM occurred more frequently in the placebo group, excluding patients that developed acute OM will improve the outcome (i.e., reduce the number with persistent effusions) in that group, reducing the observed difference between the amoxicillin and placebo groups in the study. The rule "once randomized always analyzed" applies here. This rule is particularly important when censoring, loss to follow-up, or exclusion may be related to treatment, as in this case.

1d. As noted above, numbers in the table are biased against amoxicillin due to differential late exclusions. But even neglecting that, there is a trend toward benefit even for the tympanometry endpoint. The expected benefit is pretty small (<10%) because most of these effusions are sterile anyway. So, although this study does not provide strong evidence of benefit, it does not at all rule out a benefit of the magnitude expected from previous studies. We will discuss "negative" studies at length in Chapter 11.

   Note: Since 1990, the debate has shifted from treating OME (the topic of this study) to treating acute OM, because of randomized trials showing that most cases of acute OM resolve without antibiotics and because of increasing concern about use of antibiotics contributing to selection of resistant organisms.

2a. The RR is usually risk with treatment divided by risk without treatment. These authors inverted the usual quotient, putting the control group on top. But they also did something else wrong – (see below).

2b. Putting the risk in the control group over the risk in the treatment group, the relative risk = 38%/14% = 2.7, not 3.8 provided in the abstract.

2c. As TBN pointed out in a Letter to the Editor (*N Engl J Med.* 1991; **325**: 1654–5): "It looks as if odds ratios were calculated throughout the paper and then mislabeled as relative risks. When a disease or outcome is common, relative risks and odds ratios are not interchangeable." (What do you think of the authors' response? "The issue raised by Newman is relevant, and he is correct in saying that what we calculated were odds ratios (Table 6). As defined by the Dictionary of Epidemiology, 'the term relative risk has also been used synonymously with odds ratio... The use of the term relative risk for several quantities arises from the fact that for rare diseases, all quantities approximate one another.' We use the term 'relative risk' instead of 'odds ratio' or 'cross product ratio' or 'approximate relative risk' because it has frequently been used interchangeably with these terms in the literature. Nevertheless, the P-values... are correct and unaffected by this confusion in semantics.")

3a. It is not clear how patients were selected for treatments, but it does not appear to have been random. Perhaps the 53 controls were too sick to get alpha interferon!

3b.

| | Death or liver transplant | No death or liver transplant | Total |
|---|---|---|---|
| **Interferon Alpha** | 8 | 95 | 103 |
| **Untreated** | 5 | 48 | 53 |

$R_C = 5/53 = 0.094$

$R_T = 8/103 = 0.078$

This difference in risk 5/53 vs. 8/103 is totally consistent with chance ($P = 0.72$).

$RR = 0.078/0.094 = 0.82$ (95% CI 0.28 - 2.39)

3c. The conclusion is technically correct, but the abstract is potentially misleading. Many readers will think that this study suggests that treatment with alpha interferon improves clinical outcomes. Notwithstanding the "Background" section of the abstract, which says that the clinical benefits of treatment with interferon have not been established (implying that this question will be addressed in the current study), the authors did not compare clinical outcomes in treated versus nontreated groups. They compared patients *within* these groups (i.e., in the treatment group, they compared patients with clearance of HBeAg to those without clearance.) They showed that, within the group treated with interferon, those with clearance of HbeAg do better than those that never achieved clearance. The *clinical outcomes* you can compare in the abstract are death and liver transplantation. These occurred in 8/103 treated patients and 5/53 untreated patients – little suggestion of any benefit.

This study suggests that treatment with interferon alfa is associated with higher rates of clearance of HBeAg, but the design used to draw this inference (following two different convenience samples, no random allocation or blinding) is weak, and clearance of HbeAg is a *surrogate outcome.*

A key point is that, even if treatment allocation were randomized and were shown to increase clearing of HBeAg and even if clearing of HBeAg were shown to correlate with improved clinical outcome, we would not know whether treatment with interferon improves outcome. The reason is that the outcome in those with clearing of HBeAg is not what is relevant. The relevant outcome is what happens to the *everyone* who is treated. Thus, you would want to see an improved outcome in the entire treated group compared with the entire control group. The reason for this important point is that, unless you see improvement in the group as a whole, you can't tell whether treatment simply sorts patients into those who would have done well anyway (those who clear virologically) and those who would have done poorly. It's our old friend "once randomized always analyzed" helping out again. If you divide the subjects into those who do and do not respond to treatment and then compare outcomes among those who do and do not respond, the treatment is likely to look beneficial!

4a. The main outcome is (very) subjective: a $\geq 50\%$ reduction of headache within 15 minutes.

4b. If (as seems likely), the lidocaine caused numbness of the nose, this would interfere with the blinding. Lack of blinding is a particular problem when (as is the case here) the outcome is subjective. (The problem would be worse if the subjects knew the study was comparing a local anesthetic to placebo. If all they knew was that two different treatments were being compared it might not be as clear to them whether they were getting study drug vs. placebo.)

4c. We disagree with the conclusion. The best estimate of the relief provided by intranasal lidocaine would be the *difference* between the lidocaine and placebo groups, which was $55\% - 21\% = 34\%$, not 55%. (The point of doing a double-blind trial is to compare treatment with placebo!) Also, $\geq 50\%$ reduction is not quite the same as "relief," and the probable lack of blinding may lead to inflation of the apparent benefit.

5a. $11.8\% - 9.4\% = 2.4\%$

5b. $NNT = 1/ARR = 1/2.4\% \approx 42$

5c. 2 pills/person treated per day $\times$ \$5/120 pills $\times$ 42 people need to treat $\times$ 30 days/cardiovascular death prevented = \$104/cardiovascular death prevented.

5d. The RRR was 14%, so the RR would be $1 - 14\% = 0.86$.
The risk in the tPA group would be the risk in the SK group $\times$ the RR: $0.86 \times 7.3\% = 6.3\%$.

5e. $ARR = 7.3\% - 6.3\% = 1.0\%$.
(Alternatively, could also do $14\% \times 7.3\% = 1.0\%$.)

5f. The $NNT = 1/ARR = 1/1\% = 100$.

5g. Additional cost of tPA = \$3400 − \$560 = \$2840.
$NNT = 100$
$NNT \times Cost = 100 \times \$2840 = \$284,000$ per death prevented. (Aspirin is a better deal!)

6a. $RR = (1 - 40.2\%)/(1 - 26.7\%) = 59.8\%/73.3\% = 0.816$.
$RRR = 1 - RR = 0.184 = 18.4\%$
$ARR = 73.3\% - 59.8\% = 13.5\%$

6b. $1/ARR = 1/.135 = 7.4$.

6c. The cost per pill is \$180/60 = \$3, and treatment twice a day for a week requires 14 pills, so the cost per week is $14 \times \$3 = \$42$. Since 7.4 patients need to be treated for each one that responds, the cost per responding patient is $7.4 \times \$42$, about \$311.

6d. If each responder costs \$311/week and has 2 more CSBMs per week, the cost per additional CSBM is about \$311/2, or \$155.

## Chapter 10 Problem answers: alternatives to randomized trials

1. The greatest strength of causal inference would come from comparing autism rates in children of Rh− and Rh+ mothers before 2001. If there is any difference, it would be useful to determine whether it persists for infants conceived after thimerosal was removed from Rhogam.

Note that you wouldn't want just to compare the risk in offspring of mothers who received Rhogam to those who did not, because confounding factors, like reliable attendance at prenatal visits, might be associated with getting Rhogam and also with the diagnosis of autism. (You could, however, make this comparison if you did it both before and after thimerosal was removed.) The least satisfactory comparison would be between everyone exposed to thimerosal and everyone not exposed, including both time periods, because the exposure to thimerosal (which varied over time) would be confounded by changes in diagnostic criteria (which also varied over time).

2a. The predictor variable should be screened/not screened and/or frequency of screening with DRE.

2b. The denominators should be men at risk of prostate cancer who either were or were not screened. Denominators could also be person-years of follow-up following screening or failure to screen. The key point is that the denominator should *not* be restricted to men who develop prostate cancer.

2c. Possible ways of controlling or evaluating confounding/selection bias are:

   i)  Try to control confounding by multivariate adjustment by age, number of health maintenance visits, smoking, family history, race, etc. if data are available.

   ii) Try to control confounding using propensity score analysis: look at other predictors in the dataset of receiving DRE, then create a propensity score for DRE and stratify, match, or control for it in multivariate analyses.

   iii) To assess the likelihood of confounding, look at other predictor variables that might be affected by volunteer bias (e.g., number of measurements of serum cholesterol) and see if they are associated as strongly as DRE with decreased deaths from prostate cancer. If so, the apparent benefit of DRE is likely to be due to confounding or selection bias, especially if it is diminished after adjusting as suggested under (i) and (ii) above.

   iv) Alternatively, you could assess the likelihood of confounding by examining whether DRE also appears to protect against other outcomes one might expect to be affected by selection bias – that is, see if DRE is associated with decreased deaths from other causes, like heart disease and lung cancer. If such nonspecific benefits are found, confounding or selection bias is likely.

3. The question is whether it is intermittent ibuprofen use itself, or something associated with it (e.g., headaches) that might alter the risk of colon cancer. Asking about acetaminophen use acts as a control exposure. If it, too, is associated with reduced colon cancer risk, confounding by indication would be a greater concern.

4a. Confounding by indication could make the vaccine appear less effective than it really is. This would occur if older, sicker people (i.e., the ones most likely to die during the flu season and therefore the group in whom the vaccine was most indicated) were over-represented in the vaccinated group.

4b. Volunteer bias could make the vaccine look falsely good. This would occur if patients in better health or with better health habits or access to care were over-represented in the vaccinated group.

4c. The answer to this problem is analogous to the example of looking at deaths due to colon cancers beyond the reach of the sigmoidoscope in the study of sigmoidoscopy discussed in the chapter. The investigators could see if the flu vaccination was associated with reduced mortality during seasons other than the flu season (i.e., the summer months). Because we specifically refer to unmeasured and unmeasurable confounders, propensity scores and other multivariate techniques won't work for this problem.

5a. The propensity score for each subject in the study was the *predicted probability* (from a multivariable model) that he or she would be treated perioperatively with lipid-lowering agents. This is to control for confounders that affect both the likelihood of receiving therapy and mortality risk.

5b.

    i) The left-most column is the mortality for people at lowest probability of receiving lipid-lowering therapy, who nonetheless did receive it, so there are not very many of them. In fact, the legend to the figure tells you that only 0.5% of 156,114 (781 people) in that quintile were so treated! This leads to the wider confidence interval, reflected by that error bar.

    ii) The suggestion that people with the lowest propensity for treatment might be harmed should make you cautious about promoting perioperative lipid-lowering treatment in all patients not currently receiving it. The result suggests that perhaps people prescribing these medicines actually know some things that are not captured in the model, that allow them only infrequently to give medication to people who are do not appear to benefit. However, based on the footnote of the table, since even subjects in the highest propensity quintile had low (~31%) use of these drugs, if the results are real and causal, there will still be plenty of people not getting the drugs now who might benefit from them.

## Chapter 11 Problem answers: understanding P-values and confidence intervals

1a. False, P-values are conditional on the null hypothesis being true.

1b. False, the null hypothesis usually states that there is *no* difference between groups, so with sufficiently convincing data, you can reject the null hypothesis and conclude that there is a difference.

1c. True, high P-values are consistent with (but do not prove) the null hypothesis.

1d. False, although, if you did the study 100 times, you would expect that, in 95% of them, the 95% CI for the study would include the true value; once the study is completed, other information must also be considered.

2. It is correct that an abnormal test ordered as part of a 20-test panel is more likely to be a false-positive than when the test is ordered by itself, but only because it is likely to have a lower prior probability. Given the same clinical situation (i.e., the same prior probability), it makes no difference how many other tests you order at the same time.

3a. Since the numerator was 2, the upper limit of the 95% CI will be about $7/259 = 2.7\%$. (The exact upper limit is 2.76%.)

3b. The upper limit of the 95% CI for the risk difference is only a 0.5% increase in total mortality – well below the 2% increase felt to be clinically significant by the editorialists.

What seems to be an underpowered study may not be underpowered if the goal was to rule-out significant harm and the trend is toward benefit. (Similar conclusions apply to the adverse events other than death.)

3c. They might have trouble believing the results if their estimate of the prior probability of lower mortality in the sentinel-node group was very low.

4a. Given the incredibly wide confidence interval, the study provides very little information on this hypothesis. Therefore, all you can say about the posterior probability is that it is probably not much different from the prior probability.

4b. The sample size was probably very small. (This is probably because UTIs were uncommon among the women who had intercourse less than once a week, and may also be because both diaphragm use or oral contraceptive use were uncommon in this group of women who infrequently needed contraception.)

5a. Because the Bonferroni correction does not take prior probability into account and is overly conservative, we hardly ever think it is appropriate. In this case, it is definitely too conservative: the prior probability that an active drug will cause more adverse effects than placebo is never very low, and in the case of adverse psychiatric effects of a psychiatric drug, seems particularly high. This is a good example of why *not* to use Bonferroni!

5b. We disagree. What the treating physicians thought in this double-blind study is irrelevant. If treating physicians could determine causality, there would be no need to do randomized, double-blind trials. The strength of evidence for causality is based on the magnitude of the excess of events in the treated group compared with the placebo group and the likelihood of alternative explanations for that excess. (In a properly randomized and blinded trial, the only alternative explanation to causality is chance.)

6. The Bonferroni correction is a conservative correction that makes it harder to reject the null hypothesis. This is like requiring a test to be more abnormal before calling it positive. It will tend to decrease both true-positive and false-positive results, decreasing sensitivity and increasing specificity.

# Index

AAA. *See* abdominal aortic aneurysm
abdominal aortic aneurysm (AAA), reliability of
  testing for, 37–38, 261
  with screening tests, 135–136, 273–274
absolute risk increase (ARI), 198
absolute risk reduction (ARR), 198
  confidence intervals and, 231
ACI-TIPI. *See* Acute Coronary Ischemia – Time
  Insensitive Predictive Instrument
Acquired Immune Deficiency Syndrome (AIDS),
  dichotomous tests for, 66, 263
acute coronary ischemia, 3
  diagnosing of, 3
Acute Coronary Ischemia – Time Insensitive
  Predictive Instrument (ACI-TIPI), 175
acute myocardial infraction (AMI), randomized
  trials for, 203–204, 282
adjustment from anchor, in probability,
  245–246
alternative diagnosis, 227
alternatives to randomized trials
  for autism factors, 217, 282–283
  for colon cancer, 217–218, 283
  for flu vaccines, 218, 283–284
  for prostate cancer, 217, 282–283
American Cancer Society, 240
American College of Obstetricians, 240
American College of Radiology, 240
AMI. *See* acute myocardial infraction, randomized
  trials for
anchoring bias, 246–247
antidepressants
  randomized trials with, confidence intervals in,
    237–238, 285
appendicitis
  double gold standard bias and, 115, 273
  in multiple tests, 180–181, 277–278
  reliability of testing for, 34, 256–257
area under an ROC curve (AUROC), 70–72
  discrimination in prognostic tests and, 143
ARI. *See* absolute risk increase
ARR. *See* absolute risk reduction
as-treated analysis, 189–190
asthma, screening tests for, 135, 273
AUROC. *See* area under an ROC curve

autism, randomized trials for causes of, 217, 282–283
availability, in probability, 244–245
axillary dissection, 235–236

B. *See* cost of failing to treat
bacteremia, 6, 45, 69, 71, 73–74, 79–80, 82–84, 87,
  165, 167–168, 177, 225, 229, 231
  continuous/multilevel testing for, 91–92, 268–269
bacterial meningitis
  continuous/multilevel testing for, 91–92, 268–269
  randomized trials for, 201–202, 280
bias. *See also* double gold standard bias; spectrum
  bias; verification bias
  anchoring, 246–247
  cognitive, 246
  confirmation, 246
  definition of, 244
  in diagnostic test studies, 99–107
    application of, 109
    double gold standard, 101–103
    incorporation, 100
    overfitting, 106–107
    spectrum, 102–106
    verification, 100–101
  laboratory error and, 227
  lead time, 126
  length time, 126–127
  pseudodisease, 128–129
  publication, 148
  random error v., 10
  result distortion from, 132
  in randomized trials, 191
  in screening tests, 125–129
  slippery linkage, 130–131
  spectrum, 102–106
    definition of, 102–104
    disease prevalence and, 104–105
    ESR and, 104
    in multiple tests, 162
    sensitivity in, 102
    specificity in, 102
    test in-dependence and, 105–106
    for UTIs, 105–106
  stage migration, 127–128
  sticky diagnosis, 130